How Ireland cares the case for Health Care Reform

HOW IRELAND CARES

the case for health care reform

A. DALE TUSSING
MAEV-ANN WREN

NEW
ISLAND

How Ireland Cares: The Case for Health Care Reform
First published 2006
by New Island
2 Brookside
Dundrum Road
Dublin 14
www.newisland.ie

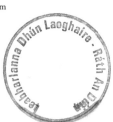

ISBN 1 905494 23 8

Typeset by New Island
Cover design by New Island
Printed in the UK by Athenaeum Press Ltd., Gateshead, Tyne & Wear

New Island received financial assistance from The Arts Council
(An Chomhairle Ealaíon), Dublin, Ireland

10 9 8 7 6 5 4 3 2 1

CONTENTS

For my mother, Carolyn Johnson Tussing – DT

For Bill and Maev, my parents, with love and thanks – MW

PREFACE

This study reviews and analyses the Irish health care system and makes systematic recommendations for reform.

This study was commissioned by the Irish Congress of Trade Unions (ICTU) in anticipation of Social Partnership negotiations with the Irish government and other parties which were scheduled to commence in November 2005. Congress contacted the authors in February 2005 and asked them to consider conducting a critical review of the health care system, with recommendations for reform, to provide Congress with a background briefing in preparation for these talks. This book is that review.

At the time of writing in early 2006, the status of Social Partnership talks is uncertain. Whatever the fate of Social Partnership talks in 2006, the authors firmly believe that the time for health care reform is now. Congress has reassured the authors that the study can still serve the purpose of helping the unions to formulate their own positions on health care and can inform the wider Irish public about the needs of the health care system.

Prior to 1987, the Irish economy regularly had double-digit inflation rates as well as unemployment rates. A large percentage of school leavers – estimated to be as many as half – emigrated to find work. Labour relations were often acrimonious, with unions demanding significant wage increases to keep up with prices, and firms raising prices rapidly because of large wage settlements.

Then, in 1987 Ireland began a series of 'Social Partnership' negotiations. The Social Partners are the main stakeholders in Irish society – the ICTU, employers, government, farmers and, more recently, voluntary groups. In 1987, the unions agreed to moderate their wage claims. In exchange, the government undertook to guarantee workers a rise in real income, delivered by reducing personal tax rates. It is thought that this historic agreement facilitated rising output, profits and eventually significantly increased employment. Basically, the main macroeconomic variables were negotiated.

1

It is widely concluded that the process was enormously successful. Commencing shortly after the first Social Partnership agreement, Ireland began to have the most rapid economic growth rate in all of Europe. After more than a decade of rapid growth, incomes are high and Ireland has become a labour-shortage economy. Though the consensus is that the so-called Celtic Tiger period is over, the Irish economy has been transformed. The Social Partnership process is generally given much of the credit for these economic successes.

The Social Partnership process is a credit to all concerned, but especially the trade union movement, whose statesmanship in that critical period may have saved the Irish economy.

The typical Social Partnership agreement lasts three years and there have been a succession of renewals since the first agreement in 1987. A relatively low-tax, low-public-spending society has emerged from years of Social Partnership. As a result, the trade union movement began to talk about taking some of the benefits of economic growth in the form of a so-called social wage, i.e. through improved public services.

After the ICTU decided to put the health care system on the table in the next round of Social Partnership negotiations, Congress engaged us to critically review the health care system and to make recommendations for their positions on reform. They were looking for immediate, short-term and long-term reform suggestions. We were asked to prepare a book-length document with a deadline of 16 October 2005. Though Congress provided us with a 'scoping document' which set out in bullet form a set of problems or issues which we had to cover,[1] we decided to be comprehensive, reviewing the leading issues and the main components of the health care system, while making sure that we covered all the items in the scoping document.

As this report makes clear, improved health and social services cannot be achieved without sustained investment and increased current spending. Reform does not necessarily require additional resources for health care, but achieving a health care system which meets the expectations of Ireland today will require Irish society to fund additional spending by means of extra taxation or social insurance, or by reduced tax incentives or state spending elsewhere.

It has not been our brief to describe how the future financing of health care might be achieved. However, we would support its achievement by equitable and progressive means. As we outline in this report, the existing state subsidies and tax incentives and the existing organisation of the health care system subsidise private care and discriminate against those who depend on the public system. We argue for an equitable, universal health care system, with care delivered according to need and funded according to ability to pay.

The affiliated unions in the ICTU include several with members in health care. The following four unions sponsored our study, each bearing 25 per cent of the cost:

- Irish Medical Organisation (IMO), representing most doctors.
- Irish Nurses' Organisation (INO), representing most nurses.
- Services, Industrial, Professional and Technical Union (SIPTU), Ireland's largest union, representing, among others, nurses, support and ancillary health care workers, social workers and other health care workers in both public and private sectors.
- IMPACT: A trade union representing public sector workers, including employees of the Health Service Executive (HSE), the new body which operates the public health services in Ireland; voluntary hospitals and other specialist health agencies; workers across the range of clerical/administrative grades; care workers; support staff; and many health care professionals like physiotherapists, pharmacists, psychologists and speech and language therapists.

A traditional trade union approach to health care might have emphasised job-related matters and jurisdictional issues. Our task has been to help the trade unions transcend these concerns and to pursue reform as citizens and potential patients, as the idea of the social wage implies.

Our agreement gave us complete intellectual freedom. We have been able to write whatever we chose, without interference or even suggestion. Therefore, it will be clear that the ICTU is not responsible for the contents of this book. Only the authors are responsible.

The authors and Congress agreed on the present project in March 2005, giving us approximately seven months to conduct the research and to prepare the manuscript. Of course, we did not begin from scratch. Both authors have had lengthy and visible relationships with the Irish health care system, and both have published books on the subject.

We determined that with such a short time to prepare a comprehensive document, we could not hope to conduct original empirical research. (Having said that, we must add that we are confident that those who follow Irish health care closely will find frequent instances of original contributions to knowledge in the following pages.) In May and then again in June 2005, the authors jointly interviewed approximately 100 people from all parts of Ireland with expertise in various aspects of the system – physicians, other clinicians, health service administrators, hospital administrators, academics, politicians and others. It was part of our understanding with our informants that our interviews were anonymous and confidential, and that we would not use quotations, data or any other information from these consultations which would identify our sources. Our report does cite relevant published literature for data and documents. Our understanding of the system and of the issues before it profited immensely from these interviews, and we are very grateful for them. We are also very grateful to the many staff of the Department of Health, the HSE, the Central Statistics Office and diverse other public and private bodies who responded patiently to our repeated searches for information.

We present our comprehensive analysis of the health and health care of Ireland, and conclude with a detailed set of recommendations.

The following persons read all or part of the manuscript: Ruth Barrington, author of *Health, Medicine and Politics in Ireland 1900–1970*; Siobhán Barry, Clinical Director, Cluain Mhuire Service, Blackrock, County Dublin, and PRO, Irish Psychiatric Association; Gerry Bury, Professor of General Practice at University College Dublin; Ian Callanan, President of the Irish Society for Safety and Quality in Health Care; Brian Nolan,

Research Professor, The Economic and Social Research Institute, Dublin; Charles Normand, Edward Kennedy Professor of Health Policy and Management, Trinity College, Dublin; Fergus O'Ferrall, Director, The Adelaide Hospital Society; Ivan Perry, Professor of Public Health, Department of Epidemiology and Public Health, University College, Cork; Paul Sweeney, Economic Advisor, ICTU; and Martha A. Wojtowycz, Associate Professor, Department of Obstetrics and Gynecology, State University of New York, Syracuse, New York. We are enormously grateful for their generous contribution of their knowledge and time, which has improved the report in manifold ways. We are indebted to Ms Hana Rhee for her help in compiling our bibliography.

Only the authors are responsible for any errors of fact, interpretation or omission which may remain.

We would also like to thank for their generous and unobtrusive help the secretariat of the ICTU and the members of the ICTU steering committee for this study: David Begg, General Secretary of ICTU; Sally Anne Kinahan, Assistant General Secretary, ICTU; Paula Carey, Social Policy Officer, ICTU; Peter McLoone, President, ICTU and General Secretary, IMPACT; Jack O'Connor, General President, SIPTU; Liam Doran, General Secretary, INO; Clare Tracey, Director of Organisation and Social Policy, INO; Fintan Hourihan, Director of Industrial Relations, IMO; John Tierney, National Secretary, Amicus; and Dan Murphy, General Secretary, PSEU. Eileen Sweeney and Fiona Elward at ICTU have smoothed our paths in many practical ways, for which we would like to thank them particularly. Finally, we wish to thank the ICTU Executive Council for the courteous hearing they accorded our presentation on this report and for affording us this opportunity to increase and share our understanding of the Irish health care system and the potential for its reform.

EXECUTIVE SUMMARY

The purpose of this study is to review the Irish health care system and make recommendations for its reform. The study was commissioned by the Irish Congress of Trade Unions (ICTU) to inform and advise it in developing its position on the health care system. It is to be made widely available to contribute to the public debate on Irish health care.

The health of the Irish people

- Life expectancy at birth for Irish men was 75.1 years in 2002 compared with the EU15 average of 75.8; life expectancy for women was 80.3 years compared to an EU15 average of 81.6. At age 65, Irish male life expectancy was at the bottom jointly with Denmark of the EU15 league table. For women at 65, Irish life expectancy was second from the bottom in the EU15 league table.
- There is pronounced inequality within Ireland between the life expectancy and experience of ill health of differing social groups. Irish people in lower-income groups suffer more illness and die younger than better-off social groups. Poor social services, diet, housing and schooling of lower-income people, in combination with social exclusion, contribute to health inequality.
- This study is driven by the core value that care should be based on need, not on income or social position. At present, this goal is not attained in Ireland. Health inequalities which derive from social causes are made worse by inequalities in access to care.
- Deficiencies in the health care system are only one reason why Irish life expectancy is lower than the Western European average. This study reviews three specific conditions which affect health in Ireland and illustrate the mixture of reasons for Ireland's low life expectancy:
  1. Obesity increasingly contributes to excess mortality in Ireland, especially among people on lower incomes. No

6

single factor explains this epidemic, and no single solution exists to attack it. The problem must be attacked in childhood, through early assessment and intervention, improved diet and a programme of sport, play and recreation. This will require investment in the public health service and linking social welfare incomes to the cost of healthy foodstuffs.

2. Ireland's incidence of breast cancer is below the EU15 average, yet the rate of death from breast cancer in 2001 was the highest reported in the EU15. This combination suggests that early detection and treatment are inferior in Ireland. When BreastCheck, the national breast screening programme, finally becomes nationwide (promised in 2007), these death rates should fall.

3. The rate of youth suicide in Ireland is the fifth highest in the EU and is particularly high among young men. Suicide is strongly associated with mental illness. Research indicates that mental health resources are over-stretched and are best developed in the areas of greatest affluence, rather than the areas of greatest need.

• Addressing Ireland's high mortality and morbidity requires better-resourced health services, available equitably across social groups and regions, with mental disorders treated as urgently as physical illness. It also requires social policy measures which address exclusion and income inequality.

Spending on health

• There is inadequate information about health spending in Ireland, and available information is often misinterpreted.

• The 2001 Health Strategy made a convincing case for significantly more resources. It represented the informed consensus and was the expressed government policy. Resources provided to date are far from the Health Strategy's goals.

• According to the OECD, Ireland's per capita current or day-to-day public spending on health was 94.4 per cent of the EU15 average in 2003, the latest year for which comparable international data are available. This is an overstatement. Careful analysis of Irish spending shows that although the

OECD has adjusted Irish data to remove non-health social spending, elements of that spending remain. This suggests that the correct 2003 figure is less than 90 per cent of the EU15 average.

- Irish current health spending is expected to have remained below the EU per capita average in 2004 and 2005.
- The most recent data show Ireland's capital investment in health care per capita to be the highest in the EU15. This high rate can only be understood in historical context. The recent increase in investment above the EU average follows decades of investing considerably below it. Over the 27 years from 1970 to 1996, Ireland invested on average each year 63 per cent of the EU average. As recently as 1990, Ireland was investing 38 per cent of the average.
- Overstatement in public current and capital spending, as well as inadequate statistical sources for private spending, mean that calculations of Ireland's total health spending are unreliable. The most recent OECD data show Ireland's total health spending as a proportion of national income to be 8.9 per cent, slightly below an EU14 average of 9 per cent and ninth of the 14 states for which data were available. This is almost certainly an overstatement.
- The proportion of national income devoted to health care has been increasing across the OECD. The OECD average rose from 7.7 per cent of GDP in 1997 to 8.8 per cent in 2003. In the US, the health share of GDP rose from 13 to 15 per cent over the same period. In France, it rose from 9.4 to 10.1 per cent; in Canada from 8.9 to 9.9 per cent; in Germany from 10.7 to 11.1 per cent; and in Norway from 8.5 to 10.3 per cent.[1]
- The authors caution that the argument that Ireland should spend less than the European average on health because its population is younger than the EU average is overly simple. This position is based on the familiar observation that older people tend to spend more money on health care, but the relationship is complex and nuanced.
- One reason the aged spend more on medical care is that end-of-life disability and illness are particularly costly. There is

reason to think that these costs occur at an earlier age in Ireland.

- The effect of an ageing population is felt more in social care programmes than in acute health care costs. International data show that Ireland under-provides for age-related social programmes. That shortcoming puts pressure on the health care system, e.g. shortcomings of community and extended care mean that older people inappropriately occupy acute hospital beds.
- Irish health care spending is inadequate, not excessive. Some recent spending may have been wasted due to bad planning and phasing and because the system required reform. Future spending increases must be carefully paced and must occur within a reformed health care system.

Authors' recommendations

- Debate on health spending should take place in a climate of honest appraisal, and a national system of health accounts should be developed as a matter of urgency to facilitate informed debate.
- Current and capital spending on health and social care need to increase to fund the capacity deficits identified in the 2001 Health Strategy in primary, continuing, community and acute care.
- This increase in spending should be implemented in a planned and paced manner, and within the framework of the 2003 Hanly Report of reform in how hospital doctors work and are remunerated, and with reform in how patients access care.
- The costing of the 2001 Health Strategy by the Department of Health should be revisited. Its statement of capacity needs should be reassessed and revised if necessary in light of population growth and the more developed understanding which is emerging of the relationships between the acute care and other sectors.
- There should be a comprehensive and realistic analysis of the investment needs of health and social services over the next 10 years, followed by a planned, phased commitment of investment.

Solidarity, decentralisation and privatisation

- The Irish health care system has been and should be based on the principle of social solidarity.
- European-style decentralisation, i.e. separation of the purchaser and provider functions in health care, holds great promise for solving problems which arise out of rigidity, inflexibility and unresponsiveness in Irish health care. Such decentralisation would provide greater autonomy to public hospitals and other providers of care. The example of other European states shows that such policies can be successful *and* consistent with democratic values, the need principle of medical ethics and social solidarity.
- However, there are dangers in decentralisation, so it must be approached cautiously and with a vigilant concern for values other than market success.
- Privatisation, meaning the substitution of for-profit forms of organisation for public or not-for-profit forms, poses still greater dangers to fundamental values. While one should not oppose privatisation in health care on principle, one should be aware of the potential it has for doing harm.
- The negatives outweigh the positives in the government's 2005 plan to permit construction of private hospitals on the grounds of public hospitals.
- Private hospitals do not offer a complete acute care service. They concentrate on elective surgery in less complex and more profitable areas. For that reason, private beds in newly constructed private hospitals on public hospital grounds will not free up private beds in public hospitals for public use on anything like a one-for-one basis.
- There will be a net increase in private beds, for which taxpayers will pay through tax breaks for private hospitals and through indirect subsidies.
- If consultants from the public hospitals are shareholders in the private hospital, they will have an added incentive (on top of the private fees they may earn there) to favour treating patients in the private hospital over devoting their time and energies to their public hospital and patients.

- The two-tier system of acute hospital care will be further institutionalised. While the plan technically reduces the practice of private care in public hospitals, private care in fact moves only an enclosed corridor or the other side of a car park away, and the new configuration retains the most objectionable features of the current arrangement.

Authors' recommendations

- The government should abandon its plan to permit and encourage private hospitals to be constructed on the grounds of public hospitals.
- The VHI should continue to be a state company so that it can continue to serve national rather than private or parochial interests. Whatever is the future of the VHI, it should not become a for-profit company.

Incentives and the health care system

- The Irish health care system has many anomalous and dysfunctional economic incentives.
- Hospital consultants are paid by salary for public patients and by fee for private patients treated in public hospitals. This means that treating a public patient does not generate any additional income for the consultant, while treating a private patient does. One would predict that consultants would favour private patients. And they do.
- Under the two-tier system, private patient care is scheduled sooner than public patient care, which has led to the existence of two waiting lists.
- Private patients are more likely to be treated personally by the consultant, while public patients are more likely to be treated by non-consultant hospital doctors (NCHDs).
- General practitioners (GPs) are paid by capitation for public patients and by fee for private patients. One would predict that GPs would favour private patients. There is no evidence that they do.
- The authors advocate hybrid systems for paying both consultants and GPs. In hybrid systems, doctors are paid for all

patients in the same way, but this is in part on a fee basis and in part on a salary or capitation basis.
- Hospitals' behaviour is also affected by how they are paid for patient care.
- Irish public hospitals receive annual budgets which are primarily incremental, which is a flawed method. Incremental budgets do not reflect demographic and social changes and are likely to perpetuate inter-regional and inter-hospital inequities. They are inconsistent with hospital autonomy and do not include any incentives for efficient behaviour.
- A growing percentage of hospital budgets is based on casemix measurement, which provides an adjustment for the complexity of hospitals' case loads, and which penalises hospitals with higher-than-average costs.
- Irish hospitals also receive revenues for patient care, which are significantly higher for private patients and provide an incentive for hospitals to favour them, which is a further flaw in the budget process.
- An unforeseen consequence of the government's decision to vote spending directly to the Health Service Executive (HSE) has been to deprive public hospitals of any increase in revenues above those estimated in the Vote.

Authors' recommendations
- Hospital consultants should treat all patients, public and private, in the same way. Hence, they should be paid in the same way for all patients. To avoid over- and under-provision of care, this should be a hybrid system, part salary and part fee per item of service. This change would be a major move in attacking the two-tier system of care.
- GPs should also treat all patients, public and private, in the same way. Hence, they should be paid in the same way for all patients. Ideally, this should be a hybrid system, part capitation and part fee per item of service.
- Hospitals should be paid in the same ways for public and private patients in order to remove any incentives for them to differentiate between them in ways that favour private patients.

- Hospital budgeting should be reformed. Hospital budgets should be set in large part on the basis of their case loads but should also have a significant discretionary component set by the HSE.
- Economically non-neutral devices, such as the doctor-only Medical Card, should be avoided.
- GPs should receive capitation rates set according to risk. Rates favouring people living greater distances from GPs' offices and favouring people aged 70 and over who do not receive Medical Cards on the basis of need should be re-examined and changed.

Financing of medical care

- The Irish health care system faces serious problems of adequacy, equity and efficiency in how care is financed.
- The proportion of the Irish population covered by Medical Cards is too low.
- Patients with new doctor-only Medical Cards face fees for treatment by professionals other than GPs, such as physiotherapists, and drug costs which are very large in relation to their incomes. Those beyond the threshold for doctor-only cards face the further unbuffered cost of GP fees.
- Capitation payment rates to GPs for people aged 70 and over who receive Medical Cards on a non-means tested basis are higher than the capitation rates for lower-income 70-year-olds and over. This creates a contributory incentive for GPs to locate in wealthier neighbourhoods. The Drugs Payment Scheme (DPS) programme caps drugs expenditures for households at €85 per month or €1,020 per year, which is too high.
- There are significant public subsidies to private care in the two-tier system of care in public hospitals. Taxpayers in the bottom half of the income distribution contribute to the private care of those in the upper half. Hospital charges for private care do not cover the true economic costs of care.
- The consultants' common contract is deeply flawed and requires revision. Consultants are paid public salaries while treating private patients. They are not accountable administratively or clinically.

13

- Irish law requires health insurers to provide community rating so that everyone insured under a given plan pays the average premium for that plan. In a society with community rating, risk equalisation is necessary whenever insurers face significantly different risks. This process transfers money from insurers with lower-risk membership to insurers with higher-risk membership.

Authors' recommendations

- Access to free primary care should be restored immediately to its historic proportion of 35 to 38 per cent of the population and extended soon to the entire population.
- Medical Card guidelines should be indexed to the median earnings of Irish workers so that they change continuously rather than intermittently and so that the level is set automatically rather than politically.
- As part of the progression to universal access to primary care, instead of doctor-only cards, a new form of eligibility should be created for those low-income people who are not eligible for Medical Cards but whose incomes place them in the bottom half of the Irish income distribution, e.g. by giving them subsidies which cover half the cost of all forms of care covered by conventional Medical Cards.
- GPs should receive the same capitation rate for all 70-year-olds and over.
- The Drug Payment Scheme should be reformed to reimburse a percentage of all prescription drug purchases by non-Medical Card holders at the point of sale, and that percentage should be higher for people on lower incomes.
- Public hospitals should set charges for private patients at the level of true economic cost.
- Risk equalisation should be effected between Bupa and VHI, and in any circumstance in which competing insurance companies have significantly different risk profiles.

Primary care

- Irish primary care needs three things: improved access, more GPs and other practitioners and modernisation.

- Two significant reports have advocated major reform in the system of primary care. The Department of Health's Primary Care Strategy and a joint report from the Irish Medical Organisation (IMO) and Irish College of General Practitioners (ICGP) advocated significant reform in Irish general practice in 2001. Both reports said general practice should move away from isolated, small practices focusing on diagnosis and treatment of illness to multi-physician team practices with an enhanced capacity for health promotion, prevention of illness and rehabilitation.
- The teams would include practice nurses, public health nurses, physio- or occupational therapists and others.
- The reports advocated that these teams practise from modern, well-equipped, high-tech primary care centres.
- From 2002 to 2005, the government seemingly abandoned its widely respected Primary Care Strategy. It did not follow up the 10 pilot projects set up under the Strategy, introduce legislation or vote funds to bring into being the modern practices and teams envisioned in its document. A primary care package announced for 2006 still fell far short of the investment envisaged in the strategy.
- The government now seems to be moving in a direction not contemplated in the Primary Care Strategy and possibly antithetical to it: the for-profit chain-store entrepreneurial model of GP practices.

Authors' recommendations

- The numbers of Irish (and other EU) students enrolled in Irish medical schools should increase, as proposed by the Fottrell Working Group, and accepted by the government.
- There needs to be an increase in the numbers of training places for the specialist training programmes in general practice.
- Steps need to be taken to make general practice an attractive career option for young people.
- The Primary Care Strategy should be revived by a new, credible plan and a committed and sustained programme of investment.

- The plan should provide for universal patient registration, investment in a modern primary care infrastructure and collaboration of clinicians within and across disciplines. It needs to address how to meld private and public sectors together in multi-disciplinary primary care centres. State contributions could include direct contribution of money or buildings.

Hospital capacity

- In the third quarter of 2005, Ireland had 2.96 acute hospital inpatient beds per 1,000 population, compared to an EU15 average of four.
- In 2001, Ireland had 3.13 beds per 1,000 population, when the government's Health Strategy identified a need for an additional 3,000 acute hospital beds over a 10-year period.
- Growth of population and the HSE's redefinition of some hospitals as non-acute have reduced the ratio of acute beds to population since the publication of the Strategy in 2001.
- The increase in inpatient beds in hospitals defined as acute by the Department of Health has been 535 since 2001.
- The government also occasionally alludes to an increase in day beds. The Department of Health's count of day beds in the third quarter of 2005 was 475 higher than in 2001. Investigation by the authors has made clear that most of this increase can be explained by the Department's redefinition of trolleys, recliners and couches as day beds, rather than by the addition of extra treatment places.
- HSE CEO Brendan Drumm has suggested that Ireland is over-equipped with acute hospital beds because of the relatively low proportion of its population which is over 65 compared to in the UK.
- In 2002, the UK had 3.7 acute inpatient beds per 1,000 population and 23.2 beds per 1,000 people aged 65 or over. Ireland had three beds per 1,000 population and 26.9 beds per 1,000 people aged 65 or over. The EU average was four beds per 1,000 population and 25.9 beds per 1,000 people aged 65 or over.
- A number of factors need to be taken into account in making such comparisons:

1. Firstly, with fewer beds than the EU average, Britain considers itself seriously under-bedded and is engaged in a substantial programme of acute hospital expansion.

2. Secondly, Ireland has a rapidly increasing population, and without added beds Ireland will fall considerably in European comparisons, either of bed to population ratios or bed to aged population ratios. Based on current population growth forecasts, without increased acute bed numbers, by 2016 Ireland's overall bed ratio would fall to 2.7 per 1,000 population, and Ireland's ratio of beds to population aged 65 and over would fall to 19.3 per 1,000.

3. Thirdly, aggregate statistics conceal regional shortages. The bed to population ratio in the Greater Dublin Area (Counties Dublin, Meath, Kildare and Wicklow) in 2005 was already low for people residing in the area. Residents of other regions occupy some 20 per cent of beds in the East. When inflows of non-residents are taken into account, there remained 2.52 beds per 1,000 population resident in the East in 2005. There remained 25.6 beds per 1,000 people aged 65 and over and resident in the East in 2005. Population growth alone would reduce this ratio to 25.1 in 2006 and 14.8 in 2021 unless the East's acute bed stock expands.

- Ireland has one of the highest rates of hospital-acquired infections in Europe. The Minister for Health has launched national guidelines on hospital hygiene and cleanliness. However, inadequate ward infrastructure and high bed-occupancy rates in Irish hospitals play a role in the high infection rate. Infection will not be controlled by hygiene alone.

Authors' recommendations

- The HSE should produce a plan for expanded hospital capacity. This should begin with a transparent, validated bed count. It should also include an assessment of the actual ratio of beds to population in each region and it should be reconciled with the regional reorganisation of acute hospital services.

- If the government is no longer convinced of the merits of the Acute Hospital Bed Capacity Review, it should initiate a fresh review as a matter of urgency. The authors are confident that, particularly in light of rapid population growth, a further review would endorse the case for significantly increasing Ireland's acute bed stock.
- Added beds should not be scattered across the state in response to local political pressures. Instead, investment in beds should take place in a carefully planned and phased manner against a backdrop of explicit identification of which hospitals should grow, which should change function and of changes in how hospitals are staffed, managed and financed.

Access to public hospital care

- Public hospitals are obliged to designate beds as public or private. Department of Health policy says private beds are not meant to exceed 20 per cent of the total, but in 2002, 33 per cent of day beds were private.
- In 2004, private patients accounted for 33.4 per cent of patients discharged from public hospitals after elective inpatient treatment, 24 per cent of patients discharged after day treatment and 23.6 per cent of patients discharged after emergency treatment. Private patients accounted for 25.6 per cent of total cases in public hospitals in 2004.
- Bed designation is not adequate to control private activity in public hospitals and to protect access for public patients. An internal Department of Health review concluded in 2003 that 'the designation process alone is not sufficient to control the amount of private activity occurring in hospitals.'
- Research verifies that public patients wait more often and longer for care than private patients. Data also show that public patients wait longer for initial outpatient appointments before being scheduled for admission and treatment.
- An OECD study showed Ireland and Portugal to have a notably greater pro-rich distribution of medical specialist care than the other 12 OECD countries studied.
- An Irish liver transplant study showed that patients without health insurance, especially those living distances from the

transplant facility, are significantly less likely to have liver transplants.

- A study of patients with coronary heart disease showed that private patients were more likely to receive important diagnostic procedures than public patients.
- The preference for private patients is not based on need. Research has shown that public patients are older, sicker and poorer than private patients.
- The National Treatment Purchase Fund (NTPF) has reduced waiting times for public patients, mainly by purchasing care for the longest waiters.
- Yet this advance has come through an odd circularity in policy: private patients are given preferential treatment in public hospitals, and the public patients whom they displace may in turn be treated in private hospitals or as private patients in public hospitals. This is neither an efficient use of public money nor an equitable way to treat patients.
- When the NTPF was created, the Department of Health ceased collecting waiting list data. The NTPF has assumed that function, implicitly assessing its own performance. This responsibility should be given to the new Health Information and Quality Authority (HIQA).
- The Comptroller and Auditor General's (C&AG) first audit of the NTPF showed that 36 per cent of NTPF cases examined were carried out in the public hospital from which they had been referred. Thus, public consultants can earn private fees from their own untreated public patients. The study shows that 44 per cent of NTPF cases were treated in public hospitals.
- The audit also showed wide variation in the rates paid by the NTPF for the same procedures. This suggests that NTPF rates paid to private hospitals may be higher than those paid to public hospitals.

Authors' recommendations

- There should be a common waiting list for patients in public hospitals, but with care to be provided promptly so that few patients appear on waiting lists and none stays long.

- If public hospitals offer patients who choose to pay for them enhanced, private rooms, they must provide them with the same care as all other patients. There should not be any private and public patients in public hospitals.
- Public hospitals with unused capacity should be funded to treat more patients within the public system, not via the NTPF.
- Until such time as there is a common waiting list in public hospitals, public hospitals with excess capacity should be permitted to compete to supply NTPF-funded treatments on the same footing as private hospitals.
- The NTPF's annual report should contain precise details of how many procedures have taken place respectively in public and private hospitals, in Ireland and abroad and of the cost per procedure in each of these hospitals

The A&E crisis

- In winter 2004/2005 the number of patients on trolleys in accident and emergency (A&E) departments nationwide regularly ran to 200 or 300, peaking in January at 422. In January 2006 numbers of patients on trolleys hit this peak again. These were patients who had been judged to require admission to acute hospitals but for whom no bed was available.
- Patients have remained on trolleys for as long as five days and nights.
- The authors have been told of one death after a patient left hospital following an inappropriately long wait for treatment in an A&E department.
- The A&E crisis is the tip of an iceberg. Its causes include cutbacks in community and public long-stay care, low capital investment in health and social services over many decades, the political system's continued failure to address how Irish society should access and pay for long-stay care in old age, failure to reform the system of hospital medical staffing, failures of internal management within hospitals and lack of integration between primary, acute and community care.
- The number of patients remaining in acute hospitals because no appropriate alternative facility can be found remains high.

This occurs not only in the case of older people, but also people who are mentally ill, terminally ill or disabled.

- There are structural changes which, by addressing other pressing problems, can also alleviate the A&E crisis:
  - ~ Acute medical units (AMUs) in all hospitals with A&E departments would improve internal efficiency. By receiving patients directly from GP referrals, such units can avoid unnecessary admissions and reduce duplication of effort.
  - ~ Addressing the need for long-stay, extended care, community care and palliative care facilities could free up literally hundreds of acute hospital beds while also providing more effectively for the needs of frail elderly, convalescing, disabled and terminally ill people.
- The 2001 Health Strategy proposed providing 5,600 extended care/community nursing unit places over seven years. This has not happened.
- At least 65 public long-stay places were closed in 2005 because of inadequate funding/staffing.
- In 2002 the government announced plans for 17 50-bedded Community Nursing Units for older people under public-private partnership (PPP). Of the 850 beds contemplated, the 450 intended for the East could have greatly alleviated the A&E problems of acute hospitals. For reasons which have not yet been publicly explained, the Department of Finance did not sanction this development.
- The government has relied on tax-incentivised private nursing home provision as its main solution to care of the elderly. Between end-2001 and 2004, extended care beds increased by 8 per cent, or 1,823, according to the Department of Health's count, and 71 per cent of these beds came in private nursing homes. In the East, where need is greatest, public and voluntary beds increased by 43 and private nursing home beds by 649.
- Private facilities do not offer the level of care or technology which patients often require when discharged from acute hospitals. When the HSE sought 100 high-dependency places in the private sector in 2005 to relieve acute hospital pressures, it only found 48.

- With appropriate supports, many older people in nursing homes could stay in their own homes. Yet OECD data show that a smaller proportion of Irish aged receive home care benefits than is the case in other countries.
- The numbers of home helps employed by the public health sector dropped by 19 per cent between 2001 and 2005, according to Department of Health data (data not available for the East).
- The 2006 Budget allocated €150 million in funding for care of the elderly, primarily in the community. There was no allocation for expanding publicly provided extended care places.
- There are no national standards and no consistent programme of inspection for home care.

Authors' recommendations

- Any existing public long-stay capacity which is not open should be reopened immediately.
- In the short term, public purchases of private nursing home care, flexibility in working practices and better hospital team-working can play a role in easing A&E pressures.
- The real solutions will take longer and require investment in public long-stay, community and acute care.
- Acute medical units (AMUs) should be developed in all acute hospitals and fast tracked in Tallaght, Beaumont and St Vincent's.
- The public Community Nursing Units for older people, envisaged in the Health Strategy, should be developed as a matter of urgency, starting in Dublin, where need is greatest.
- The state should take responsibility for providing a secure, well-funded and high-quality system of long-term care for frail elderly and severely disabled people and others unable to care for themselves.
- HIQA should be statutorily empowered to require externally validated standards in Ireland's health care system, including public and private long-stay care facilities. HIQA should have statutory powers to inspect extended care facilities and police these standards.

- The authors recommend that unmet need in care of the elderly, the mentally ill, in the community and in palliative care should be assessed and addressed in its own right and not just as a response to the acute care crisis and trolley counts in A&E.

Specialist care in acute hospitals

- The Irish system of specialist care has been described as a 'consultant-led' service, as distinct from a 'consultant-provided' service.
- Most specialist care is provided by under-trained and over-worked junior doctors, also referred to as non-consultant hospital doctors (NCHDs). They outnumber consultants by a ratio of 2.3 to 1 and work longer hours for the public system.
- The current arrangement has further disadvantages:
  - It exacerbates the two-tier system of acute care.
  - NCHDs often work without benefit of supervision by consultants, especially in smaller hospitals.
  - Many NCHD posts provide no real training.
- The Hanly Report recommends a shift to a consultant-provided service, a proposal endorsed by the authors.
- This would transform specialist care in Ireland. It would require a substantial increase in the numbers of consultants, approximately doubling the present number of posts. The Hanly Report also proposes top-to-bottom reform of the training system.
- Ireland has a hospital specialist shortage. Even when all NCHDs are included, Ireland employs fewer specialists than the EU15 average.
- One reason for this is the cap on the number of Irish (or EU) nationals enrolled in Irish medical schools. The authors support the increase in the cap, an increase in the overall number of places in Irish medical schools and an increase in state funding of medical education.
- The consultants' common contract is widely criticised, especially for two characteristics:
  - Consultants are paid a public salary for being present in

public hospitals for at least 33 hours, but they need not care for public patients during all (or any) of that time. They are permitted private practices in public hospitals, and time spent treating private patients for fees can count toward their 33 salaried hours.

 ~ Consultants are not accountable to anyone, either administratively or clinically.

- Variations of the contract permit private practice on site in the public hospital only, or also off site in private hospitals. Until 1997, consultants could choose a public-only contract, which the state then decided not to offer.
- Consultants' extraordinary degree of autonomy and excessive delegation to NCHDs raise serious management problems and have been criticised in a series of studies.
- The Brennan Commission recommended that new consultants be signed to contracts requiring that they work exclusively in the public sector. The report also recommended that consultants be unambiguously accountable, both financially and clinically, for their work.
- The authors also regard the existing system as wholly unacceptable. Clinical freedom must be preserved, but clinical freedom cannot mean an absence of clinical accountability. Clinical freedom also cannot be interpreted as meaning an absence of administrative accountability.
- In most countries, there is a peer-governed mechanism protecting the public through mandatory physician quality assurance, clinical audit and continuing medical education. Such a mechanism does not exist in Ireland.
- The Medical Council has initiated a voluntary competence assurance process. However, the Council lacks the legislative authority to make it mandatory.
- Without such a statutory requirement, the public has no protection from incompetent, out-of-date or inappropriate treatment.

Authors' recommendations

- The 1978 Medical Practitioners Act should be revised to achieve mandatory competence assurance, clinical audit and continuing medical education.

- The consultants' contract should be reformed. It is central to inequity in access to hospital care and is an obstacle to rational management in Irish hospitals.
- A reformed contract should provide for clinical and administrative accountability; should require all consultants to treat patients according to need, drawn from a common waiting list; and should require all consultants to work as rostered members of teams, answerable to a head of department or clinical director, who is in turn answerable to the hospital/hospital group's CEO.
- The option of a public-only contract should be available to all consultants and should be mandatory for newly appointed consultants.
- The Category II contract permitting off-site private practice should no longer be offered.
- Public hospital consultants should be paid in the same way for all patients, whether public or private. Ideally, it should be a hybrid method. There should be a salary component which reflects not only public care but also private care. There should be a fee component for both public and private patients.

The organisation of acute hospital care

- The 2003 Hanly Report proposed a radical reform in the configuration of acute hospitals, as well as moving from a consultant-led to a consultant-provided service. The authors endorse the main findings of this important report.
- Hanly recommended that hospitals should be organised into regional networks, consisting of Major Hospitals staffed with 24-hour, seven-day consultant coverage, with full emergency services and serving catchment areas ranging from 350,000 to 500,000 populations; and a number of Local Hospitals with more limited services. Some regions with more dispersed populations might have intermediate General Hospitals providing emergency care. Some Major Hospitals might offer either national or supra-regional specialties.

Authors' recommendations

- Implementation of the Hanly reforms for the sake of efficiency, equity and, more than anything else, for patient safety.

Too much care is provided today by under-trained, under-supervised and over-worked NCHDs.

- But hospital reorganisation must not be viewed in isolation from the many other factors which affect patients' access to and experience of care, such as primary care, community care, ambulance services, the capacity and quality of existing regional hospitals, travel distances to hospitals and the quality of roads, the quality and availability of public transport, population projections, spatial planning and the commitment of investment.
- Major Hospitals and affiliated Local Hospitals in a region should constitute an organisational entity, with a single budget, led by a single CEO and with shared consultant staff, some of whom would rotate among the hospitals to provide care.
- Each hospital network should have a governing board, with significant local and regional representation.
- Hospital networks should have gradually increasing autonomy, matched by increasing power, responsibility and accountability for the governing board.
- Within hospitals there should be a modified clinical directorate in which budget and planning powers are retained by CEOs, who then delegate them to clinical directors. Clinical directors should be chosen by hospital CEOs, or at the very least, with the concurrence of hospital CEOs.
- A reformed system of governance, funding and management will foster strong, autonomous hospitals.

Health service staffing

- A skilled labour force is central to the delivery of health and social care. Thus, planning to meet skill needs is critically important in health care. In Ireland, such planning has been notably deficient.
- Cutbacks in nurse training places in the 1990s contributed to shortages of nurses by the end of that decade. The subsequent expansion of training places has now increased numbers of graduating nurses, some of whom may not find employment in the public health sector because of an employment cap introduced in 2002.

- A cap on medical training places has given rise to serious shortages of domestically qualified doctors.
- The public service employment cap introduced in December 2002 has limited the ability of the public health sector to respond to demand. It does not apply to private health and social services, even though these are frequently substantially funded by the Exchequer. The cap has not so much restrained health care employment growth or even Exchequer cost as it has further shifted Irish health care to the private sector.
- Since the introduction of the cap in 2002, private projects subsidised by the state have included the following, all discussed in this report: private agency nurses in place of staff nurses, tax-subsidised private hospitals, NTPF funding of public patient care in private hospitals, payment of private fees to public hospital consultants for the treatment of public patients, tax-subsidised expansion of private nursing homes and state payment of home care packages to people requiring care in the community so that they can source private care.
- The cap was introduced just one year after the 2001 Health Strategy recommended substantially increased employment in public health and social care over the 10 years to 2011.
- The lack of specificity in the 2001 Health Strategy about its staffing implications led to the commissioning of a report on health care skill needs, which was published in November 2005. The FÁS *Healthcare Skills Monitoring Report* attempted to forecast demand and supply for 29 health care occupations in the years to 2015. It identified considerable current and future skills shortages and recommended an expansion of training places to address present and/or future shortages of doctors (consultants, interns and GPs), dentists, children's nurses, dieticians, chiropodists, radiographers and radiation therapists. In other occupations, the report concluded that expanded training places might not be necessary if measures were effective to adjust skills mix, improve retention rates, promote immigration and increase productivity.
- The FÁS report is predicated on assumptions that the government will expand health service employment to meet the health care demands of a rising population and will implement

the Health Strategy and Hanly reforms. FÁS therefore implicitly assumes that the government will end its cap on public health sector employment.

- FÁS calculated that for Ireland to meet the EU15 average of 3.26 doctors per 1,000 people for the current population, the number of doctors employed would require a 41 per cent increase. To meet the less ambitious target of merely increasing the number of doctors in line with population and implementing the reforms recommended in the Hanly Report would require a 33 per cent increase by 2015. Either requires a substantial increase in training places for Irish (and other EU) trainees.

- FÁS also called for increases in training places for children's nurses, dieticians, diagnostic radiographers and radiation therapists.

- FÁS did not call for increases in training places for general nurses, social workers or physiotherapists.

- The authors consider it unwarranted and premature to conclude on the available evidence that an increase in training places for nurses in Ireland is not required, notwithstanding the probable emergence of a considerable nursing shortage within the next 10 years. There are three issues on which conclusions different from FÁS's might be reached:

  1. First, FÁS reports that Ireland has the highest level of nursing employment in the EU. Denmark and Iceland have more nurses in relation to population than Ireland. While Ireland's ratio of nurses to population is high at 12.2 per 1,000 compared to an EU average of 8.5, this analysis is based on international comparisons of numbers of nurses employed and does not take into account variable rates of part-time working.

  2. Secondly, Irish numbers of other professionals, especially doctors and social workers, for whom nurses might in many situations substitute, are very low by European standards.

  3. Thirdly, FÁS is more sanguine than the authors about possibilities for substituting large numbers of health care assistants for nurses. We envisage a significantly enlarged

role for care assistants, but such an expanded role requires mandatory training (not currently required) and supervision, mainly by nurses, for care assistants.

- FÁS has not published an assessment of the current demand for social workers and bases its projections of future demand on population growth and the past trends in social work employment. In the authors' view, this approach fails to capture current deficiencies.
- There is also evidence that training places should increase for physiotherapists and speech and language therapists. In these professions, as in social work, the cap on public sector employment masks unmet demand.

Authors' recommendations

- The cap on employment in the public health services should be lifted so that health staffing can grow to meet unmet needs.
- Planning for future staffing needs should become an integral part of the operations of the Department of Health and the HSE.
- Planning should be based on assessments of need across care areas and disciplines and should be informed by regular monitoring.
- Decisions on the number of educational and training places for health and social service staff should be based on evidence of need, analysis of the inter-relationships of health care staff and population growth projections.
- The cap on Irish (and other EU) students in Irish medical schools must be drastically raised, as the Fottrell Working Group recommended, and the government accepted, early in 2006.
- The numbers of places on general practice specialist training programmes must be increased.
- The comprehensive recommendations of the Hanly Report on specialist training should be implemented.
- The Department of Health should commission and publish a specialist study on the type of work typically undertaken by nurses in Ireland and in countries at a comparable level of development to Ireland in order to assess the feasibility, safety and efficiency of the government's policy of employing more

health care assistants as complements to and/or substitutes for nurses.
- Health care assistants should have mandatory training and nurse supervision.
- The Department of Health should undertake a survey which quantifies unmet need for the services of social workers in hospitals, primary and community care.

Accountability and administration in health
- The creation of the HSE in 2005 and the prior abolition of the health boards in 2004 removed the last vestiges of local democracy in Irish health care. A unitary administrative structure has responsibility for the delivery of health services for the first time in the history of the state.
- The HSE receives almost one-third of government current spending in its own direct Vote and must remain democratically accountable, yet the mechanisms by which it is accountable are far from clear.
- The unnecessarily hasty passage of the legislation establishing the HSE has left the two critical issues of political and financial accountability unclear.
- The theory of political accountability in the new structure is straightforward. The Minister for Health and her Department remain responsible for determining issues of health policy. The HSE is responsible for the management of the health service and associated social services.
- The Minister's powers over the HSE – and therefore the public health system – are absolute within the new statutory framework. She appoints and can remove its board, which in turn appoints its CEO (although the Minister appointed the first CEO). She can direct and instruct it at every turn.
- But determining which are policy issues and which are operational matters is not clear cut and requires clarity and leadership from the Minister for Health and the government, which has been lacking.
- An example is the vexed, politicised issue of the location of hospital services. The Minister has not been explicit about this and has apparently judged this to be an operational issue, on

which she and her Department have no immediate responsibility for determining policy. The Minister's reticence on this topic contrasts with her clear, detailed and public policy direction to the HSE in July 2005 to facilitate the development of private facilities on public hospital sites.

- In relation to financial accountability, again the theory seems clear, but the practice is not. The HSE now has a separate Vote, for which the CEO of the HSE is Accounting Officer. When voting on the annual Estimates (the process by which state spending is annually allocated), the Dáil now votes separately on the HSE's funding. The CEO is answerable for this spending personally and directly to the Dáil's Public Accounts Committee (PAC).

- However, through Freedom of Information (FOI), the authors have obtained a December 2004 letter from the Minister for Finance to the Tánaiste, effectively instructing her on her role, the role of her Department and the role of the HSE (reproduced in full in Chapter 12).

- The Minister for Finance and his Department have made clear that they have no intention of dealing directly with the HSE in relation to its spending and will deal with it through the Department of Health, even though the HSE's budget does not come from that Department. Minister Cowen has informed the Tánaiste: 'I will, with my Department, operate through you as Minister and your Department when dealing with HSE matters.' One of his senior officials has been even plainer in writing to his counterpart in Health: 'In short, our Minister's and this Department's day-to-day dealings with the health system will be through your Minister and your Department. We do not intend to maintain a direct line of contact with the HSE.'

- These letters notwithstanding, the separate Vote for the HSE and the designation of the HSE's CEO as Accounting Officer will have several kinds of deleterious consequences:
    - The authority of the Secretary General of the Department of Health has been significantly diminished.
    - The HSE board's control over its CEO has been weakened.

- The HSE must maintain two separate sets of accounts.
- The HSE has no power to borrow funds.
- Any unspent funds must be returned to the Exchequer at year-end.
- It must keep all its bank accounts in credit at all times.
- It must minimise cash in hand at end-month and end-quarter because that is when Finance calculates Exchequer spending and borrowing.
- Institutions which are now wholly owned by the HSE, such as the former health board hospitals, also must not exceed their allocated expenditure for the year.
- If public hospitals earn additional, unexpected revenues, e.g. from private or public patient charges, they must return these funds to the Exchequer.
- If spending on any programme is specified in a sub-head of the Vote, then it must not be exceeded. The HSE must receive the permission of the Department of Finance to move spending from one heading to another.
- This means that the HSE is now obliged to track precisely and not exceed allocated spending on hospital and counselling services for people who contracted Hepatitis C from blood products, since this is covered by a separate sub-head.
- The centralised power over the health system now given to the Minister for Health needs to be exercised within a framework of transparency, openness and accountability.
- Regulations introduced in December 2005 governing the establishment of regional health forums and the answering of Oireachtas members' questions by the HSE are inadequate to ensure transparency.
- At the time of writing, the Health Information and Quality Authority (HIQA) had not been statutorily established.

Authors' recommendations

- The Minister for Health should be democratically and transparently accountable for the health service and its associated social services.

- The government should amend the Health Act 2004 to restore the full Health Vote to the Department of Health and the Accounting Officer role to its Secretary General.
- When the Minister issues written directions to the HSE, the Minister should be required to publish these directions at the time they are made.
- While the HSE board is required to inform the Minister of any matter that it considers requires the Minister's attention, the Minister should be obliged to so inform the Dáil.
- Regulations governing the answering of Oireachtas members' questions about the HSE should be strengthened.
- The role of the Oireachtas Committee on Health and Children should be strengthened. It should be resourced to analyse the activity of the HSE and should meet more often to review its operations. Its debates and hearings should be available on the Oireachtas website as immediately as full Dáil debates.
- Regulations governing the establishment, composition and operation of the regional forums should be revised to provide for the forums to meet more regularly and to require regional and national officials of the HSE to attend them where necessary.
- If current concerns about a democratic deficit in the operations of the HSE continue after the forums have been in operation for some time, there should be amending legislation to provide for direct elections to the forums.
- A national consultative forum should be established as a conduit for regular, formal consultation between the Department of Health and other stakeholders on national health policy once there is assurance that it will be representative of a comprehensive range of stakeholders.
- The Secretary General of Health and a senior official of the HSE should sit on the National Economic and Social Council (NESC) and the consultative forum should also appoint a representative(s) to the Council.
- The Primary Care Strategy promised to develop the involvement of local communities and voluntary groups in the planning and delivery of care. The Minister should direct the HSE to deliver on this commitment by developing local advi-

sory panels, which would directly engage citizens and their representatives in local needs identification, planning and decision making. The HSE should engage with local authorities.

- Appointment of directors to the HSE's board should not be entirely in the hands of the Minister. Their appointment should satisfy objective eligibility criteria and ensure a balanced board composition. The directors must reflect stakeholder interests, including those of employees.
- The confidentiality provisions of the Health Act 2004 should be balanced by a Whistleblowers' Charter that protects individuals who can make a defensible case that they have disclosed information in the interests of patient safety.
- Key positions in health administration should be filled by open competition and there should be further review of the common recruitment pool for the filling of vacancies in public health administration.
- The government should offer early retirement and voluntary redundancy packages to former health board staff who do not wish to remain in the HSE.
- There should be a statement of principles affirmatively expressing patients' rights, along the lines of the European Charter of Patients' Rights. It is not necessary, and given the litigious character of Irish society, not desirable, that the charter be enforceable in courts of law, unless there is specific legislation regarding any of its contents.
- Legislation creating the HIQA should be passed without further delay.
- HIQA should be statutorily empowered to require externally validated standards in Ireland's health care system. These standards should apply to all hospitals – public, voluntary and private, to primary care providers, long-stay care providers and all other health care facilities. HIQA should have the statutory power to inspect health care facilities and police these standards.
- HIQA should regularly publish health system data, including health accounts, the national bed count, discharge and treatment patterns of public and private hospitals and earnings of health care professionals (both public and private).

An agenda for reform in Irish health care

It is widely acknowledged that the Irish health care system is in crisis. It is under-resourced, inequitable and frequently chaotic. Changing it for the better will require advancing on a number of fronts together: improving resourcing, both of people and facilities, ensuring access according to need as a core value and reforming many aspects of how health and social services organise and deliver care.

The authors' vision of the future Irish health care system is not a utopia, but rather an attainable system appropriate to this country which can be reached in a decade or less if appropriate first steps are taken now. While we have made many recommendations, the following are the major objectives which any reform should aim to achieve:

- *Access*: Free primary care for all. A common waiting list for patients in public hospitals, but with care to be provided promptly so that few patients appear on waiting lists and none stays long. Public hospitals may offer hotel-like private rooms to patients who choose to pay for this, but will provide them with the same care as all other patients. In other words, there are no private and public patients in public hospitals. A state-provided or guaranteed long-term care system for frail elderly, severely disabled and others unable to care for themselves.
- *Resources*: More Irish medical students, GPs, hospital consultants, allied professionals, community care services and modern long-stay and community care facilities in addition to a planned expansion of acute hospitals.
- *Quality*: A modern primary care system, with GPs, practice nurses, public health nurses, physiotherapists, social workers and others working in teams from modern, well-equipped, computerised primary care centres in every community and large urban neighbourhood. A consultant-provided specialist service in acute hospitals. Reduced numbers of NCHDs, but sufficient in specialist training to provide an adequate continuing stream of new consultants. Mandatory medical competence assurance.
- *Management*: Improved accountability and control, including

clinical accountability, for all doctors and hospitals and other clinicians as well. Transparent and rational allocation of resources, including a reformed method of financing hospitals. Standardised health accounts comparable with those of other states, comprehending all care, both public and private.

Among the alternative investment priorities, the authors have chosen two to advance for immediate action. One is the modernisation of primary care. This is a past-due reform and its full achievement will take a decade or more. It requires a new plan and immediate investment to begin the long but exciting task of building a patient-centred, technologically advanced, inter-disciplinary primary care system. The other is expansion of long-stay and community facilities for the ageing population, not only in Dublin, where it is desperately needed, but throughout the state.

The authors believe that expansion of acute hospital capacity is also urgently needed, but that investment should be developed with care and driven by planning. It should be paced and should take place first in hospitals which can show that they are using their existing capacity in the most effective manner possible, and which are well integrated with local community, primary and long-stay services. This planning and vetting process should take no more than a year. In the meantime, both primary care modernisation and expansion of long-stay and community facilities for the aged will relieve pressure on the acute system. Private hospitals on public sites should not and cannot substitute for the expansion of public acute hospitals.

In addition to investment priorities, there are immediate access priorities. First is the low-income population just above the current Medical Card eligibility threshold. Two steps need to be taken to relieve their burdens. Firstly, full Medical Card eligibility should be restored to the 35 to 38 per cent level. Secondly, the remaining 12 to 15 per cent of the population in the bottom half of the income distribution should be given partial Medical Card benefits. In the acute system, there should immediately – tomorrow! – be a common waiting list for public and private patients.

Immediate steps are possible to relieve the A&E crisis. These include opening any available public long-stay facilities and lifting the cap on public health service employment. The government should make it a priority to publish proposals for the funding of a system of long-term care which guarantees care to all citizens in need and for which the cost is shared across the community. This measure will not immediately improve A&E, but it will provide reassurance to many older people and their families about their future care. If such a system were in place, with community support, in 12 months' time, discharge planning from public acute hospitals would be transformed. A further measure, which will take time to bear fruit but which will also reassure older people and health sector and hospital managers, would be immediately putting out to tender the 17 Community Nursing Units planned by the former Minister for Health, Micheál Martin, and vetoed by the Department of Finance.

Consultant contract negotiations have the potential to deliver an historic reform. Their outcome could control our ability to reform the acute care system for years to come. The negotiations cannot be addressed in isolation. They must be seen in the context of a holistic need to reform the Irish health care system. Without contract reform, the system will remain inequitable, unsafe and unmanageable.

The plan to erect publicly subsidised private hospitals on public hospital grounds is a crossroads issue. If it goes forward, a changed Irish acute care system, one difficult to reverse or reform, may be in place in a matter of months. Along with the priorities for modernisation of primary care, restoring Medical Cards and for nursing homes and community care, there is the priority to stop the private hospital plan. Indeed, the latter may be more crucial than the former in the coming days, because soon the private hospitals' scheme will be a *fait accompli* and we will be talking about undoing it rather than preventing it.

Improved health and social services cannot be achieved without sustained investment and increased current spending. Reform need not necessarily require additional resources for health care. Free primary care, for instance, obviates the need for much private spending on health and represents a rechanneling of payments by individuals (from private fees to tax or PRSI), not an additional cost to Irish society, except in so far as services grow and need to be funded in the sector. The benefit of such a universal, free at point of use system is that instead of flat fees which hit poorer families hard and hit people hardest when they are sickest, there is a predictable annual contribution, progressively levied and shared across the community. But achieving a health care system which meets the expectations of Ireland today will also require growth in services, which means that Irish society must fund additional spending, whether by means of extra taxation or social insurance or by reduced tax incentives or state spending elsewhere. (Appendices 3 to 5 analyse what increased health spending has and could deliver, and at what cost.)

It has not been our brief to describe how the future financing of health care might be achieved – which sectors of society should contribute more or less, now or in the future. However, we would support its achievement by equitable and progressive means. The existing state subsidies and tax incentives and the existing organisation of the health care system frequently subsidise private care and discriminate against those who depend on the public system. We argue for an equitable, universal health care system, with care delivered according to need and funded according to ability to pay. We indicate the dimensions of the investment required to deliver a better-resourced system, and explain which reforms would represent a rechanneling of payment and which would require additional resources for health care.

There are two possible paths to fundamental reform of the Irish health care system. One is the path of universal health insurance (UHI), as advocated by many reformers. The central attraction of UHI to its advocates is that it provides a clear path to enhanced equity. If consultants and public hospitals privilege private, fee-paying patients over non-fee-paying public patients, one way to provide seemingly instant equity is to pay fees for all patients. A very straightforward way to achieve that is to provide health insurance for all. UHI has several other advantages as a way to achieve an efficient, decentralised health care system.

38

One approach to UHI is a social insurance model (funded by PRSI), such as is found in Germany, France and the Netherlands.

UHI typically makes the greatest use of fee-for-service medicine of any model of health care system. The authors have tried to mitigate these effects by suggesting hybrid payments systems for both GPs and consultants. But with UHI it would be difficult to avoid increased use of user charges, prices and fees. It is known that the economic effect of such instruments is to increase utilisation throughout the system. Thus, a UHI system is predisposed to higher levels of utilisation and hence health care expenditure than other systems.

There are equitable and efficient alternatives to UHI, achieved through reforms of the existing tax-funded system. Without UHI, there could be free primary care in which the state would pay GPs by salary, capitation, fees or a mixture of methods. Without UHI, the state could ban private practice in public hospitals and invest in public care so that the majority would opt to be treated in one-tier public hospitals. Without UHI, consultants could be paid with a hybrid of salaries and fees. Such a system would move towards that in the UK or Denmark.

Those of us – the authors and our readers – who try to influence policy must guard against dogmatism about the means towards the end. Other states have achieved greater equity and efficiency than Ireland in uniquely different ways. Ireland should have confidence in designing its own solution while taking the best from other states. What is required is clarity about the destination: free and well-resourced multi-disciplinary primary care; equitable access to public hospitals; an end to the dishonest public-private mix within public hospitals, on public hospital campuses or between public and private hospitals; a well-resourced system of primary, acute, community and long-stay care; and a democratically accountable and transparent health administration.

1

THE HEALTH OF THE IRISH PEOPLE

Introduction

This study is primarily about the problems of the Irish health service and the manner in which they might be resolved. Yet it is important to keep in mind that health care is about health – the health of the Irish people – and many of the measures which would most improve our health and thereby our life expectancy and the quality of our lives have nothing to do with health services. Thus, initially in this chapter we will explore the health of the Irish people: how long Irish people live, the diseases which afflict them and the inter-relationship between health and the nature of Irish society. One of the most striking aspects of health experience in many states, and notably striking in Ireland, is the difference in health status and life expectancy between those on lower incomes and those on higher incomes. Inequalities in health are real and marked. They reflect other deep inequalities in life experience, such as inequalities in income, access to education, housing and recreational facilities. Ill health can be a consequence of the stress and life-threatening behaviours (like alcohol and substance abuse and violence) which emerge from social exclusion and a fragmented society. Modern Irish living engenders multiple stresses, caused by, for example, poor transport networks, unplanned expansion of communities, poor child care and long working hours. Alcohol abuse has soared, as young people have become cash-rich fast.

In Ireland, inequalities in health and life experience are mirrored and compounded by a health care system in which access to care is determined by income rather than need. Changing the health care system will not happen without a change in Irish values, driven by an understanding that we all pay a price for this inequity, that we live shorter lives on average and experience greater ill health than the average European. In Chapter 3, we discuss the principle of social solidarity: that health care is not just a product, but part of the glue which holds a society together. This chapter explores how health is inextricably inter-linked with how we live, how we value our health and how we value one another.

Life expectancy

Men and women in Ireland die younger than the average Western European. At birth Irish men and women have shorter life expectancies than the EU15 average.[1] For Irish men, life expectancy at birth was 75.1 years in 2002 compared to 75.8 years in the EU15 and 74.8 years in the EU25. Irish women have a shorter life expectancy at birth than the average across the enlarged EU. Irish women's life expectancy at birth was 80.3 years in 2002, compared to 81.6 years in the EU15 and 81.1 years in the EU25 (see Table 1.1).

The highest European life expectancy at birth for males is reported in Sweden, at 77.7 years, and in Spain for females, at 83.1 years. In 2002 Irish male infant life expectancy ranked eighth jointly with Belgium out of those reported in the EU15. The life expectancy of Irish baby girls ranked second last of those reported in the EU15.

Table 1.1: Irish and EU average life expectancy				
2002	At Birth		At Age 65	
Area	Males	Females	Males	Females
Ireland	75.1	80.3	15.4	18.7
EU15	75.8	81.6	16.3	19.9
EU25	74.8	81.1	16	19.6

Source: Central Statistics Office, Irish Life Tables No. 14, June 2004.

At age 65, Irish life expectancy is below both the EU15 and the EU25 average for men and women. Irish male life expectancy at age 65 in Ireland is at the bottom jointly with Denmark of the EU15 league table. For women at this age, Ireland is second from the bottom in the EU15 league table.

Between 1996 and 2002, life expectancy improved by 2.1 years for males and 1.8 years for females. This narrowed the gap between Irish and EU average life expectancy, which had widened considerably over the period since 1960 (see Figure 1.1).

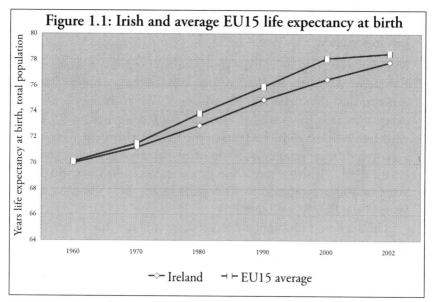

Figure 1.1: Irish and average EU15 life expectancy at birth

Source: OECD Health Data 2005.

Morbidity

Diseases of the circulatory system are the leading cause of death in Ireland, followed by cancer, respiratory diseases and injuries and poisonings. While death rates for circulatory diseases have been declining, the rates are still considerably above the EU15 average. Of the 10,984 people who died from circulatory diseases in 2003, the majority died of ischaemic heart disease. In 2001 Ireland had 146.1 deaths per 100,000 people from this condition, compared to the rate in France at 45.1 per 100,000. The average for 13 of the EU15 states for which data were available was 96 per 100,000 in 2001 (the rates are age-standardised).[2]

Cancer of the lung is the most common type of cancer causing death (20 per cent of cancer deaths), followed by colorectal cancer (12 per cent) and breast cancer (9 per cent). Lung cancer is the most common cause of death from cancer in men, while breast cancer is the most common cause for women.[3] Infectious diseases (pneumonia and influenza) and chronic obstructive airways disease are the leading causes of death from respiratory disease in Ireland.[4]

Suicide is the most common mode of death registered under 'injuries and poisonings', followed by motor accidents and falls. Most people who die from road accidents are male. For young males aged 15–24 years old, the most common cause of death is from injuries and poisonings. Official suicide mortality data from the CSO records that from 2000 to 2002 there were 494 deaths by suicide in Ireland annually on average, peaking at 519 in 2001. This represents a rate of approximately 12.9 deaths per 100,000 population and is average when compared to other EU countries. However, the rate of youth suicide in Ireland is the fifth highest in the EU, at 15.7 per 100,000 for 15–24 year olds. Currently, the highest rate of suicide is found among young men in the age group 20–29 years (35 per 100,000). This contrasts with traditional patterns and with most other countries, where suicide is more frequently observed in older men.[5]

Health inequalities

Irish people on lower incomes suffer more illness and die younger than better-off social groups. A series of recent reports have illustrated the following.

- Unskilled manual male workers are twice as likely to die prematurely as higher professional men.
- Unskilled manual male workers are eight times more likely to die as a result of accidents than higher professional men.
- Unskilled manual workers are almost four times more likely to be admitted to hospital for the first time for schizophrenia than higher professional workers.
- There is an increasing socio-economic gradient in the incidence of all psychiatric conditions from professional to unskilled manual groups.

- Unemployed women are more than twice as likely to give birth to low birth-weight babies as women in the higher professional socio-economic group.
- Perinatal and infant mortality rates are higher in families where the father is an unskilled manual worker or is unemployed.
- On average, Traveller women live 12 years less than women in the general population. Traveller men live on average 10 years less than men in the general population. Travellers' babies experience higher rates of stillbirth, infant mortality and perinatal mortality.
- The prevalences of specific conditions, such as coronary heart disease and lung cancer, are higher in geographic areas that experience higher levels of socio-economic deprivation.
- Adults and children in lower socio-economic groups have higher levels of smoking, higher body mass index and less healthy eating habits than those in higher socio-economic groups.
- Homeless people experience high incidences of ill health. A study in 1997 found that 40 per cent of hostel dwellers in Cork had serious psychiatric illnesses, 42 per cent had problems of alcohol dependency and 18 per cent had other physical problems.[6]
- The prison population suffers from a disproportionately large rate of psychiatric and drug-related problems. Almost one quarter of this population suffers from a long-standing disability or illness that limits their activity.
- On average, 39 per cent of men and women surveyed in 2003 identified financial problems as the greatest factor in preventing them from improving their health.[7]

A population health approach

The poorer health status of people on lower incomes is compounded by their difficulties in accessing care. Later chapters will examine inequities in access to health services in detail. However, the remedy for the poor health experience of people on lower incomes is not entirely or even mainly a matter of improved access to care.

Many life circumstances that depend on income affect health. Poor housing, poor public transport, poor diet, no playgrounds for children and no pre-school education will all affect the health of families. Some public health experts would nominate pre-school education as the priority investment for improving the health of poorer Irish people.

There is a substantial body of research supporting the view that inequalities in income lessen the health status of the population, including its richer members as well as its poorer ones. Unequal societies are stressful societies, with high rates of alienation, violence and substance abuse, whereas egalitarian societies have higher average life expectancies than less egalitarian ones.[8] In Ireland, relative income poverty rates are above the EU average and have risen during the boom years.[9]

In its recent publication *Just Caring – Equity and Access in Healthcare*, the Adelaide Hospital Society argues:

> Death rates caused by alcohol, violence or accidents tend to be strongly related to income distribution and to reflect the effects of increasing income inequality in society. In brief, social exclusion and low social status are major sources of stress, which is chronic in relatively less well off socio-economic groups. A survey of Tallaght's people, for example, revealed very high levels of stress: 59% of primary or principal carers surveyed had experienced stress in the year prior to the survey and, of those, 35% consulted their general practitioner because of their stress and 19% of them had received prescribed medication.[10] Chronic stress affects the endocrine and immune systems and leads to greater vulnerability to illness…Close-knit, egalitarian and inclusive societies are comparatively much healthier. Therefore, economic and social policies, such as taxation policy, should be used to promote an egalitarian and inclusive society and in the longer term this will result in a much healthier society.[11]

In the cases of the three special issues discussed below (obesity, cancer screening and suicide prevention), a complex mixture of factors determines who will be well or ill and who will receive the health care they need, when they need it. These factors include relative income, health service resourcing and inequity in access to care for reasons of income or geography. We have chosen to discuss these health issues not just because they have important effects on health in Ireland, but because they illustrate the mix of reasons for Ireland's low life expectancy.

Special issues

Obesity

Approximately 39 per cent of Irish adults are overweight and 18 per cent are obese. *The Report of the National Taskforce on Obesity* (2005) calculates that approximately 2,000 premature deaths in Ireland can be attributed to obesity annually, at an estimated cost, in economic terms, of €4 billion to the state. The taskforce has expressed its concerns 'that childhood obesity has become the most prevalent childhood disease in Europe.' While currently there are no agreed criteria or standards for assessing Irish children for obesity, some studies suggest that the numbers of children who are significantly overweight have trebled over the past decade. Extrapolation from UK data suggests that these numbers could now amount to more than 300,000 overweight and obese children on the island of Ireland, and they are probably rising at a rate of over 10,000 per year.[12] Levels of overweight and obesity in Irish adolescent girls are higher than the international average. Diseases which obese people suffer from proportionally more than the general population include hypertension, type 2 diabetes, angina, heart attack and osteoarthritis.

In developed countries such as Ireland, levels of obesity are higher in the lower socio-economic groups. Those with lower levels of education are more likely to be obese. Those who have only 'some' education have higher levels of obesity than those who have completed secondary or tertiary education. However, the rates of obesity have increased across all educational levels since 1998.

It is generally accepted that in developed countries the main barriers to healthy food choices are access to healthy foodstuffs, their affordability and one's level of disposable income. Social welfare payments are the main source of income for many low-income groups and therefore are important in determining the living standards of households in these groups. In Ireland it was found, as it was in the UK, that the foods recommended in the Irish healthy eating dietary guidelines were often more expensive than the less-healthy options. Research has found that for low-income groups there are large discrepancies between the amount of money they would need to spend in order to purchase a healthy diet, the amount of money they have available to spend and the amount of money they are currently spending.[13] A recent survey showed that 51 per cent of Irish children consumed sweets, 37 per cent drank fizzy drinks, 27 per cent consumed crisps, 12 per cent ate chips and 7 per cent ate hamburgers at least once daily.

In making over 80 policy recommendations, the National Taskforce on Obesity emphasises that issues of population health such as obesity have implications for policy-makers in many spheres: high-level government; education; social and community; health; food, commodities, production and supply; and the physical environment. The taskforce points out that the rapidity of the rise in obesity, particularly amongst the young, 'implies that factors outside the individual's immediate, conscious discretion are at play here.'

The taskforce recommends that the health services should take a more proactive approach to this problem: 'all contacts with the health services, both scheduled and opportunistic, should be used as opportunities to promote and encourage healthy eating and active living.' It suggests that the public health system, which provides immunisation in schools, should also support and promote healthy eating and active living and engage in early detection of overweight and obesity. Measurement of height, weight, waist circumference and calculation of body mass index (BMI) should be part of routine, clinical health care practice in primary care and in hospitals. The school health services should include the opportunity to have a growth assessment for overweight or underweight. Assessments should be carried out on school entry (four to five years old) and then at regular intervals throughout each child's development. This taskforce recommendation has implications for how primary care and public health services are resourced and organised.

The taskforce also recommends that the Department of Social and Family Affairs should review social welfare payments to take account of the relatively high cost of healthy foods for socially disadvantaged groups. Access to a healthy diet, e.g. fruit and vegetables, should be included as an indicator to measure food poverty as part of the National Anti-Poverty Strategy. The Department of Transport and the Department of the Environment should apply a specifically designated percentage of all road budgets to the construction of safe walkways and cycle-ways. Local authorities should ensure that sports, recreational, leisure and play facilities are equitably available and accessible to all members of the public.

Cancer screening

The rate of death from breast cancer was higher in Ireland in 2001 than in any other of the 13 pre-enlargement EU states for which data are available. The rate of 31.1 deaths from breast cancer per 100,000 Irish women may be compared with an EU13 average of 24.2 deaths. Yet Ireland's incidence of breast cancer is actually below the EU average.[14] This suggests that early detection and treatment are inferior in Ireland compared to those in many other EU states.

BreastCheck, the national breast screening programme, has yet to be offered to women throughout the state. BreastCheck offers free screening to women in designated areas aged between 50 and 64. The programme started in February 2000 and covers the East, Midlands, North-East and South-East. It is expected to open in Kilkenny in early 2006, according to the Department of Health. There is still no programme in the South and West. In May 2005, Minister Mary Harney announced plans for the development of a further two BreastCheck clinics in those regions. It is 'expected that the target date of 2007 for commencement of the roll-out to the regions will be met', according to the Department of Health.

Meanwhile, this basic public health measure – screening for breast cancer – is still denied to women in the highest at-risk age groups in a significant percentage of the country. Outside the programme, women who have become concerned about breast symptoms may be referred by their general practitioners (GPs) for screening, but many women may not have symptoms which provoke their concern, and even for those who are referred, there are waiting lists for screening in the public health system. Income and geography may deny women the early detection which could save their lives.

Suicide prevention

Suicide rates have doubled over the past 20 years at a time when society in Ireland has changed from being highly integrated with shared values to becoming more fragmented, with values no longer widely shared. As social changes have affected the nature and extent of suicidal behaviour in Ireland, efforts to address this serious public health issue require social policy as well as health policy responses.[15]

The National Strategy for Action on Suicide Prevention, published in 2005, states that suicidal behaviour, especially completed suicide, is strongly associated with a history of previous deliberate self-harm, mental health problems (diagnosed and undiagnosed) and alcohol and substance use. High-risk groups include the marginalised, those in prison, the unemployed and those who have experienced abuse. In a study of suicide in Ireland, nearly half (47 per cent) of those for whom a GP could be identified had been referred to the mental health services. According to GPs, 43 per cent of those who died by suicide were suffering from a diagnosable mental health problem at the time of their last visit to the GP.[16] The most common diagnoses in those who die by suicide are an affective disorder (including major depression), followed by a substance abuse disorder, personality disorders and psychotic disorders (including schizophrenia). The combination of a psychiatric disorder and alcohol or substance abuse greatly increases the risk of suicide.

The National Strategy for Action on Suicide Prevention recommended more multi-disciplinary, community-based mental health teams; improved early detection and treatment of psychological distress and mental health problems through community services; and increased levels of child and adolescent psychiatric inpatient resources and community services.

The Taoiseach, Bertie Ahern, stated in the foreword to the *Strategy for Action* that 'additional funding allocations will be made available over the coming years to support the strategy and to complement local and national efforts...if the comprehensive and sustained action recommended in this document takes place over the coming years, then we have cause to be optimistic that the best possible response to the problem of suicide in Ireland will be developed.'[17]

Mental health services

While the strategy for action recognises a correlation between suicide and alcohol abuse, suicide in Ireland also represents the tip of an iceberg of untreated mental illness. A study in 2003 concluded that clinical resources in mental health were overstretched and were not concentrated in the areas of greatest need, 'but paradoxically have been best developed in areas of greatest affluence.'[18] A further report has shown considerable regional disparities in per capita spending on adult mental health services and in numbers of staff.[19]

The *Report of the Expert Group on Mental Health Policy* was published in January 2006 and recommended a radical move to community-based care funded by the closure of psychiatric hospitals. (We revisit the issue of mental health services and discuss the report in Chapter 8 in a review of the effect on the acute hospital sector of deficiencies in other services.)

There is considerable evidence of inadequacies in mental health services. It has been stated in the last year by specialists in the field and in published reports that:
- In 2004, fewer than one in five psychiatrists in public practice could offer a full service to their patients one year after taking up their posts. Only 18 per cent of them could access a social worker, psychologist or an occupational therapist.[20]
- Children and adolescents can expect to wait between six and 18 months to be seen by specialist psychiatric services for a routine outpatient appointment. Young people who are recognised to be at risk of self-harm can be seen sooner as emergencies.

- Over 200,000 children have mental or behavioural problems at any one time, in excess of 100,000 have mild disorders, 81,000 have moderate to severe disorders and 20,000 have disabling disorders. Their treatment requires 236 inpatient psychiatric beds. In 2005 there were 20 beds in two units based in Galway and Dublin.[21]
- Their treatment also requires 150 consultant child and adolescent psychiatrist posts. In 2005 there were 62 such psychiatrists.[22]
- There is currently no capacity in the child and adolescent psychiatric services to provide for young people aged 16 and 17.
- Inadequate numbers of psychotherapists, family therapists, clinical psychologists, occupational therapists and other staff seriously inhibit the provision of child and adolescent psychiatric services through multi-disciplinary teams.
- Compared with other major psychiatric disorders, eating disorders have the highest mortality rate, from medical complications and completed suicides. There is no public specialist inpatient eating disorder unit. An eating disorder service at St Vincent's University Hospital in Dublin has access to three beds and has no designated staff. More than 100 new referrals to this service per year have led to a long waiting list for care. There is an urgent need to establish a specialist outpatient team providing a regional service with an inpatient facility to specialise in eating disorders.
- GMS patients have little or no access to generic publicly funded counselling services. Patients who have been sexually abused or have a major addiction can access counselling through dedicated clinics.
- A UK enquiry into maternal deaths found that suicide was the second cause of death in young mothers, the first being cardiovascular disease. In 2005 there were just three psychiatrists, each of whom had a minor sessional commitment to perinatal work, all based in the Dublin area.

Conclusion

The reasons for Ireland's low life expectancy are many and complex, but it is clear that addressing them requires better-resourced health services, accessed first by those in greatest need, available equitably across regions, and treating mental disorders with the same urgency as physical illness. It also requires a recognition that improving health means developing a more equal society that values the health of all its members, puts playgrounds before golf courses, provides for cycle tracks and public transport as it does for motorways and ensures that everyone can afford a healthy diet.

2

SPENDING ON HEALTH

Introduction

There is great uncertainty about health spending in Ireland: how much we spend, how much we should spend and whether we spend well. The fear that health spending is a black hole that consumes funds without delivering extra services seems to have undermined the 2001 Health Strategy's case for substantial, sustained investment in additional health service capacity and staffing. Yet no one has presented an analytical challenge to its assessment of capacity needs.[1] The debate about health spending is too often confused by misleading international comparisons of health spending, informed by inadequate Irish data; by a failure to appreciate the degree of misclassification within Irish health expenditure of spending on social services; the very wide range of health and social services, which the health budget must fund; and the very low base from which Irish health spending increases rose in the late 1990s.

This chapter examines Irish health spending in detail. Its international comparisons are based on the latest OECD data (October 2005 update[2]). It records that in 2003, the most recent year for which international comparisons are available, Irish per capita current health spending was 94.4 per cent of the EU15 average, a marginal drop on the 2002 position.[3] However, detailed analysis of the degree to which Department of Health returns to the OECD conform with its accounting requirement that social programmes, such as care of the elderly or disabled, should be excluded from international health spending comparisons suggests that the Department should exclude further spending. This suggests that, accurately defined, Irish per capita current health spending was below 90 per cent of the EU average in 2003. With real increases in spending on hospitals of 1 per cent in 2004 and 2 per cent in 2005, it is expected that, when available, international data will show that Irish per capita current spending on core health programmes remained below the EU average in 2005.

Irish public health spending per capita, which aggregates current and capital spending, is recorded by the OECD as 0.5 per cent above the EU average in 2003, an assessment which should also be adjusted downward for spending on social programmes and because of an overstatement of capital spending. The level of Irish capital investment in health and social services has exceeded the EU per capita average in the years from 1997, and in 2003 was twice the average. This should be seen against the backdrop of the 27 preceding years from 1970 to 1996, in which Irish investment averaged only 63 per cent of the EU average. Recent increases in investment have only begun to make inroads on decades of deficiency in health and social care facilities.

In response to arguments that Ireland's health spending per capita should be lower than average because of Ireland's relatively youthful population, we point out that the costs of ageing are primarily borne in social, not health, services and that deficiencies in social services (for which there is convincing evidence but no comprehensive international comparator) are a primary driver of Irish health care costs. Progressive ageing of the population does, however, underline the need to address Ireland's investment deficit in both health and social care facilities.

Over the period 1997 to 2003, spending in the acute hospitals programme (adjusted to take into account rising prices for goods and services in the public sector) increased by 69 per cent and delivered an increase of 38 per cent in the number of patients treated in hospitals. This raises the question of why more care had not been delivered for the substantial funds invested in recent years. We argue that steep increases in current health spending over the period from 1997 to 2002 could not deliver full value against a backdrop of capital deficiency. The

pace of spending increase was also so rapid that it presented difficulties for planners and administrators, particularly in 2001, a
year of significantly large health expenditure growth.

In later chapters, this study makes a detailed case for reform of
how hospitals are funded, managed and staffed and how patients
access care. Spending increases to date have been channeled into
an unreformed public hospital network, which is over-reliant on
highly paid junior doctors; in which average consultants' incomes
exceed specialist incomes in other Northern European countries;
and in which there are incentives to maximise treatment of
insured patients while rationing care to the uninsured.

We argue that current and capital spending on health still
needs to increase to offset the capacity deficits identified in the
2001 Health Strategy (in primary, continuing, community and
acute care), but that this should be in a planned and paced
manner, and within the framework of the 2003 Hanly Report[4] of
reform in how hospital doctors work and are remunerated and in
how patients access care. The costing of the 2001 Health Strategy
by the Department of Health was a limited exercise. We urge that
its capacity needs should be reassessed, even revised if necessary
in light of population growth and the more developed understanding which is emerging of the relationships between the
acute care and other sectors, and that there should then be a comprehensive and realistic analysis of the investment needs of health
and social services over the next 10 years, followed by a planned,
phased commitment of investment.

A simple exercise based on the Health Strategy's original 2001
costings and on a realistic exclusion of the costs of social programmes has suggested that were it implemented over 10 years,
at the end of the period Irish health spending would be approximately 9.9 per cent of national income, still below the current
levels in France, Germany and Canada – states with envied health
care provision – and also below the level contemplated in the UK
by National Health Service planners, who seek to address its
capacity deficits and deficiencies.[5] Funding the strategy would
also require funding its social care component, but this investment requirement should not be confused in international
comparisons of the *health* share of national income.[6]

How much does Ireland spend on health care?

There are a number of ways to answer this question. The combined budgets of the Department of Health (€401 million) and Health Service Executive (HSE) (€11,540 million) in 2005, published in the government's estimates for spending, come to nearly €12 billion. This is a lot of money, yet Irish health care has multiple deficiencies and problems, so it is hardly surprising that there has been a debate about value for money in health spending.

Health represented a large proportion of the government's overall spending in 2005: 28.7 per cent of current or day-to-day spending; and 9.6 per cent of capital spending, i.e. investment in plant and facilities (see the pie charts[7] below).

Health spending has increased considerably in recent years. In simple money terms, current health spending in 2004 was nearly three times the 1997 level. To attempt to assess how much of increased health spending has been required simply to keep up with rising prices and wages, it is necessary to distinguish between nominal and real increases in spending. Nominal increases are the increases in money amounts, year on year. Real increases are adjusted for price increases.

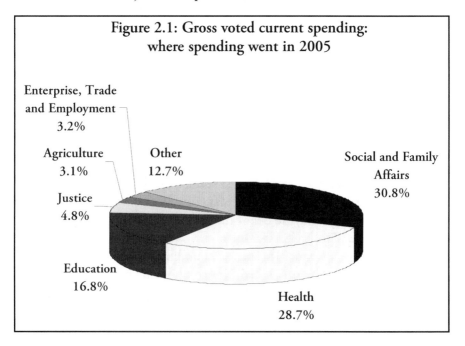

Figure 2.1: Gross voted current spending: where spending went in 2005

Enterprise, Trade and Employment 3.2%

Agriculture 3.1%

Justice 4.8%

Other 12.7%

Social and Family Affairs 30.8%

Education 16.8%

Health 28.7%

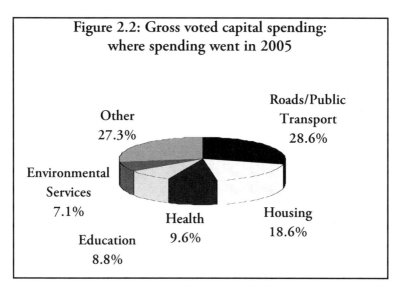

Figure 2.2: Gross voted capital spending: where spending went in 2005

Other
27.3%

Roads/Public
Transport
28.6%

Environmental
Services
7.1%

Health
9.6%

Housing
18.6%

Education
8.8%

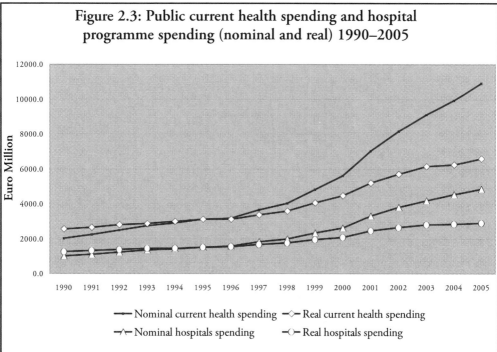

Figure 2.3: Public current health spending and hospital programme spending (nominal and real) 1990–2005

Euro Million

—•— Nominal current health spending   —◇— Real current health spending
—△— Nominal hospitals spending   —○— Real hospitals spending

Source: Revised Estimates for the Public Service. Department of Health for reconciliation 2004 and 2005 data with pre-HSE. Real spending calculated using CSO's deflator for public authorities' goods and services, and Central Bank 2005 forecast.

Figure 2.3 graphs the increase in nominal and real spending over the years from 1990 to 2005 for overall current health spending and for that part of it which funds hospitals. It will immediately be apparent that the real increase is much less steep than the nominal increase and that the increase in real spending on hospitals has been less steep again, almost flat in the last few years.

Proponents of the black hole theory of health spending sometimes equate the top line, the increase in nominal overall health spending, with the bottom line, the real increase in hospitals' budgets, and expect the two to have a direct relationship. Of course, they cannot. Figure 2.3 shows how the efficacy of health spending increases is very much affected by the rate of price increase for the public sector and by the way in which the health budget is divided up. Much so-called health spending in Ireland funds social programmes, like care of the disabled, of older people at home and in institutions. These are very necessary programmes in their own right, which have been under-funded, and when the health budget has increased to begin to address that under-funding, these increases do not directly affect the budgets for hospitals.

In 2004 less than half (46 per cent) of the current Health Vote went to the hospitals, and even this included some long-stay institutions. Acute hospitals alone (regional, county and public voluntary hospitals) received 41 per cent of the Health Vote. A further 16 per cent of the Vote funded GP services and subsidised or free medication, less than 7 per cent went to mental health services and nearly 21 per cent went to what might broadly be regarded as social services (in areas like care of the elderly, disabled, homeless and children at risk).[8] If cost of care in district and health boards hospitals, which is generally long-stay care, were included, these social programmes would come to 27 per cent of the total current health budget.

It is necessary to adjust health spending by an index of 'own prices', i.e. health care prices, to show volume increases. No index of Irish health care prices is available. An index of purchases of goods and services by public authorities is a conservative approximation. In Figure 2.3, to calculate real spending, nominal spending has been adjusted for price changes using this index.

This is a minimal deflator for health spending, given that health employers must pay nationally agreed wage increases in a highly labour-intensive sector and given the internationally acknowledged experience of rapidly rising prices in health care.[9] The real spending curve for hospitals should probably be somewhat less steep than it appears if it were to reflect the actual rate of price increases faced by hospitals. The 2005 and 2004 figures underlying this graph are approximations supplied by the Department of Health, not those published in the 2005 Estimates, which are on a new basis because of the establishment of the HSE. Among other things, the 2005 Estimates overstate the increase in gross health spending because they must take into account income earned by health agencies, which was hitherto excluded. (See discussion in Chapter 12.)

How does Irish spending compare to spending in other states?

It is true that Irish health spending has increased rapidly. It is also the case, however, that it had fallen to very low levels indeed after health and social service cutbacks in the late 1980s and early 1990s. Furthermore, the increases over the last decade have taken place at a time of rapid population growth in Ireland and of a shared international experience of rapidly rising health care spending, driven largely by advances in medical technologies, population ageing and rising public expectations.[10] It is therefore useful to examine how Irish health spending compares with spending in other countries at a similar stage of development and with similar expectations for living standards, for example the EU15. It is even more useful if this comparison takes into account the size of population in each state and is expressed as per capita spending, i.e. spending divided by the number of people living in each country.

International comparisons require care because of differences in the definition of health spending and the manner in which statistics are collected in different states. There are many obstacles to ensuring true comparability despite the OECD's efforts to develop a consistent System of Health Accounts (SHA). Ireland has been one of the slower countries to provide health statistics in the prescribed SHA manner.[11] Consequently, whereas based on earlier OECD data, the government's 2001 Health Strategy document *Quality and Fairness* estimated that total Irish health spending per capita had exceeded the EU average in 2001, an estimate repeated by others, including one of the present authors,[12] subsequent OECD revisions have changed this picture.[13] The latest OECD database, updated in October 2005, is the source for all the following comparisons.

Total health spending

Total health spending is public and private spending combined and incorporates measures of both current and capital spending. The Irish measure is of limited usefulness for international comparison because of the manner in which it is calculated. It requires an estimate of private spending, typically assumed by the Department of Health to run at some 25 per cent of the total.[14] Private spending includes private health insurers' purchase of services for their members; households' and individuals' spending on medicines, GP visits and other medical fees; and investment in private hospitals and facilities.

In its 2004 database update, the OECD explicitly warned against trusting Irish estimates of private health spending, since they are based on imprecise national accounting definitions. In 2005, the OECD again observed that 'national accounts are intended to measure the macro-level output of the national economy. They are not well suited to make detailed estimates of expenditure on health.' This is one of the reasons why we recommend that Ireland should have a system of national health accounts (see Chapter 12). Total health spending also overstates public health spending, for reasons we will discuss below.

With these caveats in mind, the 2005 OECD update shows Ireland's total health spending per capita to be below the EU average in the latest years for which comparable international data are available (see Table 2.1). Total Irish spending fell from 98 per cent of the EU average in 2002 to 96.3 per cent in 2003. It is ranked eighth of 14 EU countries. The OECD had estimated in 2004 that total Irish health spending exceeded the EU average in 2002, but revisions across the range of countries' data have changed this picture.[15]

Table 2.1: Total health spending per capita				
	2002	2003	2003	
	US$ ppp		% EU average	Ranking
Luxembourg	3,729	3,705	145.5	1
Germany	2,916	2,996	117.7	2
Netherlands	2,775	2,976	116.9	3
France	2,762	2,903	114.0	4
Belgium	2,607	2,827	111.0	5
Denmark	2,655	2,763	108.5	6
Sweden	2,595	2,703	106.2	7
Ireland	**2,386**	**2,451**	**96.3**	8
Austria	2,236	2,302	90.4	9
Italy	2,248	2,258	88.7	10
Finland	2,013	2,118	83.2	11
Greece	1,854	2,011	79.0	12
Spain	1,728	1,835	72.1	13
Portugal	1,758	1,797	70.6	14
United Kingdom	2,231	NA		
EU average	2,433	2,546	100	

Source: OECD Health Data 2005.

When measured as a proportion of national income, Irish total health spending was just below the EU average in 2003 at 8.9 per cent (see Table 2.2 – Irish spending expressed as a percentage of GNP, not GDP; see also note to table). The proportion of national income devoted to health care has been increasing across the OECD. The OECD average rose from 7.7 per cent of GDP in 1997 to 8.8 per cent in 2003. In the US, the health share of GDP rose from 13 to 15 per cent over the same period. In France, it rose from 9.4 to 10.1 per cent of GDP; in Canada from 8.9 to 9.9 per cent; in Germany from 10.7 to 11.1 per cent; and in Norway from 8.5 to 10.3 per cent.[16]

Spending on pharmaceuticals is an increasing share of health costs in many OECD countries.[17] It accounted for 2.1 per cent of national income in France and 1.9 per cent in the US in 2003, up from 1.7 per cent and 1.3 per cent, respectively, in 1997. While in Ireland there has been criticism of cost escalation in the state's funding for prescription medicines for Medical Card patients and subsidy for non-Medical Card patients' bills,[18] Ireland has one of the lowest per capita spends on pharmaceuticals in the OECD – 77 per cent of the OECD average and 75 per cent of the EU average in 2003. In 1997 Ireland spent less per capita on drugs than any other EU15 country. In 2003, only one other EU15 country spent less per capita.

Table 2.2: Total health expenditure as percentage of GDP		
	2003	Ranking
Germany	11.1	1
France	10.1	2
Greece	9.9	3
Netherlands	9.8	4
Belgium	9.6	5
Portugal	9.6	6
Sweden	9.4	7
Denmark	9.0	8
Ireland*	8.9	9
Italy	8.4	10
Spain	7.7	11
Austria	7.5	12
Finland	7.4	13
Luxembourg	6.9	14
United Kingdom**	NA	NA
EU average	9.0	

*Source: OECD Health Data 2005. * Irish data as per cent GNP. GNP is used as a measure of national income because GDP includes multinationals' repatriated profits and is an overestimation. **UK 7.7 per cent in 2002.*

Public spending

Irish public health spending is the portion of spending controlled by the government. Its two component parts – current and capital – have such different places in the international range of spending that looking at aggregated public spending can be misleading. The OECD records that in 2003, Irish public health spending, current and capital combined, was just above the EU per capita average and seventh in a ranking of 14 EU states (see Table 2.3). However, Ireland's public *current* health spending was only 94.4 per cent of the EU per capita average and ranked eighth of 14 states (see Table 2.4), while Ireland's *capital* investment in health care per capita was recorded as the highest in the EU15 at 2.5 times the average (see Table 2.5).

Table 2.3: Annual public health expenditure (current plus capital) per capita			
	2003		
	US$ ppp	% EU Av.	Ranking
Luxembourg	3,329	175.1	1
Germany	2,343	123.2	2
Sweden	2,304	121.2	3
Denmark	2,292	120.6	4
France	2,214	116.5	5
Belgium	NA	NA	6*
Ireland	**1,911**	**100.5**	**7**
Netherlands	1,856	97.6	8
Italy	1,697	89.3	9
Finland	1,622	85.3	10
Austria	1,557	81.9	11
Spain	1,306	68.7	12
Portugal	1,253	65.9	13
Greece	1,032	54.3	14
United Kingdom	NA	NA	NA
EU average	**1,901**	**100**	

*Source: OECD Health Data 2005. UK expenditure marginally exceeded Irish total public spending in 2002. *Belgium 2003 public current spending (US$ purchasing power parity 2009) exceeded Irish current plus capital combined.*

Table 2.4: Annual public current health expenditure per capita			
	2003		
	US$ ppp	% EU Av.	Ranking
Luxembourg	3,252	175.4	1
Germany	2,267	122.2	2
Denmark	2,229	120.2	3
Sweden	2,219	119.7	4
France	2,143	115.6	5
Belgium	2,009	108.3	6
Netherlands	1,856	100.1	7
Ireland	**1,750**	**94.4**	**8**
Italy	1,649	88.9	9
Finland	1,552	83.7	10
Austria	1,544	83.3	11
Spain	1,255	67.7	12
Portugal	1,228	66.2	13
Greece	1,008	54.4	14
United Kingdom	NA	NA	
EU average	**1,854**	**100**	

Source: OECD Health Data 2005. UK public current spending not available. UK public current plus capital expenditure marginally exceeded Irish total public spending in 2002. No data for 2003.

Irish health spending is still overstated in these tables despite the efforts of the OECD to ensure international comparability. The Irish entries in these tables still capture some elements of social spending. The measure of capital spending is derived from the national accounts and significantly exceeds the government's published outturn for public capital investment in 2003. The OECD records that Ireland invested €653 million in health facilities in 2003. The government's *Revised Estimates for Public Expenditure* discloses that public investment in health (including social care facilities) was €514 million in 2003, still in excess of the EU per capita average but not at the level recorded in the OECD comparisons. Overstated capital spending therefore contributes to overstatement of Irish public and total health spending in the OECD comparisons. It should further be noted that Irish returns to the OECD for capital investment in health care do not yet distinguish between investment in health and social care facilities.

Table 2.5: Annual public capital health expenditure per capita			
	2003		
	US$ ppp	% EU Av.	Ranking
Ireland	161	252.7	1
Sweden	85	133.4	2
Luxembourg	77	120.9	3
Germany	76	119.3	4
France	71	111.5	5
Finland	70	109.9	6
Denmark	63	98.9	7
Spain	50	78.5	8
Italy	48	75.4	9
Portugal	26	40.8	10
Greece	24	37.7	11
Austria	13	20.4	12
EU average	63.7	100	

Source: OECD Health Data 2005. Data for UK, Belgium and Netherlands not available.

The intricate inter-relationship between health and social spending

The OECD strips out social programmes in making international comparisons of health spending. Its System of Health

Accounts (SHA) excludes spending on institutional care for the elderly or the disabled when the care provided is not predominantly medical: 'Accommodation in institutions providing social services, where health care is an important but not predominant component, should not be included in the health function. Examples might include institutions such as homes for disabled persons, nursing homes, and residential care for substance abuse patients.'[19]

The overstatement of Ireland's health spending in earlier OECD comparisons has led to persistent overstatement of Ireland's relative health spending, even by government figures, despite partial correction of this in recent OECD publications. (See p. 84 *Health Warning – the Elusive Facts about Health Spending*)

In Ireland, the health budget funds both health and social services. The former health boards' administrative role was centralised in the new Health Service Executive (HSE) in 2005. Formerly the health boards and now the HSE administer major health programmes, such as acute hospital care and the Medical Card scheme, and major social programmes, such as care of the elderly and the disabled. Irish health service employees range from cardiac surgeons to home helps. There are advantages to this integration of care because health and social care needs are closely inter-linked. Arguing for retaining responsibility for both services in one government department, social policy analyst, Dr Virpi Timonen, has written:

> Social problems are frequently converted into health problems, and vice versa. For instance, the lack of social support can lead to worsening health problems, and a person with extensive health care needs is often also in need of social support. Many of those who use the health services are in need of social services during or after their period as a health services client: an example of this would be an older person who, following hospital treatment for a stroke, is in need of domiciliary services in order to return home.[20]

This desirable linking of health and social programmes frequently creates confusion in the analysis of trends in Irish health care spending. In the 2005 Budget, for instance, the government provided €2.8 billion for people with disabilities, an 11 per cent increase over 2004. The Minister for Finance announced a multi-annual funding package for disability services over the years 2006 to 2009. Some of this will be reflected in increased health budgets. In 2005 the health budget gained an additional €70 million in current expenditure and a capital allocation of €60 million for services for people with an intellectual disability or autism, physical or sensory disabilities and mental illness. The government said this would fund over 800 extra residential, respite and day places for persons with intellectual, physical or sensory disability or autism; over 200,000 extra hours of home support and personal assistance for persons with physical or sensory disabilities; and additional community-based mental health facilities.[21]

This overdue investment in disability services represents an increase in social programmes. When Irish health spending is compared with spending in other states, much of it should be excluded. Yet some analysts of Irish health spending appear to believe that the entire health budget is devoted to the acute hospital sector.[22]

It would appear that the OECD definition should exclude the bulk of spending under two of the seven programmes in the pre-2005 Department of Health Vote. The social programmes in the pre-2005 Vote were the Community Welfare Programme, which funds services ranging from home helps to contributions to patients in private nursing homes, and the Disability Programme, which funds residential and day care for people with intellectual and physical disabilities. In addition, it would appear that a significant proportion of funding for district and health board long-stay hospitals should also be excluded. In 2003, funding for these three areas was €2,323.7 million, some 25 per cent of all current health spending. Yet in its latest returns to the OECD, the Department excluded only €1,129.4 million, or 12 per cent of current health spending for 2003, on the basis that it funded 'non-health programmes'. This is a conservative and fairly arbitrary count, which, for instance, only attributes to non-health programmes half the budgets for contributions to patients in private nursing homes and for welfare homes for older people, and

20 per cent of budgets for district hospitals and health board long-stay hospitals.[23] In 2004 it had appeared to be the Department of Health's intention to further refine these figures in discussion with the OECD, but possibly because of the many personnel changes in the Department, this refinement has not taken place. There would certainly appear to be justification for excluding as much as 20 per cent of current spending on the grounds that it funds social programmes.

The Department of Health has confirmed that 'an OECD expert, reporting on an examination of Irish public health expenditure figures, stated that public health expenditure figures may be overstated by up to 20 per cent as against boundaries of health care used by OECD SHA (System of Health Accounts). This refers to areas such as intellectual disability and social aspects of elderly care.' The Department conceded that 'additional work is still…required to establish even greater adherence to the SHA standard in returns to OECD. If anything, a further examination of public expenditure involving areas covered by the Department of Health and Children seems likely to decrease further the percentage of that expenditure which falls under health in relation to Ireland, if the SHA standard is fully adhered to.'[24]

If 20 per cent of current spending were excluded, Irish current health spending per capita would be less than 90 per cent of the EU average in 2003. Figure 2.4 shows how Irish public current health spending per capita, which remained below the EU average in 2003, even on the conservative deduction for non-health programmes by the Department of Health, would be shown as falling even more behind the average were a more realistic proportion of spending deducted for social programmes. The graph also illustrates how the recent rapid rise in Irish health spending came from a very low base indeed.

If Irish current health spending per capita is graphed as a percentage of the EU average (see Figure 2.5, based on the present conservative exclusion of spending on non-health programmes), it can be seen how Irish per capita spending was a little over 60 per cent of the average in the late 1980s and early 1990s. The steep increase of the years since 1997 has not been consistent. Irish spending dropped from 83 to 78 per cent of the average between

1998 and 1999, when there was concern about value for money in health spending, and in 2003, a year in which public health sector employment was capped and there were significant restrictions in services, Irish per capita current spending was effectively flat relative to the average, falling from 94.5 to 94.4 per cent.

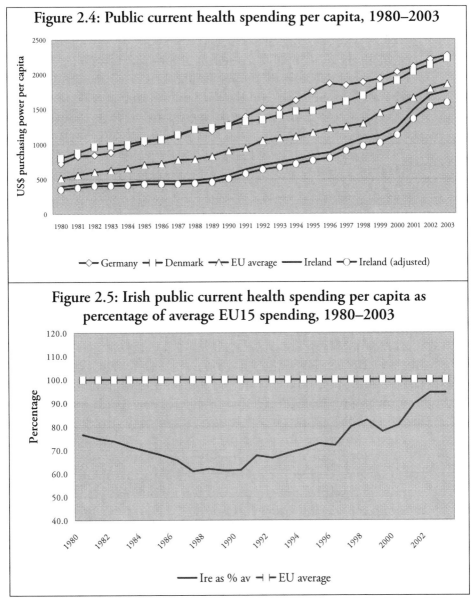

Figure 2.4: Public current health spending per capita, 1980–2003

Figure 2.5: Irish public current health spending per capita as percentage of average EU15 spending, 1980–2003

Source: OECD Health Data 2005.

The restriction in health spending in 2003 was largely influenced by the prevalent view, based on extrapolation from superceded OECD data, that Irish public health spending was on course to be higher in that year than in most other EU states.[25] It is impossible to assess yet where precisely Ireland's spending will have fallen in the range of EU states' in 2004. However, given that in 2004 the increase in hospitals' spending was little over 1 per cent higher than the rate of increase of public prices, and the increase in the overall public current health budget was under 2 per cent above that rate, the strong likelihood is that Ireland will not have advanced its place in the EU health spending ranking.

We stated above that looking at aggregated public spending can be misleading. We have seen that Ireland currently invests more in health care facilities than other EU states, even after adjustment for overstated national accounting data. But to understand the problems of the Irish health and social care system, it is critical to realise what a recent phenomenon this is and what a great deal of ground Ireland must make up in investment in health and social care facilities. The evidence is there to see – hospitals are run down, and as we shall discuss later, this makes it difficult to maintain standards of hygiene. In the long-stay sector, many public institutions are very old indeed, some in effect converted nineteenth-century workhouses. Primary care is a private enterprise in most counties, run from doctors' homes, not in purpose-built buildings. Equipment is deficient: there are too few MRI scanners and GPs cannot gain access to diagnostic facilities. All these problems are the consequence of insufficient investment over many decades when other states were investing in and building up their health and social care infrastructures.

Figure 2.6 graphs Irish investment in health per capita from 1970 to 2003, as recorded by the OECD (and therefore overstated to some degree in recent years). It shows that the recent increase in investment above the EU average follows decades of investing considerably below it. Over the 27 years from 1970 to 1996, on average Ireland invested 63 per cent of the EU average each year. As recently as 1990, Ireland was investing 38 per cent of the average. Whereas over the 24 years from 1970 to 2003 Germany invested on average 138 per cent of the EU average each year, Ireland has invested 84 per cent, our recent increases notwithstanding. There is still considerable ground to make up.

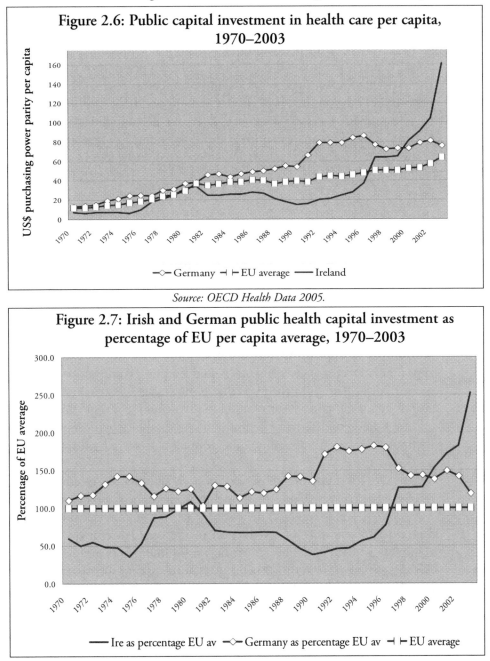

Figure 2.6: Public capital investment in health care per capita, 1970–2003

Source: OECD Health Data 2005.

Figure 2.7: Irish and German public health capital investment as percentage of EU per capita average, 1970–2003

Source: Derived from OECD Health Data 2005. Average of data range available in a given year.

Health spending and demographics

Some commentators have argued that Irish health spending should be below that in many other states because of the age structure of the Irish population. The National Economic and Social Council has pointed out that in 2002, 15 per cent of the Irish population was aged 60 years and over, compared to 20.6 per cent in France and 24 per cent in Germany and Italy.[26] Efforts have been made to assess the effect of relative demographics on how one should compare countries' health spending.[27] There are a few points about this argument which need to be borne in mind:

(a) The argument for a strong association between population ageing and rising health care costs is not an uncontested one.

There are, in brief, three theories. The first is that elderly people may continue to become sick at the same ages as previously, leading to an association of extended lifespan with extended morbidity (sickness), and consequently demands on the health care system. This argument would appear to be favoured by the NESC. The second theory is that the extension of the lifespan has an upper limit. As poor health and disability tend to appear at later ages on average, this would lead to 'a compression of morbidity'. The third theory is that both average lifespan and age of onset of poor health or disability would continue to extend, leading to deferral of disability. Thus, disability in old age becomes 'end of life' disability, not inevitably associated with a particular age.

An OECD study has observed from a number of recent reviews of international data that the third scenario best coincides with the observable trends. There was evidence from a review of a number of countries of a reduction in the prevalence of disability rates in old age. This reduction was found mainly among the age groups from 65 to 80 and was more striking for males than females.[28]

This theoretical argument has particular application in Ireland, where life expectancy is on average below the EU average. Thus, age onset of sickness and disability might be expected to be earlier in Ireland, especially for those social groups with particularly low life expectancy. We know Irish people die younger than the French, so we might reasonably conclude that they experience fatal illness or events at an earlier age on average than the French, and that the Irish health care system logically must experience the consequent 'end of life' demands for the delivery of care to a younger cohort of the population than in France.

There is evidence that just as different populations have differing life expectancies, so too do they have differing rates of health and sickness in old age. This is a difficult area for international comparison because of differing definitions of disability. However, given that caveat, the OECD has assembled reports that in Germany, up to and past 90 years of age only 40 per cent of women and 50 per cent of men are defined as having a disability, whereas in Ireland, at the age of 85, 50 per cent of women and 60 per cent of men are defined as having a disability.[29]

(b) The effect of an ageing population is primarily felt in increased demands for care – or the cost of social care programmes – and not in increased acute health care costs.

A study of proximity to death and acute care utilisation in Scotland observed that there was now 'extensive evidence that the cost of acute hospital care increases with proximity to death but that these additional costs in the last six months of life fall with age.' Analysis of people who died of cancer showed that less was spent per person as they aged. This study concluded that 'increases in costs of health care directly attributable to the ageing of populations may be small, since increases in costs of caring for older people are at least partially offset by lower proximity to death costs.'[30]

This Scottish study replicated in part the findings of an earlier study in the Canadian province of British Columbia, which found that while costs of care increased with age, proximity to death was a better predictor of cost than age:

> The additional cost of dying falls with age, even when social and nursing costs are included. In the very elderly group, the additional cost of dying comes almost equally from additional

medical costs and additional nursing and social care costs. In the younger groups it is mainly acute medical care that is used by those close to death...The findings support the assertion that the growing costs of care resulting directly from ageing are likely to be relatively modest, with the rise in social care costs being the major part overall...Despite the falling cost of dying with increasing age, it is likely the overall care costs will rise, but this change is more likely to be like a glacier than an avalanche.[31]

The distinction should also be made here, as above, between current and capital spending in health care. The progressive ageing of the Irish population underlines the need to address Ireland's investment deficit in both health and social care facilities. Other states made this investment many years ago and it is not reflected in their annual per capita health spending today. It is reflected in Ireland's spending because Irish health investment figures returned to the OECD reflect investment in both health and social care facilities. Ireland is just now beginning to address the deficit in provision and this is driving up Irish capital investment in health care to the highest level in the EU, as we have seen, and increases the aggregate of current and capital spending.

In relation to Germany, Japan and Luxembourg, the OECD has observed that the main growth of long-term care spending takes place during the initial phase of setting up new social programmes. Where a system is in place for a longer period of time, no cost explosion relative to acute care spending has occurred. Ireland is just now entering the high-cost period in long-term care provision.[32]

(c) If the costs of ageing are primarily social care costs, then it does not follow that because Ireland has a lower proportion of older people than the EU average, Ireland should have below EU per capita average health spending.

Arguments that assume Ireland's demographics should greatly reduce its demand for health care compared to other states may be posited on an assumption that international comparisons include both health and social care. But, as we have seen, this is not the case. If there were an international database which compared countries' combined per capita current spending on health and social care programmes, and if Ireland were to show approximately average spending compared to other states for these two categories of programme combined, then it would be legitimate to question why Ireland's demographics were not reflected in lower spending. But there is no such international data source, and if there were, it is highly improbable that that is the picture that would emerge.

This is because the existing international comparisons of spending on social care show that Irish spending is relatively very low in proportion to its older population. The OECD has measured the proportion of older people receiving home benefits, and at 5 per cent of the population of over 65-year-olds, Ireland's rate compares to over 20 per cent in the UK, 18 per cent in Norway and 15 per cent in Australia.[33]

(d) Ireland's low rate of social spending, particularly on care for the elderly, is a primary cause of the considerable pressures on the Irish health care system and a key driver of Irish health care spending.

In examining the arguments about demographics and health spending, the case for removing social spending from international comparison, as required by the OECD Health Database, is turned on its head. In order to compare like with like, it would be necessary to compare spending on both social and health care programmes to see where Ireland stands in the international ranking relative to its demographic structure.

The latest Central Statistics Office (CSO) population forecasts are predicated on the percentage of the population aged over 60 having been maintained at 15 per cent in 2005, but within a rapidly increasing population. The CSO estimates that the number of people aged 60 and over will have increased by 59,000, or 10 per cent, between 2000 and 2005.[34] This rapid growth in Ireland's older population has put considerable pressure on Ireland's social infrastructure. The 'non-health programmes' which should be removed from OECD comparisons of health care spending are the very programmes which must be expanded to meet the care needs of older people.

It can be said with certainty that deficiencies in Irish social programmes have placed an enormous burden on the health care system. Chapter 8 will examine the inter-relationship between deficiencies in long-stay and community care and the pressures on acute hospitals. The most obvious instance is the continued occupancy of acute hospital beds by older patients who are ready for discharge from acute care but for whom there is either no suitable long-stay place or inadequate supports to allow them to return home. Ireland's health spending has been driven upward by the need to address the consequences of decades of neglect in both health and social care, and significantly by deficiencies in social and community care programmes and institutions.

Is health spending a black hole?

In political and policy circles there is evidence of great unease about the recent increases in Irish health spending. Arguments against continuing to increase health spending range from ill-founded assertions about the level of Irish spending relative to other states', to the demographic arguments discussed above to the belief, verging on dogma, that health spending is a black hole and that it does not matter how much you spend on health because its problems will remain intractable. We have outlined how the health budget funds a wide range of services, yet in much discourse it is equated with the hospitals programme. (Appendix 4 gives some idea of the range of services and of how they have increased in recent years.) What, then, has increased spending achieved in the hospitals' programme? In 1997, the programme received €1,624 million (for acute as opposed to district and long-stay hospitals). The public and voluntary acute hospitals treated 680,245 patients as inpatients or day cases. In 2004, these hospitals received €4,105.4 million and treated 982,925 patients. When adjusted for public price increases, the increase in current spending had been 72 per cent and the increase in patients treated 44 per cent.[35] That comparison gives fuel to the black hole theory.

Value for money and Irish health spending

Later chapters will outline many areas where both reform and investment are necessary in Irish health and social care. The authors will not and could not attempt to argue simultaneously that all spending to date has represented good value and that health in Ireland requires root and branch reform, as those would be manifestly incompatible positions. Nonetheless, we do distance ourselves from the pernicious and pervasive black hole argument, which can be used to undermine each and every case for further investment and spending in health care, no matter how well founded. It is our belief that there are instances of poor value in Irish health spending and that these can be remedied by reform, but that not even wholesale reform will obviate the need for sustained investment and higher spending.

These are some instances of poor value for money which we would readily acknowledge.[36]

Pace of spending increases

There is evidence that the pace of increase in spending caused difficulties in the 1997–2002 period. The particularly large spending increase in 2001 (a nominal increase in the hospitals' budget of 26 per cent and a real increase of 18 per cent) appears to have been driven by the electoral cycle rather than a sober assessment of what the system could sensibly absorb in any one year. However, to argue that better value might have been achieved with more gradual increases of funding is not at all the same as to argue that increased funding was or is not required.

Mismatch in current and capital spending

Since increased current spending has taken place against a backdrop of serious deficiencies in capacity, this has caused diminishing returns on current spending increases.[37] Anyone who is familiar with the Irish health service can provide many examples of this phenomenon. Surgical and anaesthetic teams are under-employed when surgical patients cannot be admitted due to the occupation of available beds by patients (like elderly people with chest infections) who require medical rather than surgical treatment. Newly appointed consultants have complained that they are unable to work due to the unavailability of operating theatre sessions.[38] Large Dublin hospitals are notoriously unable to deploy their staffs to treat the optimal number of patients because of the presence of long-stay patients for whom no convalescent or rehabilitative accommodation can be found. Day case activity increased by 105 per cent over the years 1997 to 2004, from 206,541 patients treated in 1997 to 424,381 in 2004. But inpatient activity could not increase at the same rate because inpatient bed numbers remained constrained (see Chapter 7). The number of patients treated as inpatients increased by 18 per cent from 473,704 in 1997 to 558,544 in 2004 (see Appendix 4).

Paradoxically, the perception of a black hole caused staffing cutbacks in 2003, with the result that many larger hospitals closed wards, exacerbating the capacity deficiency. Simultaneously, new facilities developed at a reported capital cost of €400 million remained idle in 2003 and 2004 due to Department of Finance strictures. This recent experience makes it clear that addressing mismatches in public capital and current spending has become of critical importance in planning health service development.

Additional expansionary pressures on the hospital system

The hospital system has faced expansionary pressures which exceed those of the general public sector. Although extra staff have been recruited to provide new services, they were also needed to maintain services: to make up for junior doctors' reduced hours; to replace trainee nurses who went into full-time education and ceased staffing wards; to avoid sole rostering, where staff might be vulnerable to accusations of abuse; and to replace the dwindling religious, who frequently worked unpaid overtime or took no salary.[39]

The national nurses' strike in 1999 secured significant improvements in nurses' pay and conditions. From 1989 the excessive working hours of non-consultant hospital doctors (NCHDs) had progressively fallen and there was a concomitant increase in their numbers. In 2000 the negotiation of a new NCHD contract so increased basic pay and overtime rates that junior doctors in Ireland could earn more than in many other states. The average senior registrar earned more with overtime in 2002 – €146,076 for an 82-hour week – than the average consultant's public salary and allowances of €142,051.[40]

Medical staffing and the Hanly agenda

Later chapters will explore in detail the arguments for reform in how Irish hospitals are organised and staffed. Here we briefly examine the value-for-money implications of the traditional organisation of Irish hospitals. The political imperative to offer acute care in every county, albeit delivered by unsupervised junior doctors, has caused the health service to employ many well-paid juniors who must frequently refer up the line for appropriate clinical decisions in the 'serial failure' model of tiered on-call working, as described in one of the earlier, unpublished, drafts of the 2003 Hanly Report.

While some Irish public hospital consultants have little opportunity to augment their public salaries, others have sizeable opportunities for private practice, either within or outside their public hospital. Although there are no published data on individual consultants' private earnings, it is possible to infer that in 2002, public consultants' incomes ranged from €149,000 for those with no private practice to an average of €280,000 for those with a significant private practice. This compared to an average salary range of €80,000–€139,000 in the UK with relatively small opportunity for private practice, €88,000–€100,000 in the Danish public system and an average fee income of €162,000–€214,000 in Canada.[41]

If implemented as part of a comprehensive, well-resourced plan, the Hanly agenda to replace inadequate 'acute' care largely delivered by junior doctors in a multiplicity of hospitals with regional centres staffed by teams of consultants offering high-skilled, around-the-clock acute care should improve the quality of Irish hospital care (see Chapter 10 for caveats). Hanly proposed a substantial increase in consultant numbers and a reduction in the number of junior doctors. While Hanly eschewed industrial relations issues, it logically follows that these juniors would receive reduced pay for working shorter hours but would gain better working conditions and much-enhanced career prospects. It further follows that consultants should be required to work full time for the public sector at rates comparable to their European counterparts.

In 2002, Ireland had at most 24 doctors for every 10,000 people, compared to an EU average of 32. Irish hospital consultants regularly point out how few they are in proportion to population compared to their European counterparts. The EU average is a ratio of 18 specialists to every 10,000 people. Ireland has five consultants to every 10,000 people and 13 specialists (if one includes NCHDs).[42] We argue elsewhere for increases in medical education and staffing. It could be further argued that it would be possible to employ more consultants were their remuneration more modest, or conversely that were there more consultants, their remuneration would fall. Danish rates of remuneration could buy Ireland something approaching the EU average proportion of specialists in relation to population, for the existing hospital staffing pay bill.[43] Perhaps more realisably, implementation of the Hanly Report could increase the Irish ratio to 10 consultants for every 10,000 people, at very little extra medical payroll cost, by substituting consultants for highly paid juniors, provided newly appointed consultants required no more remuneration than their public salaries. Further increasing current health spending could further increase doctor numbers and quality of care. How much Irish doctors earn will be determined over time, partially through negotiation, but will also be critically influenced by how and whether the Irish government chooses to reform the health care system. Many well-qualified Irish medical graduates currently work in other countries for a great deal less than they would earn in Ireland, were there posts for them in Ireland. There will eventually have to be a trade-off between the numbers of doctors employed in Ireland and their earnings.

It remains the case that delivery of the Hanly agenda would require substantial investment in regional hospital capacity, ambulance services and primary care, so that communities need no longer regard their local hospital as their first port of call when in medical need. The funding of thousands more acute beds should be predicated on the implementation of Hanly – specifically, the choice of regional centres of excellence in which to locate the beds – and vice versa, an argument we will explore further in later chapters.

Dual medicine and two-tier access

The parallel existence of public and private medicine in Irish public hospitals has fostered the development of a dual medicine, in which the privately insured not only achieve more rapid access to care, but they, their insurers and their doctors face a set of incentives to maximise their treatments in subsidised public facilities. Our recommendations in later chapters for reforming this system would deliver greater value for money in Irish health care. Were Irish public hospitals to administer a common waiting list for public and private patients, as we recommend, insured patients would take their place in the queue. It can be inferred that waiting times for public patients would fall and waiting times for insured patients would rise, but those in greater need would be treated more rapidly, a not unreasonable measure of improved public health system performance. At present, the policy tool to reduce public patients' waiting times is the National Treatment Purchase Fund, which has gone some distance to achieving that end, but which has done so by purchasing private care for public patients while private patients retain preferential and subsidised access to public facilities – an inefficient use of public funds. If the Hanly reforms were coupled with a requirement that public consultants should work full time for the public sector and that the system of two-tier access to public hospital care should end, it should be possible to ensure that public investment delivers better consultant-delivered care for all patients. Such a reform package would remove the existing duality in which public doctors and hospitals are incentivised to supply more care to some patients while rationing care to others.

Unmet need

Ultimately the only true measure of value for money in health care is improved health, and it remains the case that Ireland has a primary care system which is unaffordable for many citizens and has inequalities in income and access to social services, which foster ill health. Were these issues addressed, the demands on the hospital sector would be much reduced. If the health of the nation were viewed as an asset or an investment in the future, as education has come to be viewed, then it would be logical to introduce a system of universally accessible primary care, the norm in other Western European states, whether funded by taxation or social insurance.

Conclusion: Funding the Health Strategy

The detailed costing of the 2001 Health Strategy by the Department of Health was not published (Appendix 5 describes it in detail). At the time of writing, the strategy is over four years old. As we will outline in detail in later chapters, the strategy has not been implemented. The expansion it promised has not occurred in any significant way: not in acute bed capacity, primary care, continuing care or in staffing.

A simple exercise in 2004 based on the Health Strategy's original 2001 costings, and on a realistic exclusion of the costs of social programmes, suggested that were it implemented over 10 years, at the end of the period Irish health spending would be approximately 9.9 per cent of national income,[44] below the current level in France, Germany and Canada – states with envied health care provision – and also below the level contemplated in the UK by National Health Service planners, who seek to address its capacity deficits and deficiencies (see Appendix 5).[45] Funding the strategy would also require funding its social care component, but this investment requirement should not be confused in international comparisons of the *health* share of national income.[46]

Rhetorical dismissals of the Health Strategy's analysis or costing, such as those from the Minister for Health, Mary Harney (see panel p. 84), are not a substitute for policy. The sums currently being spent on Irish health care are great; the remaining deficiencies in its services are manifest; the 2001 Health Strategy was the product of a long process of analysis and consultation. Doubtless, it can be refined and deserves to be re-examined. Its statement of capacity needs should be reassessed and revised if necessary in light of population growth, and the more developed understanding which is emerging of the relationships between the acute care and other sectors. However, it is the authors' considered view, in light of Irish circumstances and international trends in health spending, that current and capital spending on health still needs to increase to fund the capacity deficits identified in the Strategy – in primary, continuing, community and acute care. A comprehensive and realistic analysis of the investment needs of health and social services over the next 10 years should be followed by a planned, phased commitment of investment, which takes place within the framework of the 2003 Hanly Report, of reform in how hospital doctors work and are remunerated and in how patients access care. In later chapters we will examine the needs of the primary, acute and continuing care sectors, and assess progress against the Strategy's targets. In Appendix 5 we discuss costing investment and reform in health care.

Health warning – the elusive facts about health spending

How Ireland's health spending compares:

April 2005

The Minister told the Irish Medical Organisation: 'At €3,000 per capita, we spend 7 per cent more in real terms than the Blair government in Britain. This is 9 per cent per capita more than the Germans and 70 per cent more than the Italians. Only Denmark and Luxembourg are ahead of us.' (*The Irish Times*, 2 April 2005)

April 2005

The Department of Health later explained: 'The Tánaiste did not deliver a scripted speech at the IMO conference in Killarney, as often is her preference. In relation to some statistics, she was speaking from memory of an article she wrote for *The Irish Times* in October 2003.'

Facts

The Minister was referring to an outdated forecast of health spending in 2003, not 2005. Latest OECD analysis shows that in 2003, Ireland's total health spending per capita was at most 82 per cent of the German level, and ranked eighth of 14 EU states. Ireland's public current health spending per capita was 77 per cent of the German level and also ranked eighth. These assessments are probably still overstated and are the most up-to-date international comparisons available. (See Tables 2.1 and 2.4.)

Costing the Health Strategy:

May 2005

The Minister for Health told the Irish College of General Practitioners there was insufficient money to implement all the strategies and reports compiled for the Department of Health. These included the Primary Care Strategy. To implement them all would cost an estimated €50 billion, she said. (*The Irish Times*, 23 May 2005)

June 2005

In response to a request for the analysis underlying this €50 billion figure, the Department of Health replied: 'We cannot confirm the exact quotation. The Tánaiste was focusing on public health spending growth over the next 10 years, as many of the strategies produced in recent years set out policy objectives over timeframes up to 10 years.' The Department then explained that health spending (gross, current and capital) had grown 'by about 225 per cent since 1997'. 'If we grow spending at the same rate over the next 10 years that we have over the last eight, health spending would be €53 billion by 2015, as compared to €12 billion now.'

Fact

The Minister did not therefore have an assessment of the costs of implementing the health strategies. The Department says she was forecasting a continuation of health spending growth over the last eight years 10 years into the future. That is not the same thing.

3

SOLIDARITY, DECENTRALISATION
AND PRIVATISATION

Introduction

The Irish system of health care should be based on the need principle of medical ethics and on the principle of social solidarity. Medical care cannot be just another product to put in market baskets. It must be part of the glue which holds a society together.

Is Europe – is Ireland – moving away from the solidarity principle? Two important trends in health care systems in Europe are *decentralisation*, with increasing reliance on market-like institutions, and *privatisation*, the conversion of government-operated public facilities into private, autonomous facilities, organised for profit. This chapter looks at these trends in light of the need for reform in the Irish health care system. In the process, we raise the question of whether the principle of social solidarity is consistent with such trends as decentralisation or privatisation.

The Irish health care crisis

There is significant unmet demand for health care in Ireland. It manifests itself in many forms:
- waiting lists for acute hospital care;
- bed occupancy rates in Irish hospitals approaching (and sometimes exceeding) 100 per cent, far higher than the generally agreed optimum of 85 per cent;

- the accident and emergency (A&E) crisis, with patients spending night after night on trolleys in hallways and waiting rooms;
- 'bed-blockers' – patients ready for discharge for whom no appropriate institutional setting exists for further care;
- inadequate capacity in primary care, especially outside of GPs' usual working hours;
- inadequate capacity in post-acute care and beds.

While the existence of unmet demand is obvious, the exact nature of the problem is not. This is because bottlenecks in each sector are reflected in other sectors. For example, A&E patients are on trolleys largely because there are not enough acute beds, which may in turn reflect the lack of adequate post-acute or primary care facilities.

The system as a whole cannot handle the demands currently placed on it. But where the strategic bottleneck is located cannot really be inferred by identifying the place where it is manifested. That observation actually leads to another important conclusion: the Irish health care system is apparently badly organised or structured to respond to high and rising demand.

The crisis does not simply show an inadequate response to unmet demand. It shows inadequate *responsiveness*. More resources are needed, but equally, the system needs reform to make it less rigid and prone to lock-up and breakdown.

Part of the problem is that the decision-making structure is bureaucratised and politicised. The incentive structure is dysfunctional, an analysis we develop in detail in Chapter 4.

The government's strategy

One response to the crisis is the present government's policy, as announced in 2005, to allow and encourage the construction of private hospitals on the grounds of public hospitals. Public hospitals would then shift some of their private beds to public use. The promised result would be a shift in the location of private beds and a net increase in the number of public beds.

Does this structural change answer the need for flexibility and responsiveness? Whether we should call the result – more private hospitals, more public beds – 'privatisation' is not clear. We examine the government's plan toward the end of this chapter in the context of our discussion of decentralisation, privatisation and social solidarity.

Social solidarity

Health care can be defined as a commodity. Its production uses scarce resources which therefore cannot be used otherwise, so its production imposes a cost on society. It is produced using technology which changes considerably from period to period. It is also a source of employment for many. Thus, it satisfies all the definitions of a commodity. However, that by itself answers few questions about the character of medical care. Other institutions in which society places great value – education, even religion – can similarly be defined as commodities in the same strict sense.

This study is guided by the following principles, which are shared by many, if not most, people resident in Ireland. First is the *need principle of medical ethics*: 'Access to care should be on the basis of medical need or capacity to benefit from care, and should not be affected by other factors such as ability to pay or geographic location.'[1] That does not necessarily mean that health spending must be the same across persons with differing preferences or means. If individual preferences dictate and if individual means permit, person-to-person differences in health care expenditures can reflect differences in *amenity level* of bed accommodations, food and television and telephone facilities. But people with similar medical need should receive care of similar types, quality and timing.

No health care system fully meets this standard, though it must be conceded that many come closer to achieving it than Ireland. The Irish system deviates from it in important respects. One objective of this report is to move the Irish system closer to satisfaction of this standard.

Second is the *principle of social solidarity*. Health care in Ireland should be, and in fact to an extent is, governed by this principle. The health care system taken as a whole should be viewed as the shared and common heritage and wealth of all. This wealth is not alienable property which, like a home or car, can be bought and sold: it is inalienable, like education, values, culture and the democratic political system. An articulate statement of the principle of social solidarity appeared in an Organisation for European Cooperation and Development (OECD) publication describing the admirable French system: 'This plan does not call into question the principle of solidarity between those in good health and the sick, with everybody contributing according to their income and receiving care according to their needs.'[2]

In Ireland, social solidarity is not merely an abstract principle; it has an empirical existence. It exists on the revenue side of the health care system because everyone shares the burdens of taxation to support the health care system. Solidarity also exists on the expenditure side. Everyone is a public patient in the Irish system. Even those who are private patients at certain times for certain procedures are virtually certain to be public patients at crucial times in their lives. Even as private patients, they are beneficiaries of public subsidies. Ultimately, everyone shares the same health care system, though manifestly all do not benefit equally.

Medical ethics and social solidarity are not the same as socialism, public ownership or a centralised state apparatus. It is not definitionally necessary to have state-owned or state-managed institutions or a centralised command structure to achieve either desideratum. In this chapter, we explore the relations among the three issues of solidarity, decentralisation and privatisation.

The free market, bureaucratic provision and decentralisation

Several models are available for organising a country's health care system. Among them are the market, free from interference or regulation; direct state provision and control; and intermediate arrangements in which a managed form of market competition substitutes for direct, hands-on state administration.

Should we rely on the free market to determine health care utilisation?

In general, economic efficiency is thought to result from free competition among sellers and free choice by buyers.

However, this idea does not apply, or applies only with major modifications, in health care. There is a long list of reasons why that is the case.

- *Moral hazard*: Because the need for health care over time is typically unforeseeable and because its costs may be crippling, societies tend to develop health insurance of some type. Health insurance, in turn, lowers the price of health care at the point of use. That leads people to demand more health care. This is a phenomenon known in the insurance trade as 'moral hazard'. In a free market there may be too much utilisation.

- *Unclear benefits*: Even if there were no moral hazard, a free market would fail to work correctly because patients lack the knowledge or expertise to evaluate the benefits from medical care.

- *Information asymmetry*: Free markets work well only when both buyer and seller share the same information. In medical care, this frequently is not the case. Doctors know more than patients about diagnosis and treatment.

- *Physician dominance of utilisation decisions*: Because patients lack knowledge of medicine, physicians make or influence most utilisation decisions, and a free market is impossible. Indeed, in many instances patients lack the legal authority to choose their own care, not only with respect to prescription pharmaceutical medicines, but also in relation to other aspects of care. There are three more points to make in this connection:
    1. Virtually all utilisation decisions are made either by patients covered by some kind of insurance or by physicians. In other words, most decisions are made by persons who do not bear the costs of their own decisions.
    2. Physicians often have a conflict of interest when they decide on or influence patient care. The decisions they make also influence their own incomes and workloads.
    3. Because patients must rely so much on physician training and skill, most countries evaluate physicians and license those determined to be qualified. In Ireland, the Medical Council registers doctors on its General Medical Register when they become eligible to practice.

- *Possibility of externalities*: Many types of health care influence the well-being of third parties. For example, treatment or prevention of infectious illness such as pneumonia benefits not only the person cared for, but others whom that person might otherwise infect. People typically take into account only their own benefits from transactions. In a free market, benefits would be underestimated because third-party benefits, or externalities, would be ignored. If one compared the probable gain (reduced chance of disease) with the cost of inoculation, one might choose to skip the shot. But if the effect of that one inoculation on the health of family, friends and co-workers were added to the equation, the decision might be to choose the shot.

- *Health care and the health of society*: The evolution of universal health insurance in many states, including Prussia under Bismark, was driven by a recognition that good health is of value not only to the individual, but to society as well. An important externality from health care available to all takes the form of the gains from a productive, vital nation.

- *Health care may be a merit good*: A merit good is one which, even if it is a private good with no externalities, is deemed so meritorious or important by society that we make certain that all members of society can avail of it. Society is willing to ignore or interfere with individual preferences in the case of merit goods, even for goods which solely benefit the individual. Primary education is a leading example of a merit good. Indeed, we do not allow children (or their parents) the freedom to choose not to be educated. To be sure, one child's education benefits society, i.e. primary education has significant externalities, but we compel school attendance mainly for the child's own sake, i.e. primary education is a merit good. To describe health care as a merit good is to say that the buyer in a free market may make mistakes and under-value future health care.

- *Inequality*: A health care system wholly run according to market principles will privilege the wealthy, as the market accommodates those with the most resources. This tendency towards inequality is accepted for most goods, but in relation to medical care it violates the need principle of health ethics.

The other extreme – bureaucratic provision

Because the free market will not work correctly in producing, distributing and financing health care, the state inevitably plays the central role. But what should the state do? There are many alternative models of the state role. The simplest to describe is for the state to run the health care system – to own and operate the hospitals, purchase equipment and materials, employ doctors and other professionals and staff and dispense drugs and medical supplies.

In principle, this model can deal well with most of the problems just described. The state can assure that everyone has access to modern, high-quality care and that no one loses out because of their own failure to buy health insurance. It can take advice from physicians, economists and other experts in determining what care is appropriate. It can counter the problems arising from moral hazard by limiting utilisation on the supply side. Further, this system is one wholly consistent with the principle of social solidarity. It can ensure that access to care follows the need principle of medical ethics.

While this model may be the easiest to describe (or to diagram) and while it has the potential to overcome the problems arising in the free market, it may not be the easiest to administer satisfactorily. Many problems arise in this directly state-administered model of health care. For example, the state must plan the health care system in detail, making perhaps thousands of intricate decisions which in the end must be internally consistent and fit well with technology, need and social demand. Then it must carry out these decisions through a hierarchical command structure through city centres, suburbs, villages and rural lands. This in turn requires a complex vertical and horizontal bureaucratic chain of command from cabinet minister through to porter. The result is inevitably a rigid and inflexible system in which internal inconsistencies reveal themselves as bottlenecks, crises and breakdowns and which is unresponsive to changed circumstances.

Moreover, a state system is vulnerable to politicisation, where doctors, powerful veto groups, trade unions and localities have strong motives to protect characteristics of the system which favour them, and where the political process provides a means for doing so. In the end, then, a state-run system may not deliver care in an equitable manner.

A problem arising out of a bureaucratic model which is not so obvious is the difficulty the centre faces in getting accurate information. At its best, the market is the optimal device available for getting information about needs, preferences and changing technology. A command system has trouble knowing what people want and how to get it to them.

Decentralisation and the use of the market in health care

The health care systems of Europe never reached the extremes of the bureaucratic model described above, but they did have many of its features. The Irish system still approximates the bureaucratic model in relation to public hospitals.[3] The national health service model pioneered by Britain traditionally made essentially all allocation and utilisation decisions administratively. Systems based on social health insurance – like the French, German and Dutch – had multiple payers in the form of sickness funds, but most funds operated as geography-based or industry-based monopolies.

Ireland has been relatively untouched by the European trend which began in the 1990s, and has continued until today, of decentralisation and increased use of the market and of market-like institutions in response to perceived bureaucratic rigidities and inefficiencies. Policy formulation, implementation and evaluation all were the responsibilities of the same Department of Health, making it difficult to assure that all three tasks were well achieved.

Problems similar to those that exist today in Ireland led most of Europe to experiment with one or more of three types of decentralisation:

- Centralised systems such as the United Kingdom's National Health Service (NHS) received organisational reform. Budgetary institutions, including hospitals, became 'trusts' or autonomous organisations with increased freedom of action, most notably in employment policies and capital spending.

- Social health insurance systems moved to adopt inter-fund competition. In different ways and for different reasons, Belgium, Germany and the Netherlands ended the geography- or employment-based monopolies enjoyed by their sickness funds and set them in competition with each other. More fundamentally, the funds were given greater autonomy and permitted to diverge from one another in approach.
- What was common to both centralised and social health insurance systems was a set of reforms which had the effect of separating the *purchasing* of health care, the role of payer (fund or state), from the role of *provider* of care. The common characteristic linking widely divergent reforms across Europe was movement in the direction of a *purchaser-provider system* of care.

In the purchaser-provider system, a form of regulated market economy has arisen in sectors that used to be considered the responsibility of the state. The buyers in such markets are apt to be *agents* for patients, acting on their behalf. Sometimes they are groups of primary care physicians (such as the British NHS's primary care trusts). Sometimes they are autonomous agencies (such as sickness funds or insurers). The sellers are providers of health care, usually secondary or tertiary providers. The purchasing revolution is still in the developmental stage, though many European countries are already working on second-generation models. The experiment has been viewed as generally successful, though dangers must be noted.[4]

In general, agents buying care and making decisions on behalf of patients are motivated at least in part by economic self-interest, whether they are providers, payers or intermediaries. By making efficient decisions, they reduce their own costs, generate surpluses for their agencies and in some situations raise the incomes of the individuals who make them up. There is a danger that increased emphasis on the market will shift health care systems away from the logic of social solidarity toward the logic of individual interest. That danger is greater where there is significant privatisation. Ironically, perhaps, privatisation looms as one of the greatest threats to enhanced use of the market.

In general, decentralisation and the adoption of market logic in European health care systems have been achieved without significant privatisation, in the sense of devolution of public health care systems into the private sector. European models clearly show that decentralisation and privatisation are separate phenomena. But one of the dangers in decentralisation is that it may be seen to facilitate privatisation.

Another danger is that decentralisation may lead to increased use of user fees and out-of-pocket payments for heretofore free care services, which may in turn lead to under-utilisation of those services by low-income families.

A further danger is that choice-based systems favour the savvy. People in the community are not equal in their knowledge and understanding of health care, and a system which relies excessively on unguided and unaided personal initiative and choice will result in care inequalities.

With the exception of the National Treatment Purchase Fund, which does not really fit the model discussed here, the purchaser-provider model does not yet exist in Ireland.[5] However, the creation of the Health Service Executive (HSE) has separated policy formulation from implementation, possibly inadvertently readying Ireland for the adoption of a model of decentralisation, increased autonomy in hospitals, greater use of incentives and market behaviour, and purchasing.

Decentralisation and social solidarity

The Irish health care system has recently experienced significant centralisation. Local health boards, which had governed the provision of public health services for decades, were abolished in 2004 in favour of a single Health Service Executive (HSE) at the centre. The HSE was statutorily established from January 2005. Its establishment is a major reform with many uncertain implications, which we discuss and evaluate in Chapter 12. The reform seeks greater uniformity in care, reduced parochialism and localism in decision making and greater administrative efficiency. However, it may take an important element of community voice and popular control out of the health care system.

Does the centralisation of administration in the HSE advance or hinder the cause of social solidarity? The answer is not yet clear. Abolition of health boards is likely to reduce many communities' sense of 'ownership' of the health care system. But if the new structure proves responsive and adaptive and appears able to control aspects of the health care system which have seemed to the general public to be beyond control, there may be a net gain in solidarity.

Are such reforms as autonomous hospitals and the purchaser-provider model of health care delivery consistent with social solidarity? Reformers in Britain and continental Europe have tried to be conscious of the need to preserve social solidarity as they increased the autonomy and market responsiveness of both purchasers and providers, though we have noted several dangers inherent in this approach.

It might seem that market allocation and solidarity are in conflict, in that the former is thought to be based on self-interested decision making. In addition, there is no doubt that moving to an essentially market-based system lacking guarantees and protections would involve great risks. Among other things, the principle of solidarity implies that all people in similar circumstances should have:

• the same coverage (benefit package);
• care of similar quality;
• similarly timely care.

Health care systems which rely on unmanaged free competition (such as in the US) do not achieve these standards and appear to be inconsistent with the principle of social solidarity. It must be added, however, that in Ireland, centralisation of the health care system has not been used to achieve equity.

Reforms in the Irish health care system, especially if they involve devolution, autonomous purchasers and providers and market-like institutions, need to be formulated carefully, with deliberate regard for the principle of medical ethics and the principle of social solidarity.

Furthermore, it is urgent that whether there is decentralisation or whether the present highly centralised HSE system is maintained essentially unchanged, there be two sets of new protections created: (1) a charter of patients' rights along the lines of the European Charter of Patients' Rights[6] and (2) a set of institutions, such as advisory bodies, forums, patient members on governing boards, etc., for expression of the collective voice of patients and for system accountability.

It is not necessary, and given the litigious character of Irish society, probably not desirable, that a charter of patients' rights be enforceable in courts of law, unless there is specific legislation regarding any of its contents. The charter should guide the HSE, the government, lawmakers and others who write statutes and make policy. It should also guide clinicians, administrators and other personnel who make decisions affecting patients. For example, patients, doctors and others should know and agree to the principle that patients have a right to be free from unnecessary suffering and pain in all phases of their illness and treatment, but patients should not use such a statement of principles to seek monetary damages for pain. No one should forget that the patient is the beginning and the end – the *raison d'être* for the health care system.

Public and private ownership in health care

In health care, as elsewhere in economic life, we observe three basic types of ownership: *public or government ownership*, as in Ireland's HSE-owned (former health board-owned) hospitals; *private, i.e. for-profit, ownership*, as in physician practices in most countries, including, for example, GP practices in Ireland; and *not-for-profit ownership*, a middle ground consisting of entities organised, whether by government or by private persons or groups, for purposes of service rather than profit, such as not-for-profit hospitals in many countries, including Ireland's voluntary hospitals.

What we observe in the real world

Health care systems exhibit all three kinds of ownership systems.

We can make several generalisations about global patterns of ownership of various kinds of health-related institutions.

- *Physician practices*: These are almost always private, for-profit entities. An example in Ireland is GP practices. This type of organisation comes from the tradition of the professions, originally more of a vocation or a calling than a business. Physicians today remain organised in private, for-profit firms, but not because there is no perceived public interest at stake in physician behaviour. Instead, the public interest has often been served by physician peer- and self-governance. Further, physician behaviour can be led if necessary through incentives and regulation. Physicians are typically politically powerful and carefully guard their professional status and autonomy, even where they are paid by salary or capitation. However, physicians, especially those remunerated by fee-for-service, face potential conflicts of interest where their decisions on behalf of patients also affect their own incomes and workloads, as the literature on supplier-induced demand points out.[7] Methods of remuneration affect physician behaviour, as discussed in Chapter 4.

- *Insurers*: In developed countries, health insurance is offered under all three ownership types. Some health insurance is offered implicitly (British NHS)[8] or explicitly (Canada) by government. Some is offered by not-for-profit state-sponsored (the Voluntary Health Insurance (VHI) in Ireland) or non-governmental (France, Netherlands) not-for-profit organisations. Some is offered by for-profit firms (US). All three types are well represented internationally. Historically, not-for-profit insurers originally arose partly because of reluctance of for-profit companies to insure health. Private provision of health insurance is heavily regulated.

- *Nursing homes*: All three ownership types are also well represented in nursing homes. Typically, for-profit and not-for-profit private nursing homes are well regulated (though not in Ireland).

- *Hospitals*: History tells us that hospitals began as governmental or charitable organisations, and today, with few exceptions, still have public or not-for-profit ownership. However, as discussed above, there is a strong trend away from *dependent* public hospitals (as this term is defined elsewhere in this report) toward increased hospital autonomy. In effect, this means a rise in the relative proportion of not-for-profit hospitals. In most health care systems, private, for-profit hospitals, if they exist at all, operate only on the margins, with specialised facilities that do not offer the entire range of hospital products and services.

It is useful to discuss hospital ownership in more detail. Historically, hospitals in Europe and most of the world began as either public or charitable organisations. They remain so today in almost all countries. As we have seen, while other aspects of health care, such as physician practices and health insurers, have often come to be organised into private, for-profit firms, hospitals remain predominantly either public or voluntary. In Europe, in many countries, few if any private hospitals are complete facilities, and most exist primarily to provide elective surgery, with important support from public hospitals. For example:

> Hospitals in France are either public (65 per cent of all inpatient beds), private not-for-profit (15 per cent of inpatient beds) or private for-profit (20 per cent of inpatient beds). Private for-profit hospitals mainly deal with minor surgical procedures, whereas public and private not-for-profit hospitals focus more on emergency admission, rehabilitation, long-term care and psychiatric treatment.[9]

This description could also be applied to the Irish for-profit hospital sector, which currently supplies some 12 per cent of acute inpatient beds and which offers elective surgical treatments, which are not generally complex. We discuss this sector in more detail in Chapter 7.

According to the economics literature, there are two main reasons for the strong tradition that few hospitals are organised as for-profit firms.

- Patients deal with health care providers under conditions that economists label 'information asymmetry'. Lacking technical clinical knowledge, patients must place themselves in the hands of health care providers as an act of enormous faith. In part because of information asymmetry, health care is heavily regulated. Physicians must attend approved medical schools and must submit to examinations before practising. They must show continued competency through ongoing medical education. There is a strong tradition of peer governance in the medical profession. The state and the profession go to great lengths to reassure patients regarding physician care.

- Hospitals are also generally licensed (though not in Ireland) and regulated, but such phenomena as examinations and peer review are harder to apply. Hospitals tend to be organised as public or voluntary organisations to reassure patients that decisions in relation to their treatment are made for predominantly medical rather than for private profit reasons.

- The economics literature also contains the argument that externalities – costs borne by and benefits received by others than the main parties to a transaction – are significant in the hospital arena. When for-profit organisations buy or sell in conventional markets, externalities are ignored and non-optimal results occur. For-profit organisations systematically ignore external costs and external benefits. For example, many public hospitals stand ready to treat an outbreak of infectious illnesses, though such readiness is not profitable. The treatment of the occasional patient cannot be justified in profit terms, but the externalities can be large and significant. What this means is that not all of the benefits that are generated by a local hospital can be sold, or can be sold for their full economic cost. Hospitals serve communities not only by providing hospital services, but by standing by, ready to provide services when and as needed. Hospitals cannot easily sell this stand-by service.

For these reasons, though private hospitals may always have important roles to play, they will rarely be central or fundamental in any health care system.

There are other features of private hospitals that necessarily limit their roles in the Irish health care system. We discuss some of them next.

Private hospitals are more costly than public hospitals

A group of Canadian scholars has recently published a review of all known existing studies comparing the costliness of care in private, for-profit hospitals with that in not-for-profit (public and voluntary) hospitals. The results were published in the official journals of the Canadian Medical Association[10] and the American Medical Association.[11] They clearly show that private hospital costs for similar care are systematically and significantly higher than not-for-profit care. The studies also suggest poorer outcomes, including 2 per cent higher mortality rates, accounting for more than 2,000 excess deaths in one year.[12]

A study published in *The New England Journal of Medicine* showed that US communities with large for-profit hospitals had higher costs for Medicare, the health care programme for the aged.[13] In an accompanying editorial, the journal concluded that private hospitals are more costly.[14] Private hospitals spent more on administration and paid higher salaries to senior management officials.

'Cherry-picking'

The typical community hospital combines essential but unprofitable or financially risky services with more profitable ones, the latter supporting the former in a process known as 'cross-subsidisation'. Understandably, private hospitals have included only the latter services and not the former, a tactic universally known as 'cherry-picking'. This gives some of them the illusion of greater profitability. But someone has to pay for the less-profitable services, so there is no gain to society. The extra money which in community hospitals goes to support unprofitable services goes instead into the pockets of private investors in for-profit hospitals. Likewise, private hospitals are known to concentrate on younger and healthier patients, thus once again distorting measures of their efficiency.

Contrary to its reputation for entrepreneurial venture, private money in health care has traditionally stood aside until government or charity has proved the field viable, and then they have cherry-picked. In Ireland, where there are private beds in public hospitals, cherry-picking is part of the process of public subsidisation of private care. Costly and complex care is typically public care. Private patients in public hospitals become public patients for costly aspects of their care.

Public hospitals as the safety net

Similarly, the public hospital is the safety net that protects a community with a private hospital. If a private hospital performs badly or closes, the community will of course look to the state, and particularly to the HSE or the public hospital to come to their aid.

Two-tiered system of acute care

By law, every Irish citizen is statutorily entitled to public hospital care (subject to an overnight charge of €55 in 2005 levied for a maximum of 10 nights per annum) and to treatment by hospital consultants without payment of fees. Patients who avail of such care are 'public patients'. Patients can instead choose to be 'private patients' and pay fees to hospital consultants and added charges to hospitals. Typically, private patients will have already bought private insurance to cover all or part of the added charges.

It is well known that public and private patients are treated differently in at least two important respects. Where there are waiting lists for hospital admission for treatment by specialist physicians, there are generally separate waiting lists for the two classes of patients, with the wait for private patients significantly shorter. For example, see the 2002 Eastern Regional Health Authority survey, which showed the average waiting time for private patients in public hospitals in the East to be 3.4 months, and that for public patients to be 6.7 months.[15] Moreover, private patients are more likely to be attended to personally by the consultant, while public patients are likely to be treated by junior hospital doctors, in most cases less qualified.

These differences have led us and others to say that there are two tiers of acute care in Ireland. The existence of two tiers violates the need principle of medical ethics. It constitutes one of the best-known and most serious flaws in the Irish health care system. Since in general public patients are lower-income and private patients are higher-income persons, the two-tier system of care exacerbates economic inequality in Ireland and extends it to the sensitive and important domains of care of the sick and of life and death. One of the principal priorities facing the Irish system is the reduction and eventual abolition of the differences between the treatment of public and private patients.

The two-tier system of care is not a natural phenomenon, but has been created by the state. Public hospitals have been permitted to designate some beds as private. Consultants have been permitted to treat private patients in those beds for fees while drawing substantial state salaries for treatment of public patients. The state has permitted separate waiting lists and has thus encouraged patients who qualify for public care to buy private insurance. Half the population is now covered by private insurance, an extraordinary phenomenon in a state in which all qualify for public care.

The government's private hospital plan

As discussed earlier, the government has announced a plan to add public beds by encouraging the construction of new private hospitals. The 2001 Health Strategy accepted the existence of an acute bed shortage and promised 3,000 new beds over 10 years 'designated solely for public patients'. The government reaffirmed this promise as recently as July 2005. As of June 2005, the government claimed 720 new beds toward the 10-year goal. This claim is examined in detail in Chapter 7.

Since 2002, generous tax incentives have existed to encourage the construction of private hospitals. According to the Department of Health, this has already led to the construction and planning of a number of private hospital developments. No one claims, however, that these private developments address the promise of 3,000 new public beds.

In July 2005, the government announced a new plan to permit construction of private hospitals on the grounds of (and adjoining) public hospitals. Public hospitals would convert up to 1,000 private beds to public use, in effect 'moving' (policy-makers favour the word 'decanting') the private beds from public to private hospitals. The consequence would be a net increase in public beds, with no public capital expenditure.

In Ireland, private hospitals are not licensed or regulated. Although the Independent Hospital Association of Ireland says that many private hospitals have voluntary external accreditation, this is not the same as state licensing or regulation. Incentivised private hospitals have to satisfy certain initial requirements, but no one would use the word 'regulation' for the requirements. Putting new private hospitals on public grounds gives the Department of Health new leverage. If developers want to build on public campuses, they must undertake to satisfy certain detailed requirements, one of which is to accept the Hanly Report principles of 'consultant-provided, team-based' working arrangements.

At the same time, the government states that public hospitals will charge private hospitals fully for any services the former provide the latter. Private patients in public hospitals will begin to pay the economic cost of their health care.

Evaluating the government's plan

What's good about the government's plan, and what's bad? There seem to be four important potential benefits of the plan:

- The plan moves toward the achievement of a goal long advocated by reformers, namely ending the practice of private care in public hospitals.
- The plan yields more acute hospital beds, including more public beds.
- The plan results in leveraged regulation of private hospitals, enabling the Department of Health to plan for the hospital sector as a whole.
- Consultants will find it harder to satisfy contracts merely by being present in public hospitals while treating private patients.

These are not inconsiderable gains and should not be brushed aside. But what's bad about the plan?

- Private beds in newly constructed private hospitals on public hospital grounds will not free up private beds in public hospitals for public use on anything like a one-for-one basis.
- Cherry-picking will be facilitated.
- The two-tier system of acute hospital care will be further institutionalised and locked into the system.
- While the plan technically reduces the practice of private care in public hospitals, private care in fact moves only an enclosed

103

corridor or the other side of a car park away, and the new configuration retains the most objectionable features of the current arrangement.

- If consultants from the public hospitals are shareholders in the private hospital, they will have an added incentive (on top of the private fees they may earn there) to favour treating patients in the private hospital over devoting their time and energies to their public hospital and patients.

These problems are in turn elaborated below.

The image of private bed construction generating public beds on a one-for-one basis is a false one. While to qualify for tax relief private hospitals must have at least 70 beds, be able to provide medical or surgical services year round and be equipped with operating theatres and outpatients' clinics, in fact private hospitals will not be complete hospitals.

Private hospitals have always emphasised elective surgery over all other care, including medical, i.e. non-surgical, treatment. They will not have A&E services, will not offer the multi-disciplinary care which patients may require when recovering from major surgery and will not have high-cost specialised services such as stroke units. About 68 per cent of acute inpatient admissions in public hospitals are from A&E, many of them older patients with medical conditions who do not require surgery.[16] It is not clear how many of these patients can be cared for in private hospitals.

Public hospitals will continue to provide certain services to private as well as to public patients, including obstetrics, high-complexity cases and paediatric surgery.

An accurate picture of a private hospital on public hospital grounds is of a partial hospital only, which will rely on the public hospital for services and draw on the salaried consultant staff of public hospitals for most physician care. A central question about the government's plan is whether the addition of private beds in new private hospitals will liberate beds for public patients on a one-for-one basis. The answer is certainly 'no', but it is not clear what the true ratio will be. *There will be a net increase in private beds, which taxpayers will pay for.*

Placing private hospitals adjacent to public hospitals will facilitate cherry-picking, making it easier for private hospitals to rely on tax-supported services for costly patients. As noted, private hospitals rarely have their own A&E departments and usually lack services and equipment for some severely ill or injured patients. As compared with free-standing private hospitals on their own grounds, private hospitals adjacent to public hospitals will find this kind of cherry-picking facilitated, making it easier for private hospitals to rely on tax-supported services for costly aspects of patient care.

The public hospital is the safety net that protects a community with a private hospital. If a private hospital performs badly or closes, the community will of course look to the state, particularly to the HSE or the public hospital, to come to their aid. The 2005 experience with the Leas Cross private nursing home confirms that where there are private facilities, the investors are not the only ones bearing a risk.

It is small wonder that stockbrokerage firms have advised investors that private hospital developments are good investment prospects in Ireland.

The proposal to build new private hospitals with state help does nothing at all to break down the two-tier system of acute care. On the contrary, it strengthens the hold of that system and makes it more difficult for future governments or generations to abolish it. For example, one widely advocated reform is that in public hospitals there be a single waiting list for care, rather than separate waiting lists for public and private care, as is currently the case. This goal cannot be achieved when private beds are in separate hospitals.

On balance, then, the government's plan is not a good idea. The authors believe that the government should abandon its plan to permit and encourage private hospitals to be constructed on the grounds of public hospitals.

Who pays for private hospitals?

The Irish people will pay for all hospital beds, whether they are public or private.

Given the tax incentives to private hospitals which have existed in Ireland since 2002, what is the cost to the Exchequer, and therefore to the Irish people, of private hospitals? Our own calculations show that the costs are about 44 per cent of the investment, or about 40 per cent if we use the present value (discounting future returns by a conservative rate) (see Appendix 2). For every €100 million invested, the Irish people contribute €40 million. To this must be added the value of the land on which the hospital will be located. The campus of a public hospital must be an extraordinarily valuable site for the construction of a private hospital. One can only wonder what value it would bring at auction!

As economists, we must make the point that the cost to the Irish nation of new hospital construction does not depend on whether it is public or private. The expenditure displaces just as much consumption expenditure, other investment and government spending, regardless of which label we put on the hospital.

The Irish people ultimately pay for any hospital. There is no one else available to pay the cost.

Privatisation and solidarity

Some critics of the trend toward privatisation in Irish health care lump privatisation and increased use of the market together as a single trend. One critic recently wrote, 'The tilt toward private hospitals is applying a market model to the bureaucracy of the public sector.' Another wrote that the government apparently believes 'that what Irish health care needs is an injection of private capital plus market-style competition.' The experience with decentralisation in Europe shows that privatisation and decentralisation are not the same thing.

The difference between decentralisation, as the term has been used above, and privatisation is profit. There is a strong and important trend in the direction of decentralisation in European health care systems in which providers and others act as agents for patients in purchasing care; in which hospitals and other central institutions are granted considerable autonomy, particularly with regard to personnel decisions, product line and capital spending; and in which newly autonomous organisations compete with one another in markets. But in general, these changes have been accomplished without privatisation, i.e. without changing public and not-for-profit organisations to for-profit organisations. Management in these autonomous bodies reports to a governing board, but it is not a board of directors representing shareholders; and while management must attend to the bottom line, they do not need to focus on the value of the organisation's stock shares.

Privatisation cannot be ruled out. Private firms have many advantages over both public and not-for-profit organisations, particularly in conventional settings where significant externalities and cross-subsidisation are absent, and where market incentives will not produce biased or inequitable results across social classes, geographic areas or industries.

The chief advantages of for-profit firms in the health care area, as elsewhere, particularly in a competitive setting, is that the daily concern with profits and stock value leads them to be particularly conscious of the need to control costs, and makes them particularly alert to the need to satisfy and accommodate the shifting demands of buyers. But these advantages come with some high costs.

The apparent reason European states have avoided privatisation is that they fear it would conflict with the principle of social solidarity. There is no necessary or logical opposition of privatisation to solidarity. In most health care systems, for example, even those with obvious allegiance to the principle of solidarity, physician practices are established as for-profit firms. But, as we have noted in relation to hospitals, for-profit firms do not do well in the presence of significant externalities, where the whole community benefits from the treatment of a single patient; they tend to cherry-pick where there is significant cross-subsidisation; and they depend on public agencies as a safety net in times of difficulty. In the specific case of Irish hospitals, the plan to develop private hospitals on the grounds of public hospitals and then 'decant' private patients from the latter to the former tends to lock in the two-tier system of acute care.

Privatisation of the VHI

A free market in health insurance produces dysfunctional results. One would hope that competition among insurers would focus on producing the best product at the lowest price, as in other markets. Yet competition in health insurance markets tends to also focus on *risk selection*. Insurers are aware that a very large fraction of their annual claims comes from a small number of very sick people. Risk selection is based on the idea that if the insurers can identify the most risky customers in advance and find a way to avoid insuring them, then that can have a large effect on profits. For-profit insurers must avoid *adverse selection* – insuring clients whose risk of illness is greater than is apparent – and must seek a low-risk portfolio of insured lives.

Risk equalisation is a technique which adjusts for differences in the level of risk of subscribers of competing insurance companies and makes risk selection much less likely. As is discussed in detail in Chapter 5, the authors support the use of risk equalisation in the Irish health insurance market, as between VHI and Bupa.

There is discussion of privatising the VHI. The VHI began as a semi-state body and its net equity is owned, in effect, by the government. Discussion concerns transferring ownership to the insured, as in a 'mutual' form of organisation; to an autonomous and self-perpetuating board of trustees, as in the typical not-for-profit organisation; or to private shareholders, as in a corporation. In the last case of a private corporation, the government could sell the VHI for cash.

The authors believe that the VHI should continue to be a state company so that it can continue to serve national rather than private or parochial interests. Whatever the future of the VHI is, it should not become a for-profit company.

A privatised VHI in a community rating setting without risk equalisation could be a dangerous combination. It would have a powerful motive to shed numbers of high-risk, older persons, as well as younger persons with chronic conditions such as diabetes, and to limit the numbers of such persons newly insured as a survival strategy. Irish law[17] requires health insurers to provide open enrolment and lifetime cover, but insurance companies are often able to manipulate benefit packages and other terms to adjust the profiles of their insured populations. One assumes that the present management of VHI would not engage in such behaviour; but with a privatised VHI, who could say what policies it would follow?

Solidarity, decentralisation and privatisation

There is no inherent logical contradiction, then, among the principle of social solidarity, decentralisation of the health care system and privatisation. But in fact, from the real-world choices that present themselves, both decentralisation and privatisation offer both opportunities and dangers.

Decentralisation as found in European systems, taking the form of separating the purchaser and provider functions and providing greater autonomy to public hospitals and others, holds great promise for solving the many problems of the Irish health care system, problems arising out of rigidity, inflexibility and unresponsiveness. The example of other European states shows that such policies can be successful *and* consistent with democratic values, the need principle of medical ethics and social solidarity. However, there are dangers as well, and decentralisation must be approached cautiously and with a vigilant concern for values other than market success.

Privatisation and decentralisation do not mean the same thing. Indeed, in important circumstances, they may stand in conflict with one another. Privatisation, in the sense of substitution of for-profit forms of organisation for public or not-for-profit formations, poses still greater dangers to fundamental values. One should not be doctrinaire and oppose such privatisation in health care on principle, but one should always be aware of the potential privatisation has for doing harm, especially in those circumstances where externalities, cross-subsidisation and the potential for inequalities are likely to exist. For this reason, we advocate that the government should abandon its plan for private hospitals on public hospital grounds.

4

INCENTIVES AND THE HEALTH CARE SYSTEM

Introduction

Economic theory and everyone's experience clearly show that economic incentives do affect behaviour in health care. Patients respond to the prices they pay for health care. Providers respond to the amounts they are paid, especially to the ways they are paid. Hospitals face a range of economic incentives and clearly respond to them in predictable ways. Health care is no different from any other sector of the economy in being very responsive to economic incentives.

This is *good*, in that it gives policy-makers a powerful set of instruments to affect behaviour and outcomes. Consequently, in every country, policy-makers manipulate incentives – and especially the *ways* in which providers are paid – as a central part of policy.

But this is also *bad* to the extent that in the past, policy designers have built systems without attention to the effects of incentives, and have inadvertently created dysfunctional incentives. The Irish health care system is replete with dysfunctional incentives, as we will see.

Theory and common experience show that ways of paying providers have huge effects on behaviour and outcomes. Because of this, all societies and many entities within societies manipulate methods of paying providers to achieve social or organisational goals.

Doctors

There are three main ways in which doctors (or groups of doctors) are paid for patient care: fee-for-service (FFS), salary and capitation. All three methods are present in Ireland.

FFS means that the doctor is paid a fee, usually according to a set fee schedule, for each item of service performed. For example, Irish general practitioners (GPs) are paid fees for treating non-Medical Card patients. Many GPs charge approximately €50 for an uncomplicated office visit. Particular procedures during the office visit may add to the fee. Consultants charge private patients fees for care. Of course, fees may be paid by the patient or on behalf of the patient, by an insurer. In Ireland, most consultants follow the fee schedule promulgated by Voluntary Health Insurance (VHI). FFS is the traditional way in which professionals, including lawyers, accountants and others beyond doctors, have historically been paid. When doctors are paid on an FFS basis, their incomes depend crucially on how many services they provide.

Salary, of course, means that one is paid a set amount per time period. For example, consultants and non-consultant hospital doctors (NCHDs) are paid salaries by the state. Necessarily, salaries are paid by employers, not by patients, and not usually by insurers. The payment of a salary almost always indicates an employer-employee relationship.

When doctors are paid on a salary basis, their incomes are independent of how many services they provide. Of course, many employers will monitor employee behaviour closely and try to adjust salary levels to reflect productivity, but there is no automatic or mechanical relationship between activity and income.

Under capitation, doctors are paid a given amount per month (or other time period) per patient registered with them. Irish GPs, for example, are paid on a capitation basis by the HSE Primary Care Reimbursement Scheme (formerly the General Medical Services Payments Board) for their patients who have Medical Cards. The difference between salary and capitation is that under salary, doctors are paid a given amount per time period, whereas under capitation, doctors are paid a given amount *per patient* per time period. But salary and capitation have two important things in common – under both, physicians' incomes do not depend on whether or how often patients come to them for care, and they do not depend on the amounts and types of care doctors decide to provide. Capitation payments may be made by the state or by insurers, but they are not made by patients. It is worth pointing out that capitation requires a system of *patient registration*, which is not required under FFS or salary.

Effects

The effects of these methods of remuneration are well known and important. When doctors are paid on an FFS basis, they provide more services than when they are paid on a salary or capitation basis. Utilisation of physician services is at its highest under FFS.[1]

Consider a doctor who is seeing a patient for an illness or condition. The doctor prescribes a pharmaceutical drug and is trying to decide whether to ask the patient to come back for a check-up after the course of treatment has begun. It is important to note that a return visit will impose both time costs and actual money costs on the doctor and his or her practice. If the doctor is paid on an FFS basis, then the doctor will be compensated for every visit, whether it is a patient-initiated first visit or a return visit. If the doctor is paid on a salary or capitation basis, then there will be no further income associated with a return visit. The doctor's decision about a return visit will not usually be affected by method of remuneration, but it is affected often enough to produce a large and significant difference in utilisation according to type of pay.

In a sense, this highlights the fact that when doctors are paid on an FFS basis, they face a potential conflict of interest when they decide on patient care. Their decisions affect patient well-being, but at the same time affect their own incomes and workloads.

There are further effects. Doctors who are paid on an FFS basis have a motive to *hold onto their patients* and not refer them to others because patient care is a source of income. Doctors who are paid by salary or capitation have a motive to *refer their patients to others* if that cuts their workloads without cutting their incomes.[2]

Doctors who are paid on a capitation basis *bear the insurance risk* for care of their patients. Their incomes are unaffected by patient health. Like an insurance company, a doctor paid on a capitation basis bears a cost if patients get sick and avoids a cost when patients are well. Like insurance companies, doctors paid on a capitation basis have a motive to avoid patients who are likely to be sick. (They fear *adverse selection*.) An insurance company which pays doctors on a capitation basis shifts some of the risk to the doctor. The same is true of the state when it pays on a capitation basis, as well as (though less directly) when doctors are paid by salary. They also bear costs when their patients are sick and avoid costs when patients are well.

There is one more difference that stems from methods of remuneration. Doctors who are paid on an FFS basis may not need monitoring or supervision, since their reward system encourages them to be productive. Not only will they earn higher incomes if they do more work, but if their patients become dissatisfied with them and shift to other providers, their incomes will fall. They are said to be governed 'by the market' (though of course that presupposes enough competitors – and enough competition – to provide that kind of governance). By contrast, it is said that doctors who are paid by salary must be supervised, because there is no automatic market reward or penalty for high or low quantity and quality of work.[3]

It is in this area that an anomaly is found in Ireland: consultants are paid by salary for their work in relation to public patients, but they are not supervised. In fact, the common consultant contract specifically prohibits their supervision. It is an unusual phenomenon, perhaps unique in all the world. There is no market system of control, and yet no supervision!

In the consultants' common contract there is this definition of a consultant:

> A consultant is a registered medical practitioner in a hospital practice who, by reason of his training, skill and experience in a designated specialty, is consulted by other registered medical practitioners and undertakes full clinical responsibility for

patients in his care, or that aspect of care on which he has been consulted, without supervision in professional matters by any other person. He will be a person of considerable professional capacity and personal integrity.[4]

The definition of 'professional matters' in reference to which the consultant is not to be supervised has been interpreted expansively to preclude clinical audit, whether by administrators or peers, and even how the consultant spends the contracted hours for which he or she is paid. This feature of the consultants' contract is controversial, and we will have more to say about it elsewhere.

Capitation lies somewhere between FFS and salary in the need for supervision. Productivity will not affect the income of a doctor paid by capitation *unless* his or her patients become dissatisfied and transfer to other doctors.[5] The presence of some market control reduces the need for supervision.

Which is best?

Table 4.1 below summarises the known effects of methods of remuneration on physician behaviour.

But which payment method is best? The answer is that there is no single answer. In situations in which there is excessive utilisation, we may want to shift to salary or capitation. But if we suspect utilisation is too low, then we may want to shift to FFS.

Table 4.1: Theoretical effects of method of remuneration on physician behaviour			
	FFS	Salary	Capitation
Utilisation Referrals Need for monitoring	Higher Discouraged Low	Lower Encouraged High	Lower Encouraged Moderate

In developed countries, most patients have free care or insurance which covers much of needed care. Hence, patients face prices for medical care which are systematically lower than the costs of producing it, a fact which leads to increased patient demand for care, the phenomenon called 'moral hazard'. To counteract this built-in tendency for over-utilisation, there will often be a preference for salary or capitation to create an opposing tendency. However, relying exclusively on salary or capitation might result in an even more serious problem: underprovision of care.

In choosing a method of remuneration, or a mix of methods, policy-makers will also want to take into account the effect of payment technique on quality of care.

Most health economists have come to believe that a hybrid system, under which a given provider is paid in more than one way for a given patient or episode of care, is best.[6] For example, a consultant specialist might be given a salary, based on time present and working, together with a fee for each patient treated, with the fee varying by procedure. Ideally, the proportion of a doctor's income accounted for by salary (or capitation) and by FFS would be 'fine-tuned' to achieve optimal behaviour. In practice, however, frequent adjustments would probably be annoying to all concerned, so it is best to try to get it right the first time. Hybrid methods, as defined here, do not exist in Ireland.

Such hybrid methods, which can be optimal, have to be distinguished from *mixed methods*, where providers are paid in different ways for different patients, which are almost always harmful. Some of the most egregious examples of dysfunctional incentives in Ireland are found in this category.

There are two main examples in Ireland of mixed methods of remuneration.

- *GPs* are paid by capitation for GMS or Medical Card patients, and by FFS – by the patient – for the rest of the population. This combination encourages doctors to treat FFS patients and discourages them from treating GMS patients. No research is known to have been done which verifies that Irish GPs do in fact privilege private patients, as the theory predicts they will do.
- *Hospital consultants* are paid by salary for public patients and by fee for private patients. This system of mixed methods is sufficient to explain why consultants privilege private patients, leading to the existence of the two-tier system of acute care, though other factors may be at work as well. Under the two-tier

system, private patient care is scheduled sooner than public patient care, which has led to the existence of two waiting lists, a list of public patients waiting months or even years, and a shorter list of private patients waiting shorter periods of time. Another feature of the two-tier system of care is that private patients are more likely to be treated personally by the consultant, while public patients are more likely to be treated by junior NCHDs.

The two-tier system of care is discussed in much greater detail elsewhere in this report. Here we will only note that given the designation of public hospital beds as public or private, it can be sufficiently explained by the mixed system of remuneration.[7]

	Hybrid	Mixed
Table 4.2: Hybrid vs. mixed systems of remuneration		
Definition	A given provider is paid in more than one way for care of a given patient.	Providers are paid in different ways for different patients.
Effect	Can be optimal.	One group of patients is favoured over another.

Hospitals

The ways hospitals receive their money also has enormous implications for hospital behaviour, especially for patient care. There are many techniques used around the world. Here we focus on four methods: charges, capitation, casemix-based budgeting and annual budgets, which may be transparent, incremental or obscure.

Charges

Hospitals may charge patients (or third-party payers) fees according to hospital resources used in their care. Charges for hospitals are analogous to FFS for doctors. A hospital which receives all or some part of its income from charges has an incentive to provide more services. The hospital has a motive to admit patients, provide them with services for which the hospital is compensated and increase length of stay (LOS).

A variation of charges occurs where hospitals are paid (at least in relation to inpatient care) according to numbers of patient days, a standard and simple way of measuring the output of inpatient care. In this instance, hospitals have an incentive to admit patients and to extend LOS, but not necessarily to provide other costly services.

An interesting side point is that insurance companies will of course also respond to the incentives structure they face, and these incentives may be opposite to those of hospitals. When subscribers need costly acute care, there is an incentive for the insurer to encourage them to use the facilities of the public hospital rather than a private hospital.[8]

Capitation

Hospitals may be paid by third-party payers on a capitation basis, similar to the technique used to pay physicians. The hospital agrees to provide all of the payer's patients' hospital care (as defined in a contract) in exchange for a flat amount of money per patient per time period. This technique is not very widespread. However, the British National Health Service (NHS) has long provided hospitals with budgets according to a formula in which the most important factor has been the population of the catchment area served by the hospital. This is a variation on capitation as a payment method.

Casemix

A technique that is increasingly being adopted around the world is for a payer to pay hospitals a fixed amount per discharged patient, the amount to depend on the diagnosis or care category of the patient. Each diagnosis is given a code for diagnosis category (or diagnosis-related group, DRG), and hospitals are paid according to DRGs. Ideally, the hospital is paid according to the standard cost of treating a patient, which may or may not be the cost incurred by that hospital in treating the patient. Ireland has adapted this method in a technique called casemix.

In Ireland, 62 of the largest hospitals (including two private hospitals) provide data, and 37 of the 62 have a fraction of their budgets based on casemix.

It's a complicated process. Here's a brief explanation of how it works: the Department of Health collects DRG and other data on care they provide from all participating hospitals through the Hospital Inpatient Enquiry (HIPE) (administered by the Economic and Social Research Institute). Each DRG is assigned a certain number of casemix units (units of care) according to complexity. Hospitals are paid by the government according to the care they provide (according to DRGs). Thus, hospitals with more complex caseloads receive more money. The payment rate is a blend of the hospital's own costs (currently 60 per cent) and a national rate paid to all hospitals, based on average or standard costs (currently 40 per cent).

If a hospital's own costs are the same as the average of all hospitals' costs, it will neither gain nor lose through this payment technique. If their costs are higher than that, they won't have quite enough money to cover their costs, which puts pressure on hospitals to cut costs. If their costs are lower than that, they will have a little money to spare, which will be an inducement to control costs.

The key is that, to the extent that the casemix method is applied, hospitals are paid according to standard costs of peer hospitals, rather than according to their own costs.

The system now covers in-patient, day and paediatric care. The method applies only to the part of the hospital's budget relating to patient care.

The system is being phased in gradually through increases in the 'blend rate', the percentage of their patient-care budget to which the casemix adjustment is applied. As noted, the blend rate in 2006 is 40 per cent. In 2005 the blend rate was 30 per cent.

When casemix adjustments began in 1993, there were only 15 participating hospitals, and they faced a blend rate of only 5 per cent, a rate which applied only to in-patient care. The number of participating hospitals and the blend rate have both grown over the years. A&E care was included for the first time in 2005.

The proportion of budgets accounted for by casemix is expected to rise further in the next few years, with all hospitals and all encounters covered.

Casemix-based budgets are to hospitals what risk adjustment is to insurance. Indeed, casemix budgeting is a form of risk adjustment.

Annual budgets

Where the state or a body such as the HSE provides each hospital with an annual budget not based on hospital activity, i.e. not a variant of charges, that constitutes a third method by which hospitals get their money. Annual budgets may be transparent, incremental or obscure.

(a) Transparent annual budgets

Where hospital budgets are arm's length and formula driven, annual budgets are transparent. Typically, the population size of the catchment area served by the hospital, almost always age adjusted, is the main term in the budget formula. Adjustments may be made for morbidity (or casemix) differences, teaching hospitals, unique departments or services or other factors. Three things always *absent* in the formula are budget amounts from prior years, payment for services delivered (charges) and administrative discretion. Budgets are not add-ons to prior years' amounts, but are calculated each year on the basis of recent (usually the preceding year's) data. Annual budgets are not simply charges in changed clothing, and are not based on patient days or any other measure of services provided. A truly transparent process avoids administrative discretion, though in practice some discretion is required to deal with changes and differences in circumstances that formulas cannot comprehend. A transparent annual budget process, therefore, is likely to be a variant of capitation as a method of funding hospitals.

(b) Incremental budgets

In incremental budgets, the most important piece of information in calculating a hospital's annual budget is the set of budget numbers for the prior year. To the extent that this kind of budgeting is used, it locks in place the relative differences among hospitals (and regions), whether efficient and equitable or not.

(c) Obscure annual budgets

Where there is administrative discretion, the basis for budgetary allocations will be formally obscure. Where incremental budgets are used, there is a large obscure component. Annual increments lock in place, at least in relative terms, inter-hospital (or inter-regional) differences established in some past year or years. The basis of these primordial differences is likely to be obscure, hence every year's budgets will be based on obscure principles.

Administrators often like this approach to budgeting because it maximises their discretion and hence power. Sometimes these budgets will be directly negotiated between the hospital and the regional or central funding agency, and the outcome will depend in part on the connectedness and bargaining skills of hospital personnel.

Effects

The effects of these methods of setting the budgets of hospitals are well understood, having emerged from considerable study over the past three decades. The subject of the economic consequences of method of hospital funding is one of the most-studied questions of health economics.

Charges and methods which resemble charges (for example, annual budgets based on patient bed-days of care) encourage high levels of utilisation. They encourage hospitals to admit patients, to keep them in beds longer (increase LOS) and to provide them with services.

Casemix and DRG systems, as well as transparent annual budget methods, are alike in that hospitals cannot increase revenues (though they will increase their costs) by providing patients with more services or increasing LOS. Thus, both should be associated with greater economies, and shorter average LOS in particular.

When hospitals admit patients with complex or severe problems, they bear higher costs. They are less likely to avoid or resist such high-cost patients where they are compensated for complexity through something like DRGs and casemix payments. Where hospitals receive flat annual budgets, they will fear adverse selection and will be motivated to avoid costly patients.

Obviously, it is hard to generalise about the effects of obscure annual budgets. If there are any economic effects at all, behaviour may depend on the hospital's view of the underlying bases of these budgetary allocations. For example, if hospital personnel believe that staff hiring or equipment acquisition will more or less automatically generate budget increases, they will be encouraged to spend money in these directions.

Which is best?

The best method of paying hospitals is the method that results in the most efficient use of resources, where ideally efficiency is measured in health outcomes per euro of expenditure. As with physician remuneration, it would obviously be wrong to conclude that the system which most discourages costly expenditures is necessarily best. A system which discourages hospitals from providing patients with needed and valuable care would clearly not be optimal.

As with physicians, hybrid systems are possible, under which, for example, hospitals would get partial reimbursement for costs of patient care (partial charges), together with a casemix or transparent annual budget system for the remainder of the budget.

In addition, as with physicians, mixed systems are harmful. Where hospitals are paid fees in relation to one group of patients (private patients) but receive no fee income (or nominal fee income) for another group of patients (public patients), e.g. as in the two-tier Irish system, hospitals will have an incentive to privilege the former group of patients. That is the case even where hospitals are well funded for public patients. Such a mixed system will never be equitable.

Autonomous vs. dependent hospitals

There is a worldwide trend toward autonomous public hospitals. There are two main characteristics of autonomous hospitals. Firstly, 'the money follows the patient'. Hospitals receive income, either from patients or from someone else on patients' behalf, in relation to patient care. Secondly, hospitals are free to make their own decisions about size, mix of services, personnel, capital outlays, etc. Public hospitals are treated analogously if not identically to the way private hospitals are treated. Their autonomy can be limited by regulation in the public interest in the same manner and to the same extent as is the case for private hospitals.

The advantages of autonomous hospitals are that they can respond to incentives in terms of demand and/or technology in efficient ways, they are more responsive and sensitive to patient needs and interests and under ideal circumstances they should not under- or over-spend their budgets. They are less subject to political influences because they are freer of central or regional control. A disadvantage is that they may seek to grow or thrive at the expense of each other, and may be more inclined toward empire building than co-operation or collaboration.

The opposite to autonomous hospitals is dependent hospitals. They receive their budgets from the state, do not make their own capital or operating expenditure decisions, except in detail, and act as extensions of the central or regional state body which exercises control over them. The main advantage of dependent hospitals is that they are more socially accountable. Since there is a very considerable public interest in hospital services, that is not an unimportant advantage.

Irish hospitals

Irish hospitals are discussed in detail in later chapters. The discussion here will be brief, in order to locate Irish hospitals in the present discussion.

There are three components in the budgets received by most Irish hospitals: budget allocation, casemix and revenues.

Budget allocation

Irish public hospitals receive an annual budgetary allocation which is primarily incremental. There is an administrative discretion component, primarily to deal with changes in services or equipment from the prior year. This approach has been criticised by the Department of Health's Composite Report, which argues:

> One consequence of this incrementally based estimates process is that financial allocations largely reflect their historic funding positions. There have been significant demographic and social changes over the years that have implications for health service

delivery but which are not reflected in the allocations (for example: changes in the size and age profile of the population). Funding should be determined in a manner that captures these changes in society.[9]

There are other criticisms of incremental budgets. They may perpetuate inter-regional and inter-hospital inequalities, they are inconsistent with hospital autonomy, they do not include any incentives for efficient behaviour and they are fundamentally obscure in that they annually adjust amounts with large arbitrary components.

Casemix

As discussed above, a growing proportion of budget amounts is based on casemix measurement. A hospital whose care was average in costliness has no adjustment. Where the costliness of the care provided by the hospital is high relative to that of peer hospitals, there is a subtraction from the budget. Where the cost-liness of the care given by the hospital is low relative to that of peer hospitals, there is an addition to the budget. The incentives are positive. Hospitals are in effect paid according to the *general* or average cost of treating a particular condition; those able to treat it at less cost than that gain financially, and those who do so at greater cost lose. Thus, hospitals share financially from any cost-saving they are able to achieve. Casemix-adjusted budgets are consistent with increased hospital autonomy.

Revenues

Irish public hospitals have three kinds of revenues. The largest consists of charges imposed on private patients. These charges cover approximately half the true economic costs of providing services to these patients, so there is a substantial subsidy com-ponent. There are also nominal charges imposed on public patients. The Irish system of charges, then, satisfies our definition of a mixed system. It provides an incentive for Irish hospitals to favour private patients. Some Irish public hospitals also receive revenues for treating patients on long-time waiting lists under the National Treatment Purchase Fund (NTPF). In general, hospitals are not meant to be paid to treat patients from their own waiting lists, but an audit by the Comptroller and Auditor General has revealed that 36 per cent of treatments occur in the same hospital on whose waiting list the patient languished for months or years without treatment[10] (this is discussed in greater detail in Chapter 7). This practice creates unfortunate incentives. If a consultant specialist leaves a public patient on the waiting list long enough (while of course receiving a salary, supposedly for treatment of that public patient), he or she may receive a fee for treating that patient privately.

Revenues from patient care clearly permit the money to 'follow the patient', but new Irish budgetary procedures under the HSE may defeat that principle. Estimated revenues are included in the annual allocation to each HSE-owned (or formerly health-board owned) hospital. If revenues exceed this estimate, the hospital may not retain the additional revenues, which will revert to the Exchequer. Voluntary hospitals, however, may retain additional revenues. To the extent that that is the case, revenues do not really follow the patient, and the HSE's allocation decision is the final word. Hospitals are, in effect, allocated their own revenues.[11]

The two most glaring flaws in the Irish hospital budget process are, firstly, the use of incremental budgeting, with large obscure components, and secondly, differentiation between private and public patients in ways that provide an incentive for hospitals to favour the former. Moreover, since only a fraction of hospital budgets reflects severity and complexity, Irish hospitals may have an incentive to resist admitting high-cost patients.

Other providers

The examples of doctors and hospitals will suffice to show the principles which can apply to any providers. Where providers are paid on the basis of units of service provided, they are inclined to provide more units of service. Where they are paid in a way which does not consider volume of service, they are inclined to provide fewer units of service.

Pricing of health care

As is discussed in Chapter 3, leaving health care to the market is not likely to result in an efficient use of resources. But that is not to say that the rules of supply and demand do not work for medical care. They work very well. When health care is costly, buyers cut down on its use, even where health or life may depend on prompt, adequate care. When users of health care can choose among providers or methods of care, they take price into account and move in the direction of lower-price care. The 'law of demand' applies in medical care as it does elsewhere.

In practice, prices are most likely to influence the patient's choice to make an *initial visit* to a doctor or other provider, when symptoms make the patient think that she or he is ill or pregnant. Once the patient is in the hands of the doctor, the doctor strongly influences subsequent utilisation decisions, leaving a smaller role for prices and the market.

Insurance devices

When people have health insurance (including free or subsidised state provision of medical care), they may face *co-insurance, co-pays* or *deductibles*.

Where there is co-insurance, the patient pays a percentage of the cost. For example, if a doctor's fee is €50 and a 20 per cent co-insurance rate applies, the insurer pays €40 and the patient pays €10. The patient treats the care as costing €10 and adjusts demand accordingly. A co-pay is the same except that it is stated in money terms rather than as a percentage. Patient demand for care is increased by the insurance but reduced by co-insurance or co-pay. Where there is a deductible, insurance covers only medical expenditure beyond a given amount per time period (usually a year). For example, if outpatient care is covered subject to a €200 annual deductible, the patient pays the first €200 each year of outpatient care costs; after that, the insurer pays for all care.

Many economists and policy-makers are attracted to co-insurance and co-pays, even where amounts are nominal, because it is believed that they make patients 'think twice' about seeking medical care for trivial problems.

Insurers love deductibles because they reduce, often drastically, the number of claims they have to process. From the economist's standpoint, the attraction of deductibles is that by implication they designate some amount of medical spending as routine and normal for every person, and provide insurance only for amounts beyond those norms.

The Irish Drugs Payment Scheme uses an unusual version of the deductible. An individual or family must pay the first €85 per month for approved drugs and appliances. After that amount has been reached, the state pays for all such expenditures. This is a rather typical application of the deductible device, with two exceptions: the deductible amount is very high (equivalent to €1,020 annually) and the deductible period is only one month, instead of the usual one year. (Those covered by Medical Cards have drug costs covered in full and are not eligible for the Drugs Payment Scheme.)

When applied to primary care, co-insurance, co-pays and especially deductibles have one very important disadvantage: they discourage the first contact a person might make with a doctor or other provider. Consequently, patients may postpone or even deny themselves needed care and are less likely to avail of asymptomatic preventative and screening care. When ill, they may enter the medical care system as patients when their medical problems have progressed so much that their recovery is slower, more costly or even impossible.

Importance of relative prices

Relative prices are extremely important and can powerfully influence care choices, often in arbitrary and inefficient ways. Several examples from Irish health care follow.

The majority of the population pays for GP care but is eligible for free or heavily subsidised out- and inpatient care in acute hospitals. Moreover, half the population has health insurance cover for inpatient care. The effect is to encourage costly care in the overloaded acute hospital system and to discourage less costly primary care in the community.

With the new doctor-only Medical Card, GP care is free to some, but they must pay for care from allied health professionals, such as occupational therapists. The effect is to encourage patients to seek medical care from doctors where occupational therapy (or care by other professionals) would be more appropriate and less costly.

Because public inpatient care is free or heavily subsidised to the whole population and private inpatient care is free to the insured, and because prescription drug coverage is subject to a high monthly deductible, surgical treatment is often less costly than medical treatment where the two are alternative ways of treating a given condition.

One more incentive problem may be mentioned. Medical Card holders, including those who hold doctor-only Medical Cards, get free GP care. Except for those with doctor-only Cards, these men, women and children get free care from many allied health professionals as well as free prescription drugs. Their entitlement to these benefits arises from the fact that their incomes are below the threshold for eligibility. Therefore, a few euros' increase in their incomes can have an enormous impact on the prices they face, with GP visits going from free to around €50 per visit. Private insurance does not usually cover most of these costs. A family whose income is low but above the eligibility threshold for Medical Cards will face a very high cost for routine care, and an enormous cost if someone in the family is ill. At the same time, drug costs rise significantly and families have to decide whether to have prescriptions filled. For many families, an increase in their incomes is not a blessing but rather a curse. It brings not an improvement in their living standards but a worsening, not health and happiness but illness and concern.

Incentives anomalies in Ireland

Reflecting on the Irish health care system, Professor Muiris FitzGerald, Dean of the School of Medicine, University College, Dublin, has observed that there 'are virtually no incentives, except perverse incentives, within the health care system.'[12] Our discussion has revealed many incentives anomalies in the Irish health care system:

• Mixed methods for paying GPs are capable of generating bias against patients with Medical Cards.

- Mixed methods for paying hospital consultants are known to produce bias against public patients. Because of inefficient incentives, public patients are likely to wait longer for care and are less likely to be treated personally by the consultant.
- Consultants are paid salaries but are not supervised.
- Budget allocations for public hospitals use an incremental technique, with large obscure components. For that reason:
  - They may fail to take account of significant demographic and social changes.
  - They may perpetuate inter-regional and inter-hospital inequalities.
  - They are inconsistent with hospital autonomy.
  - They do not include any incentives for efficient behaviour.
  - They are fundamentally obscure in that they annually adjust amounts with large arbitrary components.
- Mixed methods of paying hospitals create differentiation between private and public patients in ways that provide an incentive for hospitals to favour the former.
- Relative prices facing patients induce inefficient and dysfunctional behaviour.
- For Medical Card holders, small income increases generate enormous adverse eligibility consequences, perhaps discouraging low-income people from seeking to earn more.

A final anomaly, also discussed further in Chapter 5, is found in the extraordinarily high capitation rate paid to GPs who treat those patients aged 70 and over, who qualify for Medical Cards on the basis of age alone and not on need. The high rate has profoundly disturbing effects on market efficiency and inter-GP equity.

An irony is that those who preside over these anomalies, in particular present and past Ministers for Health and Ministers for Finance, are nominally, by their own statements, friends of a free market. The market does not automatically provide optimal outcomes. It assuredly will not yield optimal outcomes when policy-makers ignore the adverse effects of incentives when they design programmes.

Fortunately, such anomalies can be addressed. Because providers, patients and others do respond to the incentive structures they face, it is possible to improve resource utilisation by enlightened attention to incentives.

Recommendations

The authors strongly recommend that the incentive effects of health care policies routinely be considered in the future whenever new or changed policies are considered.

Recommendations for policies which will address and correct incentives anomalies are made throughout this study. The following are some specific recommendations which deal with the anomalies discussed in this chapter:

- Hospital consultants should treat all patients, public and private, in the same way. Hence, they should be paid in the same way for all patients. To avoid over- and under-provision of care, this should be a hybrid system, part salary and part fee per item of service. This change would be a major move in attacking the two-tier system of care.
- GPs should also treat all patients, public and private, in the same way. Hence, they should be paid in the same way for all patients. Ideally, this should be a hybrid system, part capitation and part fee per item of service.
- Hospitals should be paid in the same ways for public and private patients in order to remove any incentives for them to differentiate between them in ways that favour private patients.
- Hospital budgeting should be reformed. Hospital budgets should be set in large part on the basis of their case loads, but should also have a significant discretionary component set by the HSE.
- Economically non-neutral devices such as the doctor-only Medical Card should be avoided.

5

FINANCING OF HEALTH CARE

Introduction

The Irish health care system occupies a unique place amongst the world's health care systems because of its extraordinary public-private mix. At first sight, it looks like a health care system with a large and significant private component. Over half the population, and fully two-thirds of the non-Medical Card population, buy private insurance which permits them to be private patients when they go to hospital. Twenty per cent of inpatient beds in public hospitals, 24 per cent of patients who receive elective day treatments and 33.4 per cent of people who receive elective inpatient treatments in public hospitals are private.[1] When private hospitals are included, almost one-third of all acute beds are private. More than two-thirds of all general practitioner (GP) care is privately purchased, and nearly the same proportion of prescription drug expenditure is private.

Yet taxpayers pay 78 per cent of the costs of medical care in this seemingly largely private health care system, and that amount does not include the cost to the Exchequer of tax incentives for private hospitals and nursing homes. Private insurance covers less than 7 per cent of spending, compared with over 13 per cent paid out-of-pocket by patients.[2] How is it possible that so little private money buys so much private care?

The answers are familiar to everyone. Private patients in public hospitals pay charges that are less than the economic cost of their care, so there is a substantial public subsidy to private care. Consultants are paid handsome public salaries for being present in public hospitals 33 hours a week, though they may spend any part of that time caring for fee-paying private patients. So again, there is a substantial public subsidy to private care.

The Irish system is one with much publicly financed private care. In this chapter, we discuss the financing of health care in Ireland. We also discuss eligibility under the public health services, first for those with Category I eligibility, i.e. Medical Card holders, and then for those with Category II eligibility (all others). We then discuss voluntary insurance.

Eligibility under the public health services

There are two categories of eligibility under the public health services in Ireland. An eligibility threshold is drawn annually, traditionally covering approximately the poorest 35 to 38 per cent of the population, but today (as is discussed below) at a lower proportion. All those below that line have so-called Category I eligibility and are issued Medical Cards. This eligibility entitles them to a wide range of health care, covering virtually all care, free of charge. Everyone else has Category II eligibility.

Medical Cards

To those eligible for Medical Cards on the basis of income there are added two groups who get entitlement in other ways. Firstly, there are those, mainly people suffering from costly chronic conditions, who are not automatically eligible but who are provided with Medical Cards through administrator discretion. (The power to issue such cards was traditionally vested in Health Board CEOs but is now in the Health Service Executive (HSE).) Critics have complained that this authority has been used arbitrarily and capriciously.[3] In 2001, everyone aged 70 or above became eligible for Medical Cards, a move which came as the government was in effect moving the income-based eligibility line downward by failing to increase it in line with rising incomes, thus taking free medical care away from poor people.

Medical Card holders are entitled to free GP care. Since voluntary insurance does not generally cover primary care, almost all other people pay fees for GP care out of pocket, at rates said in

2005 to average about €50 per visit. Thus, there is a considerable price difference facing Category I and Category II people when they attend GP offices. There are frequent first-person anecdotal accounts of people going without needed doctor care because of the cost. Forthcoming research suggests that 25 per cent of all non-Medical Card holders and 40 per cent of 20- to 29-year-olds have been deterred from visiting doctors when they had medical problems by cost.[4]

Medical Card holders are also entitled to free care from a range of other allied health professionals for which others must pay, such as chiropodists, physio- and occupational therapists and others. For those using these services, again, a sizeable difference in price exists between Medical Card holders and others.

Medical Card holders are entitled to free pharmaceutical drugs, though drugs are limited to those on a formulary, approved on the basis of both efficacy and cost. In any month in which they have they have spent at least €85 (individual or family) on drugs from a wider list, everyone else, i.e. those in Category II, will get reimbursement for any expenditures in excess of €85 under the Drugs Payment Scheme (DPS). It can be said that €85 is a large deductible, and indeed the effect is that most persons in Category II pay all of their own drug costs. Again, a very big difference in costs for routine care exists between those in Categories I and II.

The effect of the DPS programme is to cap drugs expenditures for households at €1,020 per year, which is too high. Moreover, the cap is set as a flat amount, so it is a higher percentage of lower incomes. The authors propose that the DPS system should be reformed to reimburse a percentage of all prescription drug purchases at the point of sale, and that that percentage should be higher for people on lower incomes

Medical Card holders are eligible for all acute hospital care, including doctor services, free of charge. Those in Category II are also eligible to be public patients in hospitals, but in 2005 they must pay nominal fees of €55 per night for inpatient care up to a maximum of 10 nights per annum.[5] Prior to increases in Medical Card eligibility ceilings, announced in October 2005, one-quarter of the population (generally speaking, the near-poor or working poor) had neither Medical Cards nor voluntary insurance; they are the ones who face these fees in hospital.[6]

All women in Ireland, not only Medical Card holders, are eligible for free maternity care, provided by a GP and by an obstetrician and a hospital.

Medical Card eligibility

Traditionally, since their inception, Medical Cards have been granted to the 35 to 38 per cent of the population most in need, as based on their incomes and numbers of dependents. In 1983, more than 38 per cent of the population had Medical Cards. By 1996 this had fallen to 34.5 per cent. By the end of 2004, the proportion of the population eligible on the basis of need had fallen to under 26 per cent. This drastic adjustment constitutes one of the most important recent changes in the Irish health care system.

In 2001, non-poor people aged 70 and over became eligible for Medical Cards. (Poor older persons already qualified for cards according to income.) Higher-income older people are now privileged above lower-income non-aged (those just above the eligibility threshold *du jour*). This is a step which seems reasonable only if it is a step towards free primary care for all. However, the opposite appears to be the case, as free primary care has been taken away from low-income people even as it has been granted to high-income aged persons.

In November 2004 the government announced a plan to introduce so-called 'doctor-only' Medical Cards for 200,000 persons just above the Medical Card eligibility threshold. The announcement stated that holders of these cards would be allowed to visit GPs without charge but would be required to pay for medicines, up to €85 per month. Apparently, they would also have to pay to visit non-GP caregivers, such as physiotherapists, whose care is covered by the standard Medical Card. Holders of these cards will also have to pay hospital overnight charges up to a maximum of 10 nights, or €550, per annum (2005 rate), and accident and emergency (A&E) and other charges.

By 2005 the Irish population had risen to an estimated 4,130,700. If 34.5 per cent of the population held Medical Cards as in 1996, that would equal 1,425,092 people (see Appendix 3 for calculations). According to the GMS, as of November 2005, 1,150,551 cards had been issued, a shortfall of 274,541 people when compared with the 34.5 per cent of population covered in 1996. If an adjustment is made for the 112,839 people with Medical Cards[7] who were aged 70 and over and would not have qualified on a need basis, that would yield a 387,380 shortfall in people qualifying on the basis of need, compared to 1996. Even if we conservatively adjust all of these numbers downward, we can confidently say that by November 2005, 350,000 low-income Irish people were not covered by Medical Cards who would have been had coverage remained at its 1996 level.

On 13 October 2005, the Tánaiste and Minister for Health, Mary Harney, announced an increase of 20 per cent in the weekly net income guidelines for Medical Card eligibility, which would put them at about €184 for an individual and about €342 for a family of four. The Tánaiste also announced that 'reasonable rent and mortgage payments, childcare expenses and travel to work expenses' would be taken into account in assessing net income for eligibility. Doctor-only card guidelines would be about €230 for an individual and €428 for a family. At the time of writing, no one had estimated how many additional people would become eligible as a consequence of this welcome move. Some of the 350,000 lost Medical Cards were expected to be made up by the rise in the threshold; but by January 2006, three months after the announced increase, Medical Card eligibility had risen by only 6,309 persons, an increase that might be fully accounted for by the rise in population over that time, and the number of people covered by doctor-only Medical Cards was 5,080.

The authors advocate that the number of people qualifying for Medical Cards on the basis of need be returned to the historic proportion of 35 to 38 per cent and that, after that change, Medical Card guidelines be indexed to the median income[8] of production workers or the median earnings of Irish workers so that they change continuously rather than intermittently, and so that the level be set automatically rather than politically.

Notch effect

As noted, as one's income rises past the threshold for Medical Card eligibility, there is a considerable impact on the cost of health care, including GP services, other primary and community care, drugs and even acute hospital services. The result is that for a fairly wide range of incomes, an increase in earnings actually results in a reduced standard of living. The effect is equivalent to an income tax with marginal tax rates in excess of 100 per cent.

It is well known in economics that fixed income eligibility thresholds for cash and non-cash public programmes can discourage people from taking jobs, increasing hours or taking promotions. The effect is referred to as a 'notch effect' (because of its impact on a graph relating consumption levels to earnings). In Ireland, the effect may be to discourage people from seeking needed health care as well as to discourage them from seeking employment.

A notch effect can be mitigated by adopting a gradual reduction in benefits as earnings rise in place of the fixed eligibility threshold. For example, if the state would pay a percentage of GP and other fees and of drug expenses for near-poor persons, the notch effect would be lessened. One possibility is a 'demi-Medical Card', which might cover half of the money expenses paid by this population for services and products provided free to Medical Card holders. Other configurations are possible; the demi-Card is just the easiest, at least to describe.[9] The money difference between Medical Card eligibility and ineligibility is enormous and harmful to this low-income population.

Of course, universal free GP care would also mitigate the notch effect. Universal health insurance, covering primary care and drugs, would abolish it.

Capitation rates

GPs are paid on a capitation basis for Medical Card patients. The GMS pays a flat amount per patient, the amount depending on age, gender and distance from the doctor, irrespective of utilisation. In 2004, the rates ranged from €38.76 per year for a boy aged five to 15 living up to three miles from the doctor's office, to €190.05 for a woman aged 70 or over living more than 10 miles away.[10] The higher rates for female and older patients correspond to greater GP costs in treating them, mainly as a result of different visiting rates.

When doctors are paid on a capitation basis, they in effect bear the insurance risk of caring for their patients. Just as an insurance company in effect gains from clients who have few claims and loses from those who have substantial claims, doctors paid by capitation gain from patients with little utilisation and lose in relation to those with high utilisation. Therefore, the variability in capitation rates according to gender and age acts as a form of risk adjustment or risk equalisation. In the absence of such a structure, doctors with disproportionately large numbers of aged patients would be financially disadvantaged, and some doctors would find they had to limit the numbers of such patients they took on.

There seems to be no present justification for varying capitation rates by distance between the patient's home and the GP's office. That feature of capitation rates appears to reflect a need during the adjustment period when fee-for-service gave way to capitation. Its present need should be investigated.

In general, then, apart from the distance adjustment, the capitation structure is efficient and results in equity between GPs. There is an exception, however. There is a special capitation rate of €495.07 per year for people aged 70 years or more who have been issued a Medical Card on the basis of age alone, i.e. who do not qualify for a card on the basis of income. Low-income people aged 70 or over attract a capitation rate of €108.74 to €190.05, depending on gender and location, so non-poor aged attract a capitation rate which is about 2.6 to 4.5 times as high as that for poor aged. Since poor people are known to have higher morbidity (sickness), the higher rate is not meant to compensate GPs for higher costs of treating this population. Instead, apparently the rate was the result of a negotiation process and was meant to overcome GPs' opposition to the 70-and-over Medical Card. One would guess that patients with the 'gold card', as GPs are said to call the 70-and-over Medical Card holders, are especially lucrative to GPs.

And the 'gold card' does not result in inter-GP equity. Low- and high-income aged persons are not proportionately distributed across GP practices. Instead, low-income aged are concentrated in certain rural areas and in lower-income urban areas such as the north side of Dublin. Higher-income over-70s are said to be concentrated along the south-east coast. Dr Muiris Houston has reported that 'general practitioners treating older medical card patients in deprived areas of Dublin are earning less than half the income of doctors working in better-off areas of the capital.'[11] Two Dublin physicians were reported to have conducted an analysis showing that practices in the inner city and in south-west Dublin earn as little as 56 per cent of the average national Medical Card income. 'In the case of one practice, its annual income per patient was €140 compared with a south-east coast practice whose medical card income per patient was €400, reflecting the high number of "wealthy" medical card patients aged over 70 living in its catchment area.'

Besides creating inter-GP inequities, this practice can yield economically inefficient outcomes. Doctors whose 70-plus patients attract lower capitation rates may discourage those patients from enroling with them. More seriously, in the long run GPs may seek to locate in the more lucrative areas populated by 'gold card' aged and avoid locating in areas populated by the less remunerative patients. As Ireland is acknowledged to have a GP shortage, this could be a serious issue.

Mixed remuneration for GPs

As noted, Irish GPs are paid by capitation for Medical Card or GMS patients and by fee-for-service (FFS) for private patients. As discussed in more detail in Chapter 4, in incentives terms this is an unfortunate combination. GPs have an economic incentive to privilege private patients over public patients. While there is no research indicating that GPs in fact do privilege private over public patients, it seems a mistake to choose incentives known to be inherently harmful and destructive. Much research and widely discussed data show that similar incentives facing consultants clearly do harm, exactly as predicted.

If, as many advocate, Ireland adopts a GP service which is free to all at the point of use, there is a strong case to be made for capitation for all at age/gender appropriate rates. Experience with FFS in the GMS prior to 1989 showed that the combination of fees for doctors and free care to patients had inadequate checks for excessive utilisation. Patients paying about €50 per visit are sure to resist excessive visiting, but patients paying nothing are not.[12]

Systems which nominally rely wholly on capitation, such as general practice in the British National Health Service (NHS), actually have numerous fees for out-of-hours care, home visits and special services. Nonetheless, a system which relies wholly on capitation almost certainly goes too far in the opposite direction of discouraging utilisation. A hybrid system, in which GPs receive a partial capitation fee for each patient plus a partial fee for each visit or service provided, can achieve a better outcome and is advocated by the authors.

Hospital care

Hospital patients are either public or private patients. All patients in private hospitals are private patients.[13] Patients in public hospitals may be either public patients or private patients. What does it mean to be a public patient in a public hospital? What does it mean to be a private patient in a public hospital?

All residents of Ireland are eligible to be public patients. Medical Card holders get all services free of charge. Others pay a fee (€55 per day in 2005) for a maximum of 10 days per annum.[14] For this they are normally provided a bed in a public ward, and are entitled to the range of appropriate hospital services, e.g. operating theatre, radiography, pathology, etc. They are also provided with consultant-led specialist physician services. They may be treated personally by consultants, but they may instead be treated by non-consultant hospital doctors (NCHDs), usually doctors in training. If a public patient must be placed on a waiting list for care, it will specifically be a public patient waiting list. Private patients are placed on separate, shorter waiting lists. It is worth pointing out that private waiting lists are not open to public scrutiny. National oversight of public patient waiting lists has been transferred from the Department of Health to the National Treatment Purchase Fund (NTPF), but no one has oversight of the private lists.

Private patients of hospitals are in general also private patients of consultants. Traditionally, private patients in hospitals could be assumed to be insured by Voluntary Health Insurance (VHI) or Bupa, the two health insurers in Ireland. A third firm, Vivas, entered the market in 2004. (See the discussion of voluntary insurance below.) However, there is growing evidence that a large number of uninsured people are going into debt to pay for private care and circumvent public waiting lists.[15]

A private patient in a public hospital gets care that can differ from that of a public patient in three important ways. He or she is normally provided a bed in a private (one-bed) room or a semi-private (up to five-bed) room rather than in a public ward. Even children, when they are private patients, may be placed in cubicles on wards, separate from public patient children, whose beds are generally separated only by curtains. A private patient is much more likely than a public patient to be treated personally by a consultant and he or she is likely to be treated sooner. If placed on a waiting list, it will be a shorter, private patient waiting list.

These differences have led observers, including the authors, to describe the system of acute hospital care in Ireland as constituting a two-tier system. The existence of the two-tier system violates the need principle of medical ethics. Medical care is distributed on the basis of ability and willingness to pay as a private patient, and not medical need. There are two further characteristics which make the two-tier system truly outrageous:

- Private patients in public hospitals do not pay the full economic costs of their treatment. It is accepted that they pay 50 to 60 per cent of the full costs.[16] Since taxpayers provide hospitals with their budgets, the remainder is subsidised by taxpayers. This means that private patients are privileged by the system over public patients, and public patients help pay for their own subordination. (The Brennan Commission reported that on numerous occasions, private patients have not been charged at all for certain services provided in public hospitals, with public hospitals forgoing €1 million annually in fees.[17])

- Secondly, this exploitative treatment is the principal reason over half of the population buy private health insurance in a country in which everyone is eligible to be a public patient.[18] It would be unfair to those who buy private insurance to say that they do so to get special privileges. Instead, it seems more proper to say that they do so to avoid the mistreatment that public patients suffer. Instead of saying that they buy insurance to be on the top tier, we can more fairly say they do so to avoid being on the bottom tier. They are able to do so at bargain prices because of the subsidisation of private care.

Studies have shown[19] that no insured person, but 22 per cent of the uninsured, had a wait for treatment in excess of one year. Analysis in 2002 showed that the average wait for care in a public hospital was 3.4 months for a private patient and 6.7 months for a public patient.[20]

Public patients must wait longer than private patients for the initial consultant appointment after referral by a GP, which will precede being entered on a waiting list, so the actual care disparity is greater than the statistics indicate.[21]

National Treatment Purchase Fund

The National Treatment Purchase Fund (NTPF) was created by the government in 2002 to respond to the problem of long public patient waiting lists. Adults who have been on waiting lists for a year or longer and children who have been on lists for at least six months are provided care as private patients in other hospitals, with the government paying the fees. The hospital where treatment occurs may be public or private; it may be within the state or in Northern Ireland or Britain. According to the NTPF, in some regions all patients meeting these time standards have been given treatment, and waiting times are now being reduced to six and three months for adults and children, respectively.

The NTPF reduces strains on the acute system but does not deal with the underlying problem of the inability of the public hospital system to meet demands routinely placed on it. Collectively if not individually, it rewards consultants for favouring private patients by providing them with still more private patients from whom to earn fees. The NTPF states that it tries to avoid paying consultants to treat their own public patients, but concedes that this may happen occasionally. A 2005 audit by the Comptroller and Auditor General (C&AG) has revealed that 36 per cent of treatments do occur in the same hospital which failed to treat the patient in a timely manner in the first place.[22] In virtually all cases, consultants treat as private patients each others' public patients whom they have failed to schedule for prompt treatment.

The NTPF refuses to provide information on fees paid to consultants for care, stating that the information is commercially sensitive.[23] Thus, it is impossible to weigh claims regarding the efficiency of the process. But as we discuss in Chapter 7, that same C&AG audit has shown a stunning range of prices paid by the NTPF for treatment, suggesting overpayment in at least some instances.[24]

Specialist care

Public patients in public hospitals are provided 'consultant-led' specialist physician services. They may be treated personally by a consultant, but they may also be treated by an NCHD, usually a doctor in training. Public patients are much more likely than private patients to be treated by NCHDs, often without consultant supervision. Thus, consultant leadership may in some circumstances be very limited or non-existent.

On 1 January 2005, there were 1,947 approved permanent consultant posts and 4,170 approved NCHD positions in the public sector in Ireland. Not only is it the case that NCHDs are far more numerous than consultants, but they work longer hours in the public hospital system as well.[25] Thus it is clear that NCHDs deliver the majority of 'frontline services' (as the Hanly Report[26] puts it) in acute hospitals.

Private patients are much more likely to be treated personally by the consultant. Consultants will be paid a fee by the patient or by the patient's insurance carrier. Fees for treatment by consultants apparently do not diverge much from a fee schedule maintained by VHI, but fees for visits to consultants' rooms frequently do not qualify for reimbursement and may be high, i.e. over twice a GP's typical fee.

Both consultants and NCHDs are paid salaries by the state (not by the hospital). In 2005, NCHD salaries ranged from about €31,000 for the most junior of interns to around €75,000 for the highest grade of senior registrar. The Hanly Report revealed that NCHD salaries are dwarfed by their overtime pay. The long hours of NCHDs, as discussed earlier, resulted in over-time pay in 2002 which was 61 per cent of NCHD income. The average NCHD worked 77 hours per week in that year, receiving a salary of €43,231 and overtime pay of €66,842, for an average combined income of €110,073.

Consultant salaries depend on Category I or II (see discussion below), specialty and region, and range from about €120,000 to €160,000. Unlike NCHDs, consultants are allowed private practices and are able to earn fees. No data exist on the private practice income of consultants, but it is reasonable to believe that it varies by specialty and geographic area, and that it ranges from zero for consultants in some low-income areas to millions for consultants practicing in high-income areas.

Wren used insurance data to estimate private consultant income for 2002.[27] Only aggregate data were available. When paediatricians, geriatricians, psychiatrists and academic physicians, all of whom have limited opportunities for private practice, are excluded, the average private income for consultants was €130,000, roughly equaling their mean salaries and effectively doubling their incomes. However, this is a mean; it is virtually certain that private consultant income is very unequally distributed.

Consultants' common contract

The consultants' common contract, discussed more fully in Chapter 9, is one of the most problematic and controversial issues in the Irish health care system. It is widely criticised, especially for two characteristics:

- Consultants are paid a public salary for being present in public hospitals for at least 33 hours, but they need not care for public patients during all (or any) of that time. They are permitted private practices in public hospitals, and time spent treating private patients for fees can count toward the 33 hours obligated.

- Consultants are not accountable to anyone, either administratively or clinically.

There are two main categories of consultant contract currently available. The vast majority (60 per cent in 2005) of consultants chose Category I, according to which they are permitted private practice only in the hospital to which they are assigned. In 2005, 31 per cent chose Category II, which provides a somewhat smaller public salary, but under which consultants can conduct their private practices anywhere, including private hospitals.

The remaining small minority holds full-time academic posts (6 per cent) or still holds 'public-only' contracts (2 per cent), which were offered prior to 1997. Under the latter, consultants who were willing to forgo private practice received a somewhat higher salary. The state decided not to offer the public-only contract after 1997.

There are notable variations between regions and specialties in the distribution of contract types. In contrast to the rest of the country, the majority of consultants based in Dublin public hospitals hold Category II contracts, including about 90 per cent of consultant anaesthetists and consultant surgeons. Nationally, 98 per cent of consultant paediatricians, psychiatrists and physicians in emergency medicine hold Category I contracts.[28]

Mixed remuneration for consultants

As noted, consultants are paid by salary for their work for public patients and by fee for private patients. This is an unfortunate combination. Consultants have an economic incentive to privilege private patients over public patients. Moreover, unlike the case with GPs, it is very clear that consultants do systematically privilege private over public patients. Indeed, this is a source of the two-tier system of care which has been so widely and thoroughly criticised.[29] Given the fact that the state has dictated that there be private beds and private patients in public hospitals, hospitals' and consultants' incentives to earn additional income creates the differential treatment which we refer to as the two-tier system.

A solution is to pay consultants in the same way, and at the same rate, for both classes of patients. The most widely discussed method for achieving this result is the adoption of universal health insurance. We discuss this proposal in Chapter 13. The idea is that consultants would receive fees – at the same levels – for both classes of patients. This would almost certainly produce the desired result. But FFS for all is a system known to be associated with higher levels of utilisation overall. When you pay doctors according to the quantity of care they provide, they provide more care. An all-fee system of paying consultants will, at the very least, require the adoption of added cost control techniques.

Another possibility is to pay comprehensive salaries which cover both public and private patients. This solution is rarely discussed, perhaps because it is conceded that Irish consultants are likely to strongly oppose it, even though salaried hospital specialists are the norm in some countries, and staff some hospitals in many other countries. It could also arise out of universal health insurance. An all-salary system would have desirable incentives consequences, but it might have harmful negative effects on productivity.

As with GPs, the optimal payment technique for consultants is a hybrid, with partial salaries (covering care of all patients) and partial fees (for all patients). Instead of a system where salaries cover some patients and fees cover others, as is currently the case, which results in a two-tier system of care, the best alternative is one which combines salaries and fees in another, more efficient and equitable way, with each doctor paid in the same way for each patient. The authors endorse such a hybrid system.

Voluntary insurance

Voluntary health insurance in Ireland is essentially hospital and inpatient consultant care insurance. The insurers currently active in the country make a benefit available which will cover a fraction (half or less) of the costs of outpatient care, including GP care, but this coverage comes at considerable additional cost and is chosen by only a small number of people.

VHI

Voluntary Health Insurance (VHI) was created in 1957 for the deliberate purpose of protecting Irish people on higher incomes who were not eligible for free or subsidised health services. It is governed by the Voluntary Health Insurance Board, whose members are appointed by the Minister for Health. A 'state-sponsored' body, VHI has had a unique relationship to the state, which has never provided VHI with any direct financial assistance, but which stands ready to cover losses. From the start, however, the state gave VHI massive indirect aid by giving taxpayers relief on premiums. By subsidising private care, the state also significantly brought down VHI premiums. These two indirect subsidies assured the rapid growth of VHI.

In the 1980s, when a significant percentage of the population were not eligible for free care in public hospitals, VHI still concentrated on covering those people without eligibility. Yet even then a substantial number of people with eligibility for free public care bought VHI cover. Tussing, writing in the early 1980s[30] when VHI membership stood at only 25 per cent of the population, noted, 'VHI is now too large, from an efficiency standpoint, and this translates into inefficiently high demand for costly private care.'

Since that time, the central mission of VHI has changed from insuring those without public eligibility to providing a means by which the insured can protect themselves from having to *use* their public eligibility.

Until 1996, VHI had a complete monopoly on the sale of health insurance in Ireland, but European Union (EU) law required that the Irish market be open to domestic and EU competitors, and in 1996, Bupa (Ireland), a subsidiary of the leading British provider of voluntary insurance, entered the Irish market. A third firm, Vivas, of Irish origin, was launched in 2004.

Risk equalisation

The entry of additional health insurers in competition with VHI raised the vexed issue of risk equalisation.

Irish law[31] requires health insurers to provide open enrolment, community rating and lifetime cover, requirements approved by the EU. Under community rating, one's age, gender or other personal characteristics which might influence future health and hence insurance claims cannot influence the premium one pays. Everyone insured under a given plan pays the average premium for that plan.

Community rating refers to a system under which everyone in the community pays the same insurance premium for the same set of benefits. The opposite of community rating is experience rating, under which older and other riskier customers pay higher premiums. Community rating involves cross-subsidisation from the younger and healthier members of the community, who over-pay in relation to their risk levels, to the older and less healthy members, who under-pay. This cross-subsidisation is an important manifestation of the principle of social solidarity.

In a society which uses community rating and which has a competitive health insurance market, risk equalisation will be necessary whenever insurers face significantly different risks. This is the case today in Ireland. VHI, largely as a consequence of its long existence, has insured many older Irish people. Bupa, in part because it has entered the market only recently, has insured primarily younger people in this country.

Risk equalisation is a process which transfers money from insurers with lower-risk membership to insurers with higher-risk membership. Why is risk equalisation necessary?

- *Avoid risk selection*: Risk selection occurs where insurers make an effort to avoid insuring high-risk people. Risk selection is obviously harmful, but risk equalisation reduces the need for and also the opportunity for risk selection.
- *Avoid 'cherry-picking'*: Cherry-picking occurs in markets in which there is cross-subsidisation and in which some competitors seek business from those who over-pay, i.e. those who subsidise others. Cherry-picking in insurance markets ultimately makes community rating impossible because its logical extreme occurs where one insurer has most of the low-risk clients and another insurer has most of the high-risk clients.
- *Assure efficient market*: The gains from market competition arise from the process of competitors trying to outdo each other by providing the best possible product at the lowest pos-

sible price. The existence of risk selection and cherry-picking undermines market competition by shifting it away from value for money and towards trying to influence risk by choosing clients according to risk. Risk equalisation is necessary for an efficient market.

A Health Working Paper released in 2004 by the Organisation for Economic Cooperation and Development (OECD) looked at the question of risk equalisation in Ireland in detail.[32] The authors stated:

> 66. In recent years, there has been a heated policy debate in Ireland around the implementation of the RE [risk equalisation] scheme provided for under the 1994 legislation...
>
> 67. Opponents of risk equalisation find it incompatible with principles of competition and believe it will discourage insurers' efforts at containing cost. They also indicate that RE seeks to prevent a threat to the market that, in their view, is only hypothetical at the moment. In the absence of such a scheme, however, there is the potential that insurers could compete on the basis of attracting a more healthy pool of clients. In fact...there are some differences in the age and health status profiles of enrolees of the two insurers. Thus, the two insurers are not currently operating or playing upon a 'level playing field'.
>
> 68. With respect to the impact of such a scheme on competition, many experts believe that risk equalisation is a necessary buttress for fair competition within a community-rated environment. In the absence of adequate risk equalisation within an individual market subject to community rating and open enrolment, there will be large incentives for risk selection, and potential adverse effects on equity and market efficiency. There is also a general consensus in the health economics literature and among other experts supporting the importance of RE schemes in order to prevent risk selection.[33]

In June 2005, the Tánaiste, in her role as Minister for Health, rejected the decision of the Health Insurance Authority (HIA) to require Bupa to make risk equalisation payments to VHI. This decision was widely criticised, including by the present authors in their November 2005 report to the Irish Congress of Trade Unions, which was a previous version of this book.[34] In December 2005 she reversed this decision, linking her action with new legislation affecting the structure of VHI.

Bupa initiated a challenge to the Tánaiste's decision in the courts and stated that should risk equalisation become final, they would leave the Irish market.

Irish legislation providing for risk equalisation became effective in 1996 before Bupa entered the market, so Bupa were well aware that the HIA would almost certainly recommend risk equalisation. The HIA recommended an annual transfer of €33.4 million. Bupa appealed unsuccessfully to the HIA to reverse its decision, stating that such a large payment might lead it to leave the Irish market.

Then, as noted, the Minister initially decided not to go ahead with risk equalisation. She cited the unresolved nature of VHI's ownership, as discussed in Chapter 3. She also cited Bupa's threat to leave the Irish market and emphasised the need to maintain competition in the Irish health insurance market. VHI has about 80 per cent of the market, and Bupa only 20 per cent.

This was simply a mistake on her part, a failure to understand what competition means. Without risk equalisation, competition in the Irish health insurance market leads destructively to pressure on VHI to engage in risk selection. True competition, where those who seek health insurance can choose according to value and price, *requires* risk equalisation.

The government's initial decision against risk adjustment reflected the confusion of *competition* with *numbers of competitors*, a confusion commonly addressed in basic economics classes. Numerous anti-competitive devices. e.g. 'fair trade' prices, protective tariffs and cartels, are capable of sustaining competitors without encouraging competition. In insurance, where there is community rating, there must also be risk adjustment or the desirable fruits of competition will not appear.

In August 2005, the European Commission sent a letter to the Irish government warning that it could be in breach of EU rules against improper aid to domestic competitors if it went ahead with risk equalisation. In its letter, the European Commission stated, '[w]e would be inclined to take the view that a requirement to pay under the RES [risk equalisation scheme] an amount so significant that it would force an operator to exit the market would seem to discourage other operators from entering the market and does, in any event, seem disproportionate.'

There are three obvious things wrong with the European Commission's letter:

- The European Commission does not purport to have reviewed the methods or the calculations of the HIA and found them faulty. They do not like the result but they do not say the procedure or the amount is incorrect.
- Secondly, Bupa only *said* they would leave the market, so we have to revise the EC statement to read, 'an amount so significant that it would lead an operator to *state that they would* exit the market'. Obviously that is a very different thing.
- Thirdly, if the risk equalisation calculation is correct, and if Bupa would really exit the market if it were carried out, then it follows that Bupa entered the market only to cherry-pick. That is the only tenable conclusion.

It is not clear what lies behind the European Commission's remarkably inappropriate intervention.

It is the view of the authors of the present study that risk equalisation is necessary in the Irish health insurance market, for the sake both of efficient and equitable market competition. We congratulate the Tánaiste on the wisdom of her revised decision.

Ownership of the VHI

The VHI is, as described earlier, a 'semi-state body'. Its ownership status is under review. It can continue to be a state-sponsored institution, in some sense; it can convert to the status of a mutual or provident society, owned, in effect, by its policy-holders; or it can become a private, for-profit corporation.

In announcing her decision to proceed with risk equalisation between Bupa and VHI, the Tánaiste announced two planned legislative changes. VHI would be required to accumulate reserves equal to those required of a commercial insurance carrier within six years. This change is appropriately linked to the risk equalisation decision and will help achieve a level playing field.

Secondly, VHI would be converted to a public limited company (PLC).[35] A PLC is a type of limited company whose shares are not required to be offered for sale to the public.[36]

There is no necessary logical reason to link the risk equalisation decision with the ownership status of VHI. The authors advocate that VHI continue to be a state company so that it can continue to serve national rather than private or parochial interests. Whatever the future of VHI, it should not become a for-profit company.

Tax relief on medical expenses

Irish residents can claim tax relief on unreimbursed medical expenses. Once expenses have passed €125 for a person or €250 for a household, they can be subtracted from taxable income. The effect is to provide still another added subsidy to private medical expenditures. Moreover, as the money value of tax relief is equal to the relief amount multiplied by one's marginal tax rate, and because of the progressive structure of the Irish income tax, the absolute size of the subsidy actually rises with income.

Conclusion

This chapter has shown that the Irish health care system faces numerous serious problems of adequacy, equity and efficiency in five areas: Medical Cards, GP care, acute hospital care, the consultants' common contract and risk equalisation.

Medical Cards

The proportion of the Irish population covered by Medical Cards has fallen and is too low. Those whose incomes place them just above the eligibility threshold for full Medical Cards will face non-GP professional fees and drug costs which are very large in relation to their incomes. Those beyond the threshold for doctor-only cards face the further unbuffered cost of GP fees. These near-poor families regularly face the choice of foregoing needed medical care for themselves and their children, or foregoing income rises to preserve Medical Card eligibility.

Obvious short-term solutions to these problems involve reversing the recent erosion of Medical Cards, restoring the historic percentage of 35–38 per cent of the population, exclusive of the non-income-based 70-and-over card, and restoring full eligibility to doctor-only cardholders. The authors of this study believe that the historic proportion should be re-established immediately. All those awarded Medical Cards should avail of all care for which any eligible person qualifies. There should be no 'doctor-only' eligibility, but there should be a gradual reduction in benefits as earnings rise in place of the fixed Medical Card eligibility threshold. One possibility is a 'demi-Medical Card', which might cover half of the money expenses for services and products free to Medical Card holders, paid by the population whose earnings are below average for the state, but who are ineligible for Medical Cards.

GP care

A longer-term solution advocated by the authors, one needed on efficiency grounds as well as in response to the problems set out here, and discussed elsewhere in this report, is free GP care for all, or, more fully, free primary care for all, together with more thorough drug coverage.

GP capitation rates for the Medical Card 70-and-over population are inequitable between poor and non-poor aged people, and the authors argue that they should be reviewed and adjusted so that GPs receive the same capitation rate for all 70-year-olds and over, removing this contributory incentive to GPs locating in wealthier neighbourhoods.

Acute hospital care

The principal financing issue in relation to acute care is, of course, the two-tier system of care. There are unequal and excessively long waits for care for public patients and public patients are too often cared for by less-qualified NCHDs. The Hanly Report[37] advocates a large increase in the numbers of consultants employed in the system, sufficient to satisfy the European Working Time Directive, while converting specialist care from a consultant-led service to a consultant-provided service.

There are significant public subsidies to private care. The inequities of the Irish system are underlined by the fact that tax-payers in the bottom half of the income distribution contribute to the private care of those in the upper half.

A long-standing problem in the acute care system, apart from the two-tier system (but certainly related to it), is that hospital charges for private care do not cover true economic costs of care. The government has stated an intention to change this and to impose full economic costs of care on private patients.

Systematic short- and long-term policies advocated by the authors to address the two-tier system, waiting lists, a consultant-provided service and public subsidies to private care are set forth in detail elsewhere in this report.

Consultant contract

The consultants' common contract is deeply flawed and requires revision. Consultants are paid public salaries while treating private patients. They are not accountable administratively or clinically. These features require modification. The authors' proposals appear elsewhere in this report.

Risk equalisation

As discussed above in detail, the authors believe that risk equalisation is needed among competing health insurers for equity and efficiency.

These problems and flaws all add up to a crisis of adequacy and equity. Other chapters of this report show some of these flaws in greater depth and also show efficiency problems, many of them arising out of anomalous incentives.

Recent years of sustained growth and prosperity in Ireland make it possible to address many of these issues as never before.

6

PRIMARY CARE

Introduction

Primary care is both one of the great successes of the Irish health care system and one of its greatest failures. Improved access to primary care and reformed organisation in this sector are arguably the most urgent needs of the entire health care system. Fortunately, these reforms can build on the far-seeing 2001 Primary Care Strategy (which, however, may have been abandoned by the government that issued it) and can draw strength from a well-trained, skilled and dedicated corps of clinicians, led by the Irish general practitioner, the bedrock of the system.

Primary care is predominantly a private sector activity in the Irish health care system. Professor Ivan Perry of University College, Cork, who chairs the Primary Care Steering Group, has argued that the public sector subsidises the private sector in Irish primary care.[1] The Primary Care Strategy envisions very substantial further taxpayer contributions to private primary care.

Primary care is typically the patient's first point of contact in the health care system. It provides care for the simplest and most common ailments and conditions, accounting for 70 to 90 per cent of medical care needs. Providers of primary care refer patients to specialists and other levels of care, if necessary, acting as gatekeepers for treatment of more complex and severe conditions in other settings, by more specialised professionals.

The modifier 'primary' falsely connotes that patients logically move to *secondary* care (county hospital-based specialist care) and possibly *tertiary* care (national or regional specialist care). A more appropriate modifier might be 'generalist out-of-hospital' care, as primary care does not necessarily imply any subsequent specialised care, and can occur after as well as before secondary or tertiary care. As hospital-based care declines in importance in modern medical thinking, the role of primary care necessarily expands and evolves.

The clinician most likely to treat patients at the level of primary care in Ireland is the general practitioner (GP). Other primary care clinicians might include the public health nurse, the practice nurse or the midwife. More specialised professionals at the primary level could include social workers, physio- and occupational therapists and other *allied health* professionals. These primary care clinicians may be assisted by care assistants, home helps and others.

The most highly trained – and most widely skilled – of these clinicians is the GP, and most of this chapter will concentrate on that physician, though some discussion will address the relationship between GPs and others, especially the idea of a Primary Care Team (PCT).

Access

Access to primary care was discussed more fully in Chapter 5. Almost all people in Ireland fall into either of two groups in relation to access to primary care[2]: those who hold Medical Cards, and those who do not. Holders of Medical Cards in turn are holders of full or conventional Medical Cards, who hence qualify for full free medical care of all types, including primary care, and holders of doctor-only Medical Cards, who qualify for free GP care only. At the time of writing, just over one-fourth of Irish residents hold Medical Cards on the basis of income and need, well below the historic proportion of 35 to 38 per cent. In addition, everyone aged 70 and over, regardless of income, holds a Medical Card.

Primary care can be extremely expensive. Visits to GPs can cost approximately €50 and visits to other primary care clinicians are similarly expensive. Outpatient drugs are free to Medical Card holders, but others must pay the first €85 each month before they qualify for state help. Even when family members are only moderately ill, there can be monthly costs totalling hundreds of euro. The cost difference between Medical Card eligibility and ineligibility is enormous. It is too large and it is too abrupt. It may deter some Medical Card holders from trying to earn more, for fear of losing medical care for their children, and it may deter some who are not eligible for Medical Cards from seeking needed care and from getting regular preventative and screening care.

The authors of this report advocate a primary care system free to all at the point of use. Fees for primary care deter those with moderate or even high incomes from routine asymptomatic, preventative and screening visits with clinicians, and from care early in the progress of an illness. While high fees such as those found in the Irish system may discourage unnecessary care, they may also discourage needed care.

A primary care system free at the point of use[3] cannot be built overnight. Our vision of the steps that need to be taken to develop such a priceless resource for Ireland by 2010 is discussed elsewhere in this report. A move to free primary care will benefit primarily middle- and upper-income groups and should be linked in timing of introduction to gains for lower-income groups in the acute system, as is discussed elsewhere in this report.

In the authors' view, there are two immediate needs to improve access. First, full Medical Card eligibility must be restored to those who have lost it because of the erosion of coverage under the present government. Second, help with GP bills, other primary care and drug costs needs to be given to all those in the bottom half of the income distribution to buffer the huge potential costs of Medical Card ineligibility. An example would be a demi-Medical Card, as discussed in Chapter 5.[4]

Modern primary care

Ireland needs more GPs. This fact is acknowledged by all observers and is supported by the statistics cited below. Expanding the numbers of GPs will take time and requires expanding the numbers of Irish medical students, as discussed below.

Ireland has skilled and dedicated primary care clinicians. It needs a modern system of primary care. Literature on modern primary care[5] indicates a need for the following, all of which are weak or absent in the Irish system:

- *A primary care system which addresses the health needs of a mainly healthy population rather than concentrating on intervention in episodes of illness:* Ideally, generalist care is not episodic, but rather is continuous, with seamless transitions between well care and intervention for illness. By contrast, specialist care is typically focused on an acute condition and is episodic, having a beginning and an end.
- *An emphasis on disease management for the chronically ill:* Community care for the chronically ill is also non-episodic.
- *Supportive of self-care and home care:* Self-care and home care often require technology in the home and supportive services from visiting nurses and other clinicians.
- *Stronger evidence-based medicine, with appropriate protocols and guidelines:* This is the direction of modern primary care medicine, but it requires support from academic medicine, peer organisations and the state.
- *Peer review and quality assurance:* Ireland is starting almost from scratch in the area of clinical accountability, peer review and quality assurance in primary care. It will require support and resources from the state, but as the term 'peer review' implies, clinical accountability must in general be in the hands of the organised medical profession.[6] The appropriate body is the Medical Council. However, to make peer review and quality assurance mandatory, and to give them the force of law, legislation (revision of the Medical Practitioners Act 1978) is required. See the discussion of Competence Assurance in Chapter 9.
- *Primary care infrastructure:* There is an urgent need for large investments in the primary care infrastructure, in the form of facilities and both computer and medical technology for primary care teams. The investment needs state resources, in the form of grants or long-term low-interest loans. This is one of the most urgent needs in the entire Irish health care system.
- *Supportive institutions:* The expanded primary care infrastructure needs to be supported with networked out-of-hours care, minor injury units and other primary care centres specifically

designed to relieve the burden on hospital accident and emergency (A&E) departments. At one time the typical Irish GP undertook to provide out-of-hours care for his or her own patients, with adverse consequences for the GP's own quality of life. In recent years Irish GPs have withdrawn from this activity, thus accounting for some of the pressure on A&E departments. Primary care reform must replace these services, not only to relieve pressures on hospitals, but also to provide more appropriate and efficient care. Primary care should not be provided in the A&E department.

- *Skill substitution*: Irish primary care needs to economise on its use of scarce GP time by making greater use of personnel with less advanced training in the performance of tasks not requiring physicians, including practice nurses and care assistants. The same is true, often to a greater degree, in relation to other primary care professionals, such as social workers, physio- and occupational therapists and others, many of whom are in short supply.

- *GP interface*: All of the following interfaces are in serious need of attention: GP to GP (relations among GPs in a community), GP to primary care team (as will be discussed in detail below) and GP to secondary care (which requires accommodation in the secondary care system as well as reform in the primary care system).

General practitioners

According to the Organisation for Economic Cooperation and Development (OECD) (2005), Ireland had 2,750 GPs in 2004 and 2,432 in 2003.[7] Data on GPs per thousand population are available for 13 of the 15 pre-2004 European Union members (the so-called EU15) and are reported in Table 6.1. They show Ireland, at 0.6 per thousand, to have among the lowest ratios in Europe. Only the Netherlands and Portugal, at 0.5, were lower. These data may not be perfectly comparable across countries because of varying definitions and applications of the label 'general practitioner'. Data on the ratio of doctors to population for 2003, also found in Table 6.1, showed Ireland, at 2.6 per thousand population, also to be at the low end of this EU distribution, above only the United Kingdom, at 2.2, of 11 reporting states of the EU15. This is an overstatement of the number of Irish doctors because the OECD data for Ireland are sourced from the Medical Council register and include doctors who are no longer practising. The ratio of practising doctors to population should be closer to 2.3 for 2003.[8] These statistics suggest shortages of GPs and of physicians generally in Ireland. The statistics are consistent with frequent reports of problems of unfilled need or demand.

Table 6.1: GPs and practicing physicians		
Density per 1000 population, 2003, EU15		
	GPs	Physicians
Austria	1.4	3.4
Belgium	*2.1*	*3.9*
Denmark	*0.9*	*2.9*
Finland	0.7	2.6
France	1.6	3.4
Greece	NA	NA
Germany	1.0	3.4
Ireland	0.6	2.6
Italy	0.9	4.1
Luxembourg	0.9	2.7
Netherlands	0.5	3.1
Portugal	0.5	3.3
Spain	NA	3.2
Sweden	*0.6*	*3.3*
United Kingdom	0.7	2.2
Average*	1.0	3.2

*Source: OECD Health Data 2005. Italics indicates 2002 data. NA means not available. * Average calculated by authors and may be subject to rounding errors.*

Shortage of GPs

Yet the statistics cited, which show Ireland to have fewer primary care doctors than most European states, may not be as compelling evidence of a GP shortage as other, less statistical information. The *Healthcare Skills Monitoring Report*[9] notes:

> Very little quantitative data are available to provide evidence of shortages in the number of GPs. However, there is a general consensus that a shortage exists. The Irish College of General Practitioners claims that GMS appointments are increasingly difficult to fill (especially in rural and certain deprived urban areas) and that there are insufficient graduates to replace the numbers lost through retirements. A survey carried out by Indecon in 2001 reported that 95.6 per cent of GP practices stated that they found it difficult to recruit. Fees from GMS contracts normally increase in line with social partnership agreements. Private fees, however, have increased above general inflation rates and this could be an indicator of shortages.

To correct the shortage of GPs, three steps need to be taken. Firstly, the number of Irish and other EU students enrolled in Irish medical schools needs to be increased. The authors support the finding of the Fottrell Working Group (Medical Education and Training Working Group) that the limit on the number of Irish and other EU students admitted to Irish medical schools be increased from 305 to 725 annually.[10]

This is more complex than it may appear. Non-EU students pay full fees, and medical schools have come to depend on high numbers of them as a source of revenue. Hence the total number of places in Irish medical schools will have to increase, or the state will have to replace lost revenue due to a rise in the EU proportion of students, or both. The authors advocate doing both.

If this policy is adopted and successfully carried out, it will result in an increase in the number of medical school graduates ready to enter into post-graduate specialist training, following either the general practice stream or a consultancy stream. National attention has been focused on increasing the numbers of consultants. The Hanly Report,[11] to the extent to which it deals with physician supply, focuses exclusively on consultant numbers. This is understandable, because the report was prompted by the

European Working Time Directive, which concerns working hours of hospital-based doctors, but once again, the effect may be, as has been the case so many times, to focus attention on the acute system and leave the needs of general practice and primary care less likely to be attended to.

Secondly, there needs to be an increase in the numbers of training places for the Specialist Training Programmes in General Practice in Ireland.

Thirdly, steps need to be taken to make general practice an attractive career option for young people. This involves working conditions, such as out-of-hours care arrangements, locums, retirement, etc., which the authors will leave for others to discuss.[12] In addition, it involves modernising the organisation of primary care, as described below.

Organisation of primary care

The consensus assessment of the organisation of general practice in Ireland appears to be as follows.

GP practices are often too small and are generally not organised along modern lines. While no surveys are known to have been conducted since 1997, when approximately one-half of practices were single-handed, it is clear that the proportion is still high. Many GPs lack practice nurses, full-time clerical help or regular interaction with other clinicians. Many doctors practise from inadequate physical facilities, often surgeries in their own homes. Most practices are not computerised.

In his 1985 report on the Irish medical care system, Tussing[13] found that the intellectual and geographic isolation of the Irish GP was in need of urgent attention. The situation on the ground has improved considerably since then, but modernisation of the organisation of general practice remains among the most important reforms, and perhaps the single most important reform, needed in the Irish health care system.

GPs are well trained and highly qualified. While there are concerns both about supply and organisation, one does not often hear complaints about skill, training or competence. The service they deliver is well regarded by patients.

Two influential reports

In 2001, two influential reports were published on primary care and general practice in Ireland. In January, the Irish Medical Organisation (IMO)[14] and the Irish College of General Practitioners (ICGP) released a joint report, *A Vision of General Practice – Priorities 2001–2006* (hereafter *Vision*[15]). In November, the Department of Health published *Primary Care – A New Direction,* generally known as the Primary Care Strategy (hereafter *PCS*).[16] The latter was itself an elaboration of sections of the important document *Quality and Fairness: A Health System for You,*[17] generally known by its subtitle of *Health Strategy,* which was the result of a three-year period of study and consultation by a group led by the Department of Health.

While there were important differences between *Vision* and *PCS*, which will be spelled out below, they seem to share similar perspectives regarding what the current strengths and weaknesses of the organisation of Irish primary care and general practice are. Indeed, our own briefer but nonetheless extensive consultations in the preparation of the present report found virtual unanimity in this same assessment.

These two reports will be discussed below. The authors will summarise their main points and will indicate their own appraisals of these important documents.

PCS made the following summary observations about Irish general practice:

> The current system of primary care has many inadequacies which must be addressed. It is fragmented from the user per-spective and is difficult to access out-of-hours. The current system places emphasis on diagnosis and treatment while having limited capacity for health promotion, prevention of ill-ness and rehabilitation. Primary care infrastructure is poorly developed and the services are fragmented, with limited team-work and availability of certain professional groups. Liaison between primary and secondary care is often poor and many services provided in hospitals could be provided more appro-priately in primary care.[18]

General practice fared better, however, than other profes-sionals involved in primary care:

Medical treatment services predominate and availability of other elements, e.g. social services, occupational therapy, physiotherapy, counseling, home help, etc., has been limited. Non-medical services are also provided during limited hours, except on a planned essential needs basis.[19]

There is a scarcity of many key professional groups which results in secondary care having to provide a number of services that are more appropriate to primary care.[20]

PCS criticised the lack of teamwork and regular interaction among GPs and between them and other professionals:

General practitioners and other primary care staff often work in isolation and communication between the different primary care service providers is not optimal. This leads to public services that are poorly integrated and do not comprehensively meet the needs of individuals and communities in an appropriate primary care setting.[21]

The skills and commitment of individual professionals are not employed as effectively as they could be. GPs, for example, can be isolated from many other community services. Communication and work-sharing with other primary care professionals is not always readily facilitated or supported. Primary care infrastructure is poorly developed and the services are fragmented, with limited teamwork and availability of certain professional groups.[22]

The IMO/ICGP's *Vision* differs in important respects.[23] For obvious reasons, the authors of this document are not as harshly critical of general practice as are the authors of *PCS*. In fact, *Vision* spends almost no time setting out problems and concerns. Instead, the document concentrates on reforms and recommendations, and lets them speak for themselves. But a critique of general practice, similar to that of *PCS* and of the consensus described above, is consistent with the recommendations.

Vision calls for incentives for 'accelerated development of group practices offering more services'; computerisation; GP infrastructure, staffing and equipment; programmes for prevention, chronic care, shared care, disease surveillance, electronic communication and consultation; and a somewhat different approach to teamwork at the primary care level to that of *PCS* (as will be discussed below).[24]

Though private patients of GPs are not a responsibility of the Department of Health or the Health Service Executive (HSE), *Vision* makes clear that their recommendations for incentives and planning pertain to modernisation of the entire practices of GPs, and to preventative care for the total population. They call for 'more spending on GP infrastructure, staffing, and equipment...to control the demand for hospital services, [and] incentives for programmes for prevention, chronic care, shared care, disease surveillance, electronic communication and consultation.'[25]

There are two important differences between the reform plans outlined in *PCS* and *Vision*. Firstly, *Vision* calls for universal patient registration (UPR) with a GP (not a team), while *PCS* is satisfied to urge *voluntary* registration with primary care teams. Secondly, *PCS* proposes a larger (in size) and more extensive (in terms of disciplines represented) team than *Vision* does.

Universal vs. voluntary registration

PCS states that 'practice registers are an essential component of high-quality primary care', particularly in relation to comprehensive call and recall required for screening and immunisation. Individuals are encouraged to enrol with one primary care team and with one particular GP within the team.[26]

Vision advocates UPR, defined as 'the process by which every person in the country, at regular intervals or at any other time, would confirm his or her choice of one GP, as the doctor designated to provide comprehensive primary medical care on his or her behalf.' IMO/ICGP make the point that UPR would facilitate preventative care, continuing care for persons with chronic conditions and the identification of people with special needs requiring additional resources.[27]

PCS has patients enroling with a team *and* a GP, and *Vision* has them enroling with a GP. This difference is more apparent than real if each GP is a member of only one team. The real difference between the two reform plans concerns whether registration should be universal or voluntary. The Primary Care Strategy, taken as a whole, is forward looking and progressive, and seems consistent with UPR. It is disappointing that *PCS* seems to have backed away from this important recommendation. It is the authors' view that UPR is important to assure that everyone has a usual source of care, that no one be forgotten or omitted in screening and immunisation and that primary care teams can truly co-operate on the same sets of patients.

Size and membership of the team

As noted, both *Vision* and *PCS* envision a future in which GPs and other clinicians form a team. The real and important common ground between the two documents is important. What is a team? *Vision* puts the definition succinctly but articulately: 'Real teamwork requires that team members serve a common patient list, use common patient records, and meet regularly to coordinate care.'[28] This definition is harmonious with the *PCS* view as well: members of the team are 'located at the same site or in very close proximity'.[29]

But there are differences. In the *PCS* view, members of the primary care team will include GPs, practice nurses, public health nurses, nurse midwives, health care assistants, home helps, physiotherapists, social workers and administrative personnel. A typical primary care team consists of 20–22 professional and non-professional employees, including four GPs, serving about 3,000 patients. A wider primary care network of other primary care professionals, such as speech and language therapists, community pharmacists, dieticians, community welfare officers, dentists, chiropodists and psychologists, will also provide services for the enroled population of each primary care team.[30] This scheme may be too ambitious for some areas, particularly for attainment in a single step. It may be preferable to allow flexibility, permitting local variability in the scope of primary care teams.

The reader of *PCS* comes away with an appreciation for the breadth and imagination represented in the document, but also with a deep uncertainty about how primary care teams would function on the ground on a daily basis.

Vision advocates a team of smaller scope, a 'core team' consisting of GPs, practice nurses, public health nurses and possibly a community pharmacist. *Vision* cautions the reader not to confuse community care with primary care. They rightly note that 'many secondary care specialists (doctors, nurses, and other health professionals) are now community based. Access to community care should always follow initial contact with a specialist irrespective of where the specialists are based. The concept that all community-based health professionals constitute a "primary care team" is unrealistic in terms of effective team working.'[31]

Many authorities with whom we spoke in 2005 expressed admiration and support for the general goals of these documents, without being specific about the size and scope of the teams. In a future world of team-based primary care, it is highly likely that some can be extensive and complex, as described in *PCS,* while others can be simpler and more clear-cut, as set forth in the IMO/ICGP's *Vision.*

Pilot projects

In October 2002, the Department of Health designated and provided some funding to 10 pilot primary care teams, located in various parts of Ireland. According to the Department, each site is unique with respect to circumstances and location and also regarding the structure of the primary care team.

Press accounts and reports from people interviewed by the authors strongly suggest that there is considerable variety, too, in the success of the 10 experiments. Dr Muiris Houston, writing in *The Irish Times* in July 2005, wrote that seven of the 10 pilot projects were 'dead in the water'.[32]

The Department published a 'progress report' in June 2004, which listed the 10 pilot projects and gave some information about each one. The information supplied is discouragingly meagre. It may be too early to have conducted evaluations, but the progress report does not provide basic data for each site, such as how many GPs are involved or which other professionals are members of teams.

The authors queried the Department of Health about the

pilots. In response, the Department stated, in part, 'A formal evaluation of the Primary Care Implementation Projects has not been undertaken. The HSE has confirmed that as it draws up its plans to further roll out the Strategy, it will be arranging a review of the Primary Care Implementation Projects so that learning from them can be applied during the process.'[33]

The meaning of this appears to be that, remarkably, no evaluation was built into the planning and funding of the pilots, and no evaluation is currently planned.

In the summer of 2005, the authors visited two of the pilot projects and also two other primary care practices which were not included among the 10 funded and designated pilots but which nonetheless had a number of the desired characteristics. They came away impressed with what they saw and with the enthusiasm and optimism of GPs and others in these practices, though of course they conducted no evaluations. The primary care practices had worked out varying solutions to the problems of leadership, co-ordination, public sector/private sector integration and physical settings.

Is the Primary Care Strategy dead?

In their 2005 consultations with people involved in the Irish health care system, the authors encountered two views so frequently articulated as to constitute consensus and perhaps approximate unanimity. One was that the objectives of the Primary Care Strategy were the right objectives for Ireland, meaning that modernisation of primary care was a very high priority, and that the desired modernisation was along the lines of the model set forth in *PCS*. The view that modernisation of primary care had the highest priority came even from those with responsibilities in the acute system. The other commonly expressed view was that 'the Primary Care Strategy is dead'. Our interviewees certainly did not view these two observations as inherently conflicting.

The government, after issuing the widely respected Primary Care Strategy, effectively abandoned it. They did not follow up the pilot projects, many of them seemingly successful, with evaluations or with a programme to disseminate findings, lessons, caveats and pitfalls. Nor did they create legislation or vote funds to bring into being the modern, multi-clinician, preventative, care-orientated practices and teams envisioned in their document. If the Primary Care Strategy died, its death was attributable to lack of sustenance.[34] In 2005 the government seemed to be moving in a direction not contemplated in the Primary Care Strategy and possibly antithetical to it: the for-profit chain-store entrepreneurial model of GP practices.

Yet while the Primary Care Strategy seemed to have been abandoned by the government which issued it, it had been embraced by much of its audience. As a description of the need for reform, the goals of reform and the road-map to reform, the Primary Care Strategy was powerfully persuasive. While the Primary Care Strategy might be dead as a policy, it still lives as a *strategy*.

The authors certainly do not accept every detail of the Primary Care Strategy – recall that the prescient IMO/ICGP *Vision* in many respects is more far sighted and at the same time more practical – but they, too, affirm that modernisation of primary care is among the most urgent tasks for reform of the Irish health care system, and that the Primary Care Strategy remains the right approach for this reform.

The Primary Care Strategy, and the vision that lies behind it, are not dead. They are, however, in trouble and need help.

The impediments to implementing the Primary Care Strategy

To revive the Primary Care Strategy, three things are needed: a large infusion of public and private money, a new and credible plan to replace the *PCS* document and many more GPs and other clinicians.

Money

The estimate of costs contained in the *PCS* document was as follows.[35]

> At current prices, the capital cost of developing the facility required for the range of services planned is of the order of £2

million (€2.5m) per facility. Taking an initial 40 to 60 implementation projects, and allowing for the fact that the selection
of locations will be guided by the availability of good infrastructure where it exists, it can be expected that a capital outlay
of approximately £100 million (€127m) will be required
during the initial five-year implementation phase. In the longer
term, on the assumption that between 400 and 600 core
primary care teams will be required for two-thirds implementation in 2011, the capital investment would be in the order of
£1,000 million (€1,270m) at current prices. The National
Development Plan may provide some of this investment...At
the end of ten years, the staffing costs of implementation will
entail an approximate overall investment of £484 million
(€615m) per annum.

Because construction and other costs have risen since 2001,
this estimate is likely to be on the low side today. (There is a discussion of how this estimate might be updated in Appendix 5.2.)
While the *PCS* document includes some cost estimates, the
government that issued and backed it never provided adequately
for it in its budgeting. Funding sufficient for the ambitious
strategy has never been forthcoming, which is the single most
important reason for widespread pessimism regarding its viability.
The amounts provided in 2005 are desultory by comparison. In
the end-2004 progress report on the Health Strategy, the
Department of Health reports that 'additional revenue funding of
€7m per annum and once off capital funding of €2.75m plus
€1.8m for IT support have been provided to support the implementation of the primary care strategy.'[36] When one compares
these amounts to the hundreds of millions of euro cited in the
original report as needed, one can understand why some
observers believe that the government has abandoned its Primary
Care Strategy and why others believe the strategy to be dead.

It is encouraging, however, that the Health Estimates for 2006
provided an added €16 million for primary care service development, at least €10 million of which permits the HSE to employ
an additional 300 health professionals, including social workers,
physiotherapists and occupational therapists, as front-line staff
for new primary care teams.[37] Perhaps the Department wants to

convince sceptics that the Strategy is still viable. The amounts are small, however.

The fact that in 2005 the Irish government went forward with a substantial programme of costly tax incentives for construction of private hospitals on public hospital campuses, as discussed above in Chapter 3 and costed in Appendix 2, while the Primary Care Strategy was starved of needed resources, clearly shows that the government, whatever may have been its public statements or intentions, still sees the acute hospital sector as the part of health care most needing and deserving support. As Professor Perry has argued, in Ireland 'primary care is seen as a supportive or ancillary service to the hospital service.'[38]

Like Professor Perry, the authors do not share this bias. Having reviewed the thoroughly flawed Irish health care system and having considered the claims and merits of its many components, the authors advocate sufficient funding for investment in the infrastructure of primary care to put it back on the track once contemplated in the Primary Care Strategy. In some parts of the country, health boards have accommodated primary care services – GPs, public health nurses, support staff, therapists and social workers – in modern, purpose-built buildings. There has been a notable programme of development in the North-West, which pre-dated the publication of the Primary Care Strategy, and has continued since. Notwithstanding the government's apparent reluctance to fund the Primary Care Strategy, two primary care centres in the North-West were allocated substantial investment funds in the 2005 capital allocations. It is apparent that a national capital programme to house primary care teams could be funded over a 10-year period without undue burden on the Exchequer. We develop these costings further in Appendix 5.

Credible plan

When it was published in 2001, the *PCS* contained no plan or provision for funding. As is made clear in this chapter, the *PCS*, while brilliant in concept, is substantively flawed in several respects. Furthermore, in the intervening years, the *PCS* has lost credibility. What is needed is a new plan which deals with the first two of these issues, and by so doing addresses the third.

As the new plan can build on the *PCS* (and on the IMO/ICGP's *Vision*), it can be developed in months, not years. One possibility is to follow the leadership of the Primary Care Steering Group, which has had the responsibility of advising and monitoring the progress of the *PCS*, but which cannot have had much to do.

The plan should include a long-term programme of funding but should begin promptly – immediately, if possible – because a new plan which promises to provide indefinite resources in an indefinite future will not be and should not be believed.

It should provide for universal patient registration, investment in a modern primary care infrastructure and collaboration of clinicians within and across disciplines.

The new plan needs to address and solve, as the *PCS* did not, how to meld private and public sectors together in modern, one-stop, multi-disciplinary primary care centres. This is an extraordinarily important and yet extraordinarily difficult objective. Private practitioners (GPs) must work in partnership with public sector personnel, e.g. public health nurses. Both must treat public and private patients in the same manner. The plan can draw on the experience of successful pilot projects under the Primary Care Strategy and on the experience in the North-West.

The plan should be flexible so that local primary care groups are enabled to develop and design primary care teams on the basis of their own local strengths, needs and imaginations. Local groups would submit proposals and awards would be based on a combination of value for money, practicality and vision. Funding awarded on a competitive basis could be based on the novelty or originality of a local plan, readiness for integration into primary care teams, GPs' and other providers' own investments and need.

The award process must be flexible enough to provide for operating subsidies, or perhaps even a salaried GP service, in low-income, under-served areas which may not be sufficiently profitable to warrant the levels of private investment required to bring primary care centres and primary care teams into being.

Public or private ownership

The authors do not want to prejudge the structures – architectural, leadership or ownership – which might arise either in a new primary care plan or in local initiatives flowing from it, but two observations seem appropriate.

Firstly, elsewhere in this report (see Chapter 3) the authors have set out in detail their concerns about the government's programme of tax incentives for the construction of private hospitals on the campuses of existing public hospitals. But as readers may have noted in relation to the Primary Care Strategy, the authors have advocated expenditures on primary care infrastructure for centres which will be privately owned. The difference is that the GP service in Ireland is already in the private sector. GPs are essentially self-employed operators of small, local businesses. What is proposed now is not a merger, but rather an integration with the public sector. There should be a public contribution because primary care teams are partly public and in any case serve the public interest. There should be a private contribution because a large fraction of the gains will be privately appropriated as net revenues for GPs. In the North-West the health board initially required little contribution from GPs to their enviable accommodation. Currently, in recognition that half their business is private (in the North-West, 44 per cent of the population are covered by Medical Cards), GPs in that region are required to make a once-off payment of some €60,000 for a license agreement covering a defined time of residence in the health board/now HSE-provided premises.

Secondly, the for-profit chain-store entrepreneurial model of GP practices, often presented as a collaboration with pharmacists, is not appropriate for primary care teams. Far from providing a common ground for public and private sectors to meet, they move in the wrong direction and push the for-profit entrepreneurial model further than has heretofore been seen in primary care in Ireland. While the government has appeared to have abandoned its Primary Care Strategy, it has given its blessings to developments like the one opened by the Minister for Health in October 2005, developed by the Touchstone company in Mulhuddart, Dublin. This centre lacks the multi-disciplinary approach, the public-private co-operation and the modern infrastructure of the Primary Care Strategy. Instead, GPs are set in a retail shopping environment with a Touchstone pharmacist. Forty-four such projects, involving just over 250 GPs, are currently reported to be at development stage.[39]

Such centres go in the opposite direction from the Primary Care Strategy. It is improper for the government, having issued, stood behind and campaigned on the Primary Care Strategy, to betray it with a wholly different kind of development, one which has had the benefit of no discussion document or public debate. For GPs in such developments, there is a risk of conflict of interest or perceived conflict of interest since the viability of the overall development may depend on the viability of the pharmacy, which in turn will be greatly affected by their prescribing practices.

Conclusion

Primary care is the foundation and centre of the health care system, yet it has languished, typically forgotten when the state considers reforms and resources for the system. Any person residing in Ireland is eligible to be a public patient in the acute hospital system, but fewer than one-third of the population are eligible to be public patients in the primary care system. The present government has systematically reduced that proportion during its time in office. The hospital system has been modernised, but the primary care system retains a form and structure appropriate to many decades past. The exception to this neglect is the Primary Care Strategy, but the government has failed adequately to fund the document so widely hailed as far seeing and innovative. The government offers generous assistance for private hospitals to be built on the campuses of public hospitals, but not for modern primary care centres.

Addressing the 2001 conference of the Adelaide Society, Tussing distinguished between reforms that were due and those that were overdue: 'What reforms does the Irish health care system need? It seems to me that required reforms fall into two groups. Ireland needs to catch up. And Ireland needs to move ahead…The agenda, in short, calls for 20th century reforms and 21st century reforms.'

That distinction applied to primary care reforms:

> I can see several arguments in favour of a free GP service. But…there is a higher priority for modernising the GP service…Right now, if there is additional money for the General Practitioner service, it is better spent on development of a universal patient register; public investment in new technology, especially in telecommunications; incentives and seed money for group practice; the development of modern primary health care centers; and organization of community care teams of GPs, practice nurses, and public health nurses.
>
> A free GP service, with doctors paid in the same manner for all patients, remains nonetheless a high priority in the development of the Irish health services. Modernizing the GP service is a 20th century issue. A free GP service belongs, perhaps, on the 21st century list.

Needed reforms in primary care fall into four groups: access, manpower, universal registration and modernisation.

- Medical Card eligibility on the basis of need should be restored immediately to the traditional proportion of the population, which is in the range of 35 to 38 per cent. After that change, Medical Card guidelines should be indexed to the median income of production workers or the median earnings of Irish workers, so that they change continuously rather than intermittently, and so that the level is set automatically rather than politically.
- A new form of eligibility should be created for those low-income people who are not eligible for Medical Cards but whose incomes place them in the bottom half of the Irish income distribution. The rise in medical costs associated with a rise in income that makes people or families ineligible for Medical Cards is enormous; a form of eligibility which buffers the shock of this difference, perhaps through a demi-Medical Card which provides half-benefits, is needed now.
- These two should be seen as steps toward the building of a primary care system free to all at the point of use by 2010.

- Ireland needs to take steps to increase significantly the numbers of GPs. The authors support the government's acceptance of the recommendations of the Fottrell Working Group to increase the numbers of Irish and other EU places in Irish medical schools. In addition, the authors support the announced allocations of resources to increase the numbers of places in post-graduate GP training programmes.
- There should be legislation requiring universal patient registration as an immediate step toward modern care and public-private integration.
- The government should act immediately to revive the Primary Care Strategy to modernise the organisation, technology and architecture of primary care by developing a new plan, and funding it liberally. The plan must include commitment of adequate resources over a long period of time, beginning immediately. The plan should achieve multi-disciplinary, public-private primary care teams in technologically modern primary care centres, built with state support.

These changes are at the heart of any serious plan to reform the Irish health care system. They will not only reform it, they will transform it.

7

HOSPITALS: CAPACITY AND ACCESS

Introduction

Acute hospitals are the most visible arm of the health service. No matter how great the deficiencies in primary care or care of the elderly, or how serious the financial barriers to accessing care for many citizens, the problems of acute hospitals tend to be viewed as more urgent simply because they are so visible. Yet many of the problems of acute hospitals are a consequence of deficiencies in other services, so their remedy lies outside the acute sector itself.

Nonetheless, in 2004, the problems of the Irish health service came to be regarded as synonymous with the problems of the acute hospitals, and more specifically with the problems of over-crowded accident and emergency (A&E) departments. It became apparent that any citizen, poor or rich, insured or uninsured, might find themselves, when sufficiently ill to be in need of hospital admittance, spending many days and nights on a trolley in squalid and dangerous conditions. Hospital staff – the Irish Nurses Organisation and emergency consultants – and patients' organisations have campaigned for a political solution to this unacceptable state of affairs. The Minister for Health announced a 10-point plan to address the problem in November 2004. Yet the new chief executive of the Health Service Executive (HSE), Brendan Drumm, said in September 2005 that it would take two years to solve.

It is now generally understood that overcrowding in A&E reflects inadequate bed capacity in the hospitals' wards to admit patients, and that that in turn is exacerbated by inadequate capacity in institutions for long-stay patients who no longer need acute care and by inadequate supports in the community for patients who should otherwise return home. The problems of A&E have also focused policy-makers' attention on the considerable potential for reform in hospitals' internal organisation, i.e. in how they use beds, admit patients and deploy staff. The A&E crisis is therefore the tip of the iceberg of a health and social care system which is in general crisis.

Thus, any response designed to address the A&E crisis must address the problems of the health and social care system as a whole if it is to be successful in the long term.

Irish public hospitals face problems of capacity – beds, theatres, even office space – but they also operate in an extraordinary environment of institutionalised discrimination between patients. While the A&E crisis can affect any citizen and is therefore politically perceived as the most urgent problem, it remains the case that the insured and the uninsured have quite different experiences of access to hospitals for outpatient and elective care. The two-tier system of access to public hospitals – institutionalised by means of the hospital consultants' contract of employment and the system of private bed designation – remains a socially divisive anachronism, which has no place in a civilised state.

There is a considerable modernising agenda ahead for Irish hospitals – not only in their physical infrastructure, but also in how they are managed and how their staff interact. Today, Irish hospitals are unlicensed and have no compulsory system of accreditation. Their medical staff are not obliged to undergo competence assurance or peer review. Their most senior clinicians are effectively not obliged to co-operate with hospital managers. Much of day-to-day medical care is in the hands of quite junior doctors without adequate training or supervision by fully trained doctors. Many hospitals are too small to offer comprehensive care.

Hospital reform will require the introduction of proper systems of licensing and accreditation, of competence assurance and peer review and the introduction of a new consultants' contract to provide a consultant-delivered service, in which consultants work in teams, rostered around the clock in the specialties where this is required.

Other members of staff, e.g. radiotherapists, pharmacists and social workers, must also work more flexible hours to ensure that hospitals work to their full capacity, that patients are not admitted or retained in hospital unnecessarily while tests or medications are awaited or their personal circumstances are assessed. Team-working is increasingly required in hospitals to meet patients' needs to access multiple services. This will require flexibility and adaptability, in what has been a hierarchically organised system. The problems of A&E are exacerbated by under-developed internal hospital management systems. Many hospitals do not appear to operate discharge planning for patients. Many patients are directed to and through A&E who could be more appropriately and efficiently assessed elsewhere.

Despite the disbanding of the Hanly taskforce on medical staffing, the agenda for the reorganisation of hospital networks which was advanced in its report is proceeding in many parts of the state. If the plan is fully implemented, many hospitals will have to change the range of services they offer: smaller hospitals may in effect become dedicated elective and day care facilities, while larger hospitals may intensify their acute care.

This considerable agenda for change reinforces the need for transparency in the new system of health administration and for openness and dialogue between all the stakeholders. It is the authors' impression that among hospital managers and employees of every profession and grade there is an understanding of the need to do things differently, if not always total agreement about which changes should come, or come first. However, many health sector workers – in hospitals, primary care and administration – are suspicious and battered after years in which they have worked without adequate resources in an unreformed system, and in which diverse groups have felt blamed for circumstances and events which were outside their control. This suspicion has deepened because of the prevalent belief that the Health Strategy, launched in 2001 with considerable fanfare and after a long consultative process, has been effectively consigned to the shelf. Hospital managers and staff have seen very little evidence that the government has expanded or will expand hospital capacity in the manner in which it promised in 2001 and in the 2002 Programme for Government. Political and administrative leadership is now required to reform how Irish hospitals operate, and that requires a restatement of commitment to delivering the expansion promised in the Health Strategy, or an explanation at the highest level of government of why the strategy has been abandoned and what will substitute for it. As we have already discussed, the policy[1] of developing private hospitals on public hospital grounds, although presented as an alternative route to delivering public capacity, could have seriously damaging effects on public health services. It will increase private beds at the taxpayers' expense. It could further disadvantage public patients, channel private patients into institutions which offer inferior care and undermine the staffing and management of public hospitals. Despite assertions to the contrary, it could deepen the two-tier nature of Irish hospital care. It is no substitute for a properly resourced and managed public and/or voluntary, not-for-profit hospital system.

This chapter will examine the challenges for the acute hospital sector under three headings:

• acute hospital capacity;
• hospital-acquired infections;
• discrimination against public patients in public hospitals.

Subsequent chapters will discuss the A&E crisis and the relationship between acute, extended and community care; specialist care in hospitals; and acute hospital organisation, location and management.

Ownership

Firstly, we define hospitals in terms of their ownership and activity. In Ireland, hospitals have three different forms of ownership: public, voluntary and private.

Public hospitals were formerly owned by the health boards and have now passed into the ownership of the HSE. The majority of regional, county, district and community hospitals are public. The state owns and manages these hospitals.

Voluntary hospitals were typically established by charities, churches or religious orders. The majority of the acute hospitals in the East of Ireland are voluntary hospitals.[2] The state now almost entirely funds voluntary hospitals, which are run on a not-for-profit basis.

Private hospitals are owned by individuals or companies and are run on a for-profit basis.

Activity

Hospitals can also be distinguished by the type of treatment they offer.

Acute hospitals treat acutely ill patients, as well as performing less urgent elective procedures. They offer both surgical and medical, i.e. non-surgical, care. Patients may attend such hospitals for day treatment or for inpatient care (which requires one or more nights' stay). Patients may also attend such hospitals as outpatients. Acute hospitals typically have A&E departments, from which patients may be admitted or where they may be treated as outpatients.

Elective hospitals offer only elective treatments. Private hospitals are usually in this category. There are also some elective hospitals in the public hospital network. They are staffed from neighbouring public acute hospitals and their beds are counted in the national count of public acute care beds.

District or community hospitals offer non-acute care, which may be intermediate or rehabilitative for people who will return home, or may be long-stay or extended for people who cannot live independently. They may offer minor medical or surgical treatments and may be staffed on a part-time basis by local general practitioners (GPs) or consultants.

Geriatric hospitals, which are both public and voluntary, offer extended care for older people. In the private sector, this care is offered by private nursing homes.

In addition, there are specialist hospitals like paediatric (children's) hospitals, maternity hospitals, psychiatric hospitals, orthopaedic hospitals and cancer hospitals. Although not all of these have A&E departments, all but the psychiatric hospitals are officially classified as acute hospitals in Ireland.

Acute hospital capacity

Number of acute hospitals

The Department of Health listed 59 publicly funded acute hospitals (including voluntary hospitals) which had a total of 12,571 inpatient beds available for use in August 2005.[3] This broadly defined count included maternity hospitals and specialist hospitals. It also, apparently for historical reasons, listed some hospitals which no longer offer acute care. These included a number of essentially extended care facilities like the National Rehabilitation Hospital in Dún Laoghaire, Peamount in Dublin and St Mary's, Baldoyle. The Department and the National Hospitals Office (NHO) of the HSE have engaged in a process of redefining acute hospitals. The HSE's National Service Plan for 2005 listed 53 hospitals and hospital groups in the NHO's 10 hospital networks, excluding four hospitals which the Department has counted as acute.[4] The official estimates for government spending further reduced the number of NHO hospitals, also excluding Manorhamilton hospital in County Leitrim (although the NHO includes some of its beds in its acute bed count). The remaining 52 NHO hospitals had 12,211 inpatient beds in August 2005.

Acute hospitals with A&E departments range in size from St James's in Dublin with 806 inpatient beds in 2005 to Bantry in County Cork with 76. The busiest A&E is in Tallaght hospital in West Dublin, which had 71,450 new attendances in 2004, and 73,903 attendances in total, almost as many as the three midland hospitals put together. Tallaght's A&E saw over 200 patients a day on average in 2004. In contrast, Bantry had 4,066 new attendances and 5,659 attendances in total, an average of 16 a day.

Relationship between private and public/voluntary hospitals

Private hospitals do not contribute data about their activities and staffing to the Department of Health or HSE. The Independent Hospital Association of Ireland (IHAI) represents the interests of private hospitals under the umbrella of the Irish Business and Employers' Confederation (IBEC). In 2005 it represented 14 hospitals and hospital groups, three of which were private psychiatric hospitals. These hospitals had approximately 2,300 inpatient beds in 2005, of which 570 were psychiatric beds. The hospitals varied widely in size and activity. The activities of the non-psychiatric hospitals ranged from maternity care to generally low-complexity elective surgery. Exceptions were the Blackrock Clinic and Mater Private Hospital, which between them accounted for 40 per cent of national cardiac surgery in 2004, according to the IHAI.

The character of the private hospital sector has been changing with the closure or sale of some smaller religious-owned hospitals and the opening of more high-tech hospitals like the Galway Clinic and the Beacon Clinic in Sandyford, Dublin, which has invested heavily in diagnostic equipment. There is opportunity for considerable profit in the Irish private hospital sector. The Sisters of Mercy sold the Mater Private Hospital to a management group in 2000. Five years later, the original six investors realised a gain of €44 million by borrowing on the strength of the hospital's substantial profitability. The hospital's staff have shares in the hospital and also gained from this deal.[5] A study by Goodbody Stockbrokers in 2005 listed two private hospitals in development and plans for a further 11.

Developers of private hospitals have benefited from significant tax relief introduced in 2001, effectively an Exchequer investment (see Appendix 2). In the absence of published data on their operations, it is impossible to assess their contribution to Irish health care or the value which the state is receiving for this investment.

In 2005, 1,947 consultants worked in public and voluntary hospitals, of whom 650 were also entitled to work in private hospitals. Only an estimated 227 specialists worked exclusively in private hospitals or clinics, many in more than one private hospital. Whereas the public sector employed 4,170 non-consultant hospital doctors (NCHDs), the private sector employed about 70.[6] Private hospitals had approximately 5,000 employees who did not have public contracts, according to the IHAI. Private hospitals were primarily an adjunct to the public hospital sector, where salaried public consultants personally treated private patients for private fees and without the support of junior doctors, while delegating much of their public patient care to the public hospitals' NCHDs. Future private hospital development has been predicated on a continuation of this relationship: 'This unique position, where consultants have been able, for years, to practice private medicine while retaining a fulltime position within the national healthcare service, is highly conducive to the further development of the private health care sector in Ireland.'[7]

Number of acute beds in Irish public hospitals

The number of acute hospital beds in Ireland was dramatically reduced in the late 1980s and early 1990s. Despite population growth, the number of inpatient beds remained virtually unchanged through the 1990s, from 11,809 in 1993 to 11,891 in 2000. Since, as we have seen, this official count includes beds in some extended care hospitals, which are now being weeded from the official count, the actual number of beds offering acute care was lower than official figures suggested.

Using this official count, the ratio of acute beds to 1,000 population, which cutbacks had reduced from 5.13 in 1981 to 3.29 in 1996, because of rising population, had continued to fall to 3.14 by 2000. Despite an increase in the official bed count since 2001, a proportionately greater population increase reduced the ratio to 3.04 beds per 1,000 population in August 2005. If only beds in hospitals in the NHO's networks are counted, the ratio was 2.96 per 1,000 (see Table 7.1).

A smaller number of acute beds in proportion to population has put progressively greater pressure on the acute hospital system, manifest in waiting lists for elective surgery and in unacceptably long waits on trolleys in A&E departments for patients who have been accepted for admission but for whom no beds are available.

At three beds per 1,000 population in 2005, Ireland has 27 per cent fewer beds than the EU15 average of four, according to the OECD.[8]

In most OECD countries, the number of hospital beds per capita has fallen over recent decades. The number of acute beds is not necessarily an accurate measure of a health system's capacity to provide care. With changing medical technology and growth

Table 7.1: Acute hospital inpatient beds, 1981–2005			
Year	Inpatient beds	Population	Beds per 1,000
1981	17,668	3,443,405	5.13
1986	16,878	3,540,643	4.77
1991	13,806	3,525,719	3.92
1996	11,937	3,626,087	3.29
2000	11,891	3,789,500	3.14
2001	12,036	3,847,200	3.13
2002	12,264	3,917,200	3.13
2003	12,299	3,978,900	3.09
2004	12,375	4,043,800	3.06
2005 Department count	12,571	4,130,700	3.04
2005* NHO hospitals	12,211	4,130,700	2.96

*Final line calculates inpatient beds per 1,000 population in the acute hospitals in the NHO's 10 networks. Source: Department of Health, Integrated Management Returns for bed counts. Up to 2004 the bed count is the average number of beds available in the year. In 2005 the figure is the average number of beds available in August, which is higher than the average for the year to August (12,525). Population data from Central Statistics Office censuses of population and Population and Migration Estimates (CSO April 2005) for latest forecasts.

in day procedures, it is possible to treat many more patients while reducing bed numbers, as Ireland indeed achieved in the 1990s. Canada delivers superior care with 3.3 acute beds per 1,000 population. As with all international comparisons, the ratio of beds to population should be treated with some caution. Within Ireland, bed-to-population ratios vary. Many hospitals which are nominally acute offer less than comprehensive acute care.

In October 2005, the new chief executive of the HSE, Brendan Drumm, was reported as saying: 'By any measure this country is actually over-equipped with acute hospital beds by international comparisons. We have more acute beds than Britain has. Britain has 17 per cent of its population over 65, we have 11 per cent of our population over 65 and 60 per cent of your beds are taken by over 65-year-olds. Quoting to me the need for beds without controlling it for the age of the population is bizarre.'[9] The Minister for Health, Mary Harney, was reported as responding to this statement thus: 'There will be no one happier than me if we don't have to have new beds.'[10]

	Number of acute inpatient beds	Thousands of people aged 65 & over	Beds per 1,000 people over 65	Ranking	Beds per 1,000 population	Ranking
Austria	49,084	1,252	39.2	2	6.1	2
Belgium	41,183	1,754	23.5	6	4	4
Denmark*	18,231	793	23.0	9	3.4	8
Finland	12,119	793	15.3	13	2.3	13
France	234,228	9,680	24.2	5	3.9	6
Germany	547,284	14,252	38.4	3	6.6	1
Ireland	**11,801**	**438**	**26.9**	**4**	**3**	**12**
Italy	224,075	10,778	20.8	10	3.9	5
Luxembourg	2,565	62	41.4	1	5.7	3
Netherlands	51,872	2,210	23.5	7	3.2	9
Portugal	32,255	1,722	18.7	11	3.1	10
Spain	129,523	6,982	18.6	12	3.1	11
United Kingdom	218,962	9,430	23.2	8	3.7	7
Average			25.9		4	

Table 7.2: Acute beds in relation to population and older population, EU15, 2002

*Source: OECD Health Data 2005. Irish bed count lower than domestically due to OECD definition. *Danish data for 2001. Sweden and Greece not available.*

Table 7.2, derived from OECD data for 2002, shows how Ireland's three acute inpatient beds per 1,000 population in that year compared with an EU average of four and a UK ratio of 3.7. When acute bed numbers are related to population aged over 65, as advocated by Brendan Drumm, in 2002 Ireland had 26.9 beds per 1,000 population of 65-year-olds and over, compared to an

EU average of 25.9 and a UK figure of 23.2. (The OECD records that 16 per cent of the UK's population and 11 per cent of the Irish population was 65 years old and over in 2002.) There is considerable variance in this measure across Europe, with Germany's 38.4 beds per 1,000 older people at one end of the spectrum and Finland's 15.3 per 1,000 at the other end.

A number of additional factors need to be taken into consideration in interpreting these data. The UK is engaged in a considerable increase in acute bed capacity as part of a significant expansion of the health service. In 2002, the UK government committed itself to adding 10,000 beds to 135,000 in England – a 7.4 per cent increase.[11] In 2004, the UK Department of Health restated its commitment to expanding the National Health Service (NHS) capacity and forecast that it would exceed the goal set in *The NHS Plan* of 2000 to have 100 new hospitals by 2010. The UK also expects to achieve its goal of ensuring that 40 per cent of NHS facilities are less than 15 years old by 2010.[12] The UK's provision of beds is therefore rapidly increasing and its facilities are being modernised.

Were the comparisons in Table 7.2 to convince the Irish government to take the view that Ireland has sufficient acute beds, this would be to ignore the demands of a rapidly rising population; to fail to take into account the particular demands faced by acute hospitals in Dublin and in the East; and to assume that the hospitals whose beds make up the Irish acute bed count are all truly acute, when many offer less than comprehensive services.

Table 7.3: Effect of population growth and ageing on Ireland's acute bed stock

	Number of acute inpatient beds	Thousands of people aged 65 & over	Beds per 1,000 people over 65	Ranking in EU13	Population	Beds per 1,000 population	Ranking in EU13
Ireland 2005	12,211	460.7	26.5	4	4,130.7	3.0	12
Ireland 2011	12,211	531.1	23.0	8	4,167.7	2.9	12
Ireland 2016	12,211	631.1	19.3	10	4,504.9	2.7	12

Source: Acute inpatient beds assumed to stay at August 2005 count for NHO hospitals. Population assumed to rise and age as forecast by the Central Statistics Office in its 2004 Population and Labour Force Projections 2006–2036.

Table 7.3 forecasts the consequence of failing to increase Ireland's acute bed stock over the next 10 years. If the number of beds did not increase, by 2016 Ireland would have 2.7 beds per 1,000 population and, more significantly, 19.3 per 1,000 people over 65, compared to an EU13 average in 2002 of 25.9.

Table 7.4: Effect of population growth and ageing on Dublin's acute bed stock							
						Beds available for residents of East	
Greater Dublin Area	Number of acute beds in 2005	Thousands of people aged 65 & over	Beds per 1,000 people over 65	Population 1,000s	Beds per 1,000 population	Beds per 1,000 people over 65	Beds per 1,000 population
2005	5,078	158.5	32.0	1,612.5	3.1	25.6	2.52
2006	5,078	162	31.3	1,645.0	3.1	25.1	2.47
2021	5,078	274	18.5	2,063.0	2.5	14.8	1.97

Source: Beds are those in the National Hospitals Office networks 8, 9 and 10 as measured in the Department of Health's IMR figures for August 2005, with the beds in Navan hospital as well since the population forecasts are for the Greater Dublin Area comprising Dublin, Meath, Wicklow and Kildare. Population forecasts are from the CSO's Population and Migration Estimates of April 2005, and Regional Population Projections, published in May 2005. The final two columns compute the effect on ratios of beds to population if 20 per cent of the bed stock is excluded because it is occupied by non-residents of the East.

In 2001, the Eastern Regional Health Authority calculated that although the region had 3.1 beds per 1,000 population, residents of the East in effect had only 2.45 beds per 1,000 people, since 20 per cent of all patients attending hospitals in the East were from outside the region.[13] There has been no subsequent published study of such inflows but there is no evidence to suggest they have reduced. Table 7.4 above forecasts the consequences of failing to increase the acute bed stock of the Greater Dublin Area over the next 15 years. This area comprises counties Dublin, Meath, Kildare and Wicklow and is served by the hospitals of three of the NHO's 10 networks, including the hospitals in Naas in County Kildare and Loughlinstown in County Wicklow. The only hospital in those counties from another NHO network is Navan hospital in County Meath. From comparing the August 2005 acute inpatient bed count for the hospitals in those counties with Central Statistics Office (CSO) regional population forecasts, it emerges that a ratio of 3.1 beds per 1,000 population and 32 beds per 1,000 people over 65 in 2005 would fall to ratios of 2.5 and 18.5, respectively, in 2021 were there no increase in bed stock.

These remain inflated ratios because Dublin must also accommodate inflows of patients from the rest of the country. With residents from other regions continuing to occupy some 20 per cent of beds in the East, the ratio of beds to population *resident* in the East in 2005 is 2.52 per 1,000 and would be under half the EU average at 1.97 in 2021. With this adjustment, the ratio of beds to people aged 65 and over residing in the Greater Dublin Area in 2005 is 25.6 per 1,000, already below the EU average, and by 2021 would be 14.8 – lowest in the 2002 EU range.

Chapter 8 will explore the inter-relationship between pressures on hospitals and facilities outside hospitals, in particular continuing and community care. There is considerable scope for reducing pressures on hospitals by increasing facilities and services outside hospitals and by improving hospitals' internal workings. However, it should be noted at this point in the discussion that many of the countries whose acute bed ratios to population compare favourably to Ireland's (and will compare much more favourably if there is not a rapid expansion in Irish bed stock) already have well-developed community, continuing and primary care sectors. The UK government's expansion of acute capacity is being accompanied by investment in primary care. There is objective evidence that Ireland's acute bed capacity is already inadequate to need, and will rapidly become more so with growth and ageing of the population. Addressing deficiencies in other sectors will ease pressures on the acute sector, but will not remove the need to expand acute capacity too.

Health Strategy commitment to increased bed numbers

In 2001 the government's Health Strategy *Quality and Fairness* identified a need for 3,000 extra beds in acute hospitals, which, the government promised, 'will be added to the system' over the

10-year period to 2011, with 650 'in place by the end of 2002'. That would be a 25 per cent increase, the 'largest ever concentrated expansion of acute hospital capacity in Ireland'.[14]

The strategy's target was based on a study of hospital bed requirements, largely the work of a clinical epidemiologist, Dr Mary Codd. The Codd study reported that in 2000, 23 hospitals had occupancy levels above the internationally accepted measure of full occupancy of 85 per cent. Their occupancy ranged from 85 to 123 per cent, presumably reflecting patients sleeping on trolleys.[15]

This study estimated that to reduce occupancy levels, treat waiting list patients and cope with increased demand for health care and with the effects of rising population, an additional 4,335 inpatient beds were needed. It suggested this could be reduced to 2,840 additional acute inpatient beds and 190 additional acute day beds, provided a number of measures were taken to lessen demands on the acute hospital system. These included greater use of day procedures, ensuring that private patients did not exceed the 20 per cent of beds allocated to them (see discussion of bed designation below) and providing care elsewhere for those elderly and convalescent patients who were remaining too long in acute hospitals because they had nowhere else to go.

The 2001 Health Strategy contained a commitment to significant sustained investment in care places for the elderly. The commitment to fund nearly 7,000 extra intermediate and extended care beds and 7,600 day hospital and day centre places for the elderly exceeded the commitment to expand acute bed capacity, and is discussed further in Chapter 8.[16]

Underlying the Department's forecasts of future bed needs was the expectation that population would continue to rise and age. In 2000, people over 65 years of age constituted 11 per cent of the population and 27 per cent of hospital patients, and accounted for 46 per cent of hospital bed days. However, by 2026 the proportion of the population aged 65 or over was expected to rise to over 16 per cent – the current UK proportion. The latest CSO forecasts continue to anticipate this proportionate ageing of population in 20 years' time (see Table 7.5, final column).

The Codd study based its expectations of population growth and ageing on CSO forecasts from 1999, which on their highest assumptions predicted a population of 4,050,000 in 2006 and 4,254,700 in 2011.[17] Population growth rapidly exceeded the CSO's expectations. At the time of writing in January 2006, the most recent CSO forecasts on maximum immigration and fertility assumptions predicted a population of 4,168,000 in 2006 and 4,505,000 in 2011 – increases of 116,000 and 250,000, respectively, over the 1999 forecasts (see Table 7.5).

Table 7.5: How population forecasts now exceed 2001 Health Strategy's expectations

Year	Strategy assumptions		Latest CSO forecast		Difference between forecasts		65+ as % of population
	Total pop.	65 +	Total pop.	65 +	Total pop.	65 +	%
2001	3,836,400	427,700	3,847,200	429,800	10,800	2,100	11
2006	4,052,000	452,400	4,167,700	465,600	115,700	13,200	11
2011	4,254,700	503,900	4,504,900	531,100	250,200	27,200	12
2016	4,422,600	584,500	4,854,200	631,100	431,600	46,600	13
2026	4,671,900	767,300	5,398,900	866,200	727,000	98,900	16

Source: Population and Labour Force Projections, 2001–2031 (Central Statistics Office, 2001), for 2001 Strategy expectations; and Population and Labour Force Projections, 2006–2036 (Central Statistics Office, 2004) and Population and Migration Estimates (CSO, April 2005) for latest forecasts.

Whereas Codd's analysis was predicated on there being 504,000 people 65 years old or over living in Ireland in 2011, the CSO currently forecasts that in 2011 Ireland could have a population of 531,000 aged 65 and over – 27,000, or 5 per cent, more. Looking a mere 15 years further ahead, the revised population forecasts predict a potential population of 866,200 people aged 65 and over in 2026, nearly 99,000, or 13 per cent, more than anticipated in the 1999 CSO forecast which underpinned the Health Strategy.

Ireland's recent rapid population growth is highly influenced by immigration rates, which could be responsive to changes in immigration law or economic circumstances. However, the Health Strategy's targets for health service investment and capacity building were predicated on much lower population growth. They emerge, therefore, as minimum requirements to meet the health care needs of the population. On current population growth forecasts, if Ireland wished to have the latest recorded EU average of 25.9 acute beds per 1,000 population aged 65 and over in 2016, this would require adding 4,134 acute inpatient beds over the next 11 years – a 34 per cent increase on the present NHO bed stock. To bring beds for older residents of the Greater Dublin Area to the same EU average in 2021, assuming an unchanged level of inflows of patients from outside the region, would require 3,790 additional acute inpatient beds in the region in 16 years' time – a 75 per cent increase on the NHO stock of beds in the region. The long lead times in building new hospitals suggest that the government should be actively planning this expansion now. If regional hospitals were to develop into the centres of excellence envisaged in the Hanly Report (see Chapter 10), inflows of patients from outside the region should decrease and the number of beds required in Dublin would be lower. In that event, more beds would be required outside the East.

Progress on achieving the Strategy targets for increased bed numbers

It has been stated earlier in this study that analysis and policy debate about Irish health care is hampered by the paucity of up-to-date, published, verifiable data on many aspects of the services. This has been particularly true in the case of bed numbers.

It should be a simple matter for the government to publish a clear, consistent series of numbers of beds in acute hospitals. However, this has not been the case. At the time of writing, the latest bed numbers published in the Department of Health's *Health Statistics* series on its website dated from 2002. Enquiries to the Department from the authors elicited bed numbers up to 2005. However, this bed count included an apparent very steep increase in day beds, which it emerges largely reflected an exercise in redefinition rather than an increase in facilities to treat patients, an issue we expand on below.

The authors appreciate that the Department of Health supplied more up-to-date statistical information on our request. However, had it not been for documents released under Freedom of Information (FOI) we would not have reached a full under-standing of the evolution of bed numbers over the last four years since the publication of the Health Strategy.

The 2001 Health Strategy's targets for acute care beds stated:

> Additional acute hospital beds will be provided for public patients. Over the next ten years a total of 3,000 acute beds will be added to the system...650 of the extra beds will be provided by the end of 2002, of which 450 will be in the public sector, thus providing extra capacity for the treatment of public patients on waiting lists. The private hospital sector will be contracted to provide 200 beds, all for treatment of public patients on waiting lists.[18]

The strategy did not state whether these additional beds would be inpatient or day beds, but it made plain, and the Department of Health has since confirmed, that these targets were based on the Codd study with its recommendation that 2,840 additional inpatient beds and 190 additional day beds would be required by 2011. Documents released by the Department under FOI reveal that a few months before publication, the Department proposed to include extracts from an executive summary of the Codd report as an appendix to the Health Strategy.

The proposed appendix restated the Codd report's conclusion that a minimum of '2,800 inpatient beds (plus an additional 200 day beds)' would be required to 2011. It further stated that there was an immediate need that the 'public hospital acute bed stock of 11,862 (in 2000) be increased by 650 beds over a nine month timeframe'.[19]

How many new beds have been added to the acute bed stock since the publication of the 2001 Health Strategy? The government's claims about its progress in implementing the strategy's targets have been so confusing and so inconsistent with the data that it is difficult not to conclude that the government has been happy to obscure this issue, as Figure 7.1 recounts.

There is only one official bed count. This is derived by the Department of Health from the monthly integrated management returns (IMRs) which come from health boards and hospitals. From these returns, the Department compiles a count of the

Figure 7.1: Acute hospital beds: claim and counter-claim	
2001:November	Health Strategy promises 3,000 more beds, of which 450 should come in 2002. Strategy target based on Acute Hospital Bed Capacity Review recommendation of 2,800 more inpatient beds and 200 more day beds to be provided by 2011.
2002: January	Micheál Martin announces 709 additional beds.
2003: February	Department of Health says 520 of the 709 beds were funded in 2002, not all yet open.
2003: September	Department of Health says 303 additional beds available in July 2003 compared to 2001 but, due to cutbacks, approximately 400 beds closed in September, particularly in Dublin.
2004: 19 October	Taoiseach, Bertie Ahern, tells Dáil 'while there is a longer term plan to have 3,000 beds, 900 are in place'.
2004: 21 October	Department of Health states that since 2001, the number of inpatient beds has increased by 299 and the number of day beds by 284 - an increase in total of 583 beds. Day beds include trolleys, recliners and couches.
2004: 27 October	Taoiseach tells Dáil: '900 beds have been funded...most of those will be in place in the first half of 2005...600 of these beds are now in use and 300 will come on stream in the coming months...they...may not all be beds.'
2004: 28 October	Mary Harney tells Dáil: 'none of the 900 beds is a trolley, couch, armchair or whatever the Deputy is suggesting. They are beds...We do not call a couch a bed.'
2004: November	Following a Freedom of Information request, the Department of Health releases its 'Definition of a Day Bed or Day Place': 'A "bed" or day "place" is a device or arrangement (bed, trolley, reclining chair or couch) that may be used to permit a patient to lie down, recline or recover in the course of an elective day case admission.'
2005: April	HSE National Service Plan 2005 says: 'To date, 709 additional beds have been provided.'
2005: May	Department of Health Progress Report on the 2001 Strategy says: 'Provision has been made for 900 additional inpatient/day beds. 600 had been commissioned up to the end of 2004.'
2005: May	Department of Health official bed count shows an additional 535 inpatient beds and an additional 475 day beds since 2001. But the authors' analysis shows many of these new day beds are in fact pre-existing trolleys, recliners and couches, which have been counted for the first time.

Additional inpatient beds provided in the four years 2001–2005 : 535 inpatient beds – 19 per cent of what the Bed Capacity Review recommended.

Beds still to be provided in the six years 2006–2011 : 2,265 inpatient beds or 377 per annum. This calculation does not take into account the effect of the recent upward revision in population forecasts, or the fact that the Strategy's targets were based on an inflated bed count, including non-acute beds.

average number of beds available for use during the year, taking beds that have been temporarily closed or opened into account. Unless there is an unusual event, like the large numbers of bed closures in Dublin in late 2003 due to cutbacks, the temporary bed closures are understood to follow a similar pattern each year, thus providing a reasonably consistent count. The Codd report used the IMR count of inpatient beds as its measure of bed capacity (see Table 7.1).

The only available measure of the government's progress in meeting the Health Strategy's targets is to examine IMR data for the period since 2001, as in Table 7.6 below. In this table, we have used the August 2005 IMR count as the most recent available, which captures additions to the bed stock in 2005. We also compare the January to August average IMR count for 2005 with the 2004 annual average to give a better measure of the year-on-year increase in beds available.

Table 7.6: Increase in inpatient and day beds, 2001–2005						
Year	Inpatient beds	Increase in inpatient beds	Day beds	Increase in day beds	Total beds	Annual increase
2001	12,036		771		12,807	
2002	12,264	228	812	41	13,076	269
2003	12,299	35	909	97	13,208	132
2004	12,375	76	1,133	224	13,508	300
2005*	12,525	150	1,213	80	13,738	230
2005 August	12,571		1,246		13,817	
2001–August 2005 Increase	535		475			1,010

Source: Department of Health integrated management returns, which are counts of the average number of beds available each year. 2005* is the count of the average beds available from January to August 2005 and comparable with the average counts for other years. The latest count of beds available to the authors was the August 2005 IMR count.

This table measures the change in bed numbers in the Department of Health's count of acute beds, not in the newly defined and fewer NHO acute hospitals. By this measure, the number of inpatient beds has increased by 535, or 4.4 per cent, since the publication of the 2001 Health Strategy. Also by this measure, the number of day beds has increased by 475, or 61.6 per cent, proportionally very much the greater increase. Yet the Bed Capacity Review envisaged day beds contributing only 200, or under 7 per cent, of the promised 3,000 beds.

There is an international trend for treatment to move from inpatient to day procedures. This has been accentuated in Ireland because of the virtual freeze in inpatient bed numbers through the 1990s. Day cases have increased from 8,000, or 2 per cent, of non-outpatient hospital cases in 1980 to 424,000, or 43 per cent, in 2004.[20] Hospitals' more inventive use of facilities to increase throughput of day patients has undoubtedly been a feature of Irish hospital care. The case can validly be made that day beds should contribute proportionally more to additional bed capacity than the Health Strategy envisaged. However, the authors are sceptical that this is the picture that emerges from these figures.

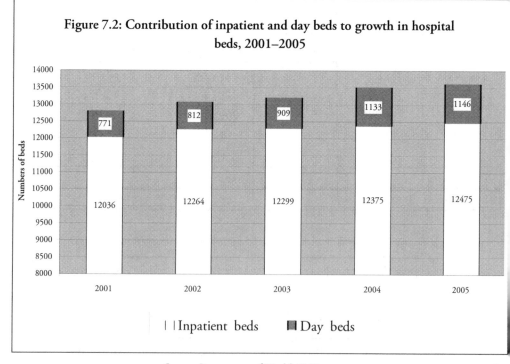

Figure 7.2: Contribution of inpatient and day beds to growth in hospital beds, 2001–2005

Source: Department of Health IMR returns.

Definition and counting of day beds

The fairly arcane issue of how day beds are defined and counted has therefore become relevant to the question of how far the government has progressed in meeting the 2001 strategy's targets. As Figure 7.1 recounts, this has been a disputed issue in the Dáil but was ultimately answered when the Department of Health released (under FOI) its definition of a day bed, which includes trolleys, recliners and couches, indeed anywhere a patient lies down, reclines or recovers 'in the course of an elective day admission'.

Department documents disclose that this definition has been clarified with hospitals in order to attempt to capture the many changing methods by which patients undergo day treatment. After the Department had observed that although its total of designated day beds was 560, the number of day beds emerging each year from the IMR count exceeded this, it undertook a bed count at every acute hospital in February 2003. This disclosed that while there were 626 conventional beds in use for day procedures at that time, there were a further 691 trolleys, recliners and couches on which day procedures were taking place. In total, this census enumerated 1,317 day places, yet the just-concluded IMR count for 2002 had only shown 812 day places.

In an internal review following this 2003 count, an official observed: 'There is no clear definition of a "day bed". Hospitals are using various types of accommodation to provide day case treatments and the Department needs to agree a definition with health agencies to allow consistent counting across the hospital system.'[21]

There followed a substantial year-on-year increase in the IMR count of day beds over the three subsequent years (see Figure 7.3). The authors have attempted to clarify how many of the 'new' day beds emerged because of this process of redefinition and how many are indeed new places. We understand that the Department does not have the information systems to distinguish these components. However, from discussion with hospital bed managers, it appears self-evident that since and indeed prior to the February 2003 bed census, hospitals have been gradually refining their own understanding of their reporting requirements under the IMR – *and this redefinition is the primary reason for the apparent increase in day places.*

Figure 7.3: Additional day places in acute hospitals – growth or redefinition?

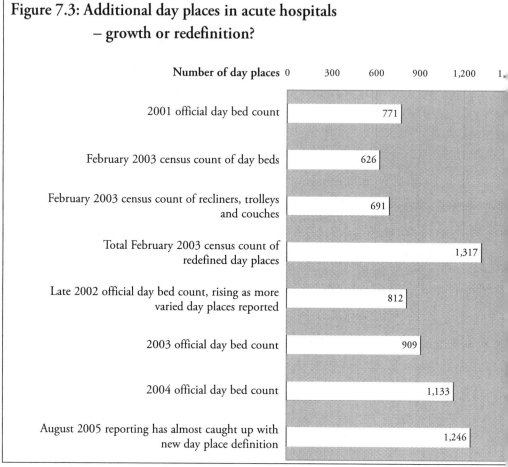

Source: Department of Health IMR returns and February 2003 bed count, released under FOI.

Of course, the authors cannot definitively state how many day places are genuinely new or redefined, but it would appear that a high proportion of the additional day 'beds' reported in the period 2001–2005 come in the latter category. As this discussion reveals, answering the questions of what constitutes a bed, and how many beds there are, is not as simple as it appears. In order to engender clarity in policy discussion, the authors recommend that the collection, collation and timely publication of hospital bed data should become a responsibility of the Health Information and

Quality Authority (HIQA), which is to be established as a key component of the reformed system of health administration (see Chapter 12). HIQA should require the Department of Health and the NHO to report regularly on when and where actual new beds have been funded, commissioned and made available for the treatment of patients. Although the NHO plans to develop its own validated census of acute beds to be published annually, the authors consider that all such data collection and publication should be a HIQA function.

Progress on achieving the 2001 Health Strategy's targets for increased acute beds – a summary

In summary, the number of acute hospital inpatient beds, as measured by the Department of Health, has increased by 535 from 2001 to August 2005, or by 19 per cent of the 2,800 additional inpatient beds recommended in the Bed Capacity Review. An accompanying apparent increase of 475 in the number of acute day beds appears to be largely the consequence of a new system of counting and not a real increase in hospital capacity.

To provide the remaining 2,265 inpatient beds recommended in the Bed Capacity Review in the six years from 2006–2011 would require an additional 377 inpatient beds per annum on average. With the redefinition of some hospitals as non-acute, the number of inpatient beds in the acute hospitals funded by the NHO is at 12,211, just 175 more than the Department counted at the time of the publication of the 2001 Health Strategy.

This failure to meet strategy targets for investment in additional acute hospital capacity is replicated in other sectors, such as care of the elderly and primary care. Yet the 2001 strategy remains government policy. The Programme for Government agreed by the coalition parties states: 'We will implement the National Health Strategy, through a coordinated multi-annual programme of service development. We will expand public hospital beds in line with a programme to increase total capacity by 3,000 during the period of the Strategy.'[22]

If the government and official policy-makers are no longer convinced of the merit of the assessment of capacity needs in the Acute Hospital Bed Capacity Review – if, for instance, they believe that changes in medical practice have further reduced the need for acute beds, or that other of its assumptions or its methodology should be revisited – it is incumbent on the government to initiate a further review as a matter of urgency. The authors have no reason to believe this is the government's view or that it is the case. While the authors recognise an argument for revisiting the Review's analysis to employ another statistical method,[23] which might or might not somewhat reduce its original estimate of the number of acute beds required, in light of the significant upward revision in population growth forecasts since the Review's publication, the authors still expect that a further review would endorse the case for significantly increasing Ireland's acute bed stock.

However, the authors would recommend against merely scattering extra beds across the 52 hospitals in the HSE's networks in response to local political pressures. This major investment should only take place against a backdrop of explicit identification of which hospitals should grow, which should change function and of changes in how hospitals are staffed, managed and financed (issues examined in detail in later chapters).

In our examination of the roles of the HSE and the Department of Health in Chapter 12, we will describe how health policy remains, firstly, the responsibility of the Minister and secondly of her Department. In light of the Strategy's place in the Programme for Government, there is an onus on the Minister to state whether she accepts its assessment of capacity needs; and if she does not do so, to publish her alternative analysis. Her programme for private hospital development is at variance with the expansion of public acute capacity promised in the Health Strategy and unsupported by published official analysis of its consequences.

Hospital-acquired infections

Hospital-acquired infections are a growing problem in Ireland. The evidence is that Ireland has one of the highest rates of MRSA (methicillin-resistant *Staphylococcus aureus*) infection in Europe.[24] This antibiotic-resistant bacterium is not generally a threat to healthy people, but in hospital patients, whose health is compromised, especially patients in intensive care units (ICU), it can cause severe illness or death. While the comparability of available international data is disputed, and while there is as yet no standardised Irish framework for the collection of such data,[25] the available evidence shows highly variable trends in MRSA across Europe, with infection rates in Ireland exceeding those in most other states. The European Antimicrobial Resistance Surveillance System (EARSS) has reported that in 2003, MRSA infection rates in Ireland were only exceeded in four of 28 European states returning data. Rates in Ireland in the years from 2000 to 2003 have been comparable to those in Britain, while rates in the Scandinavian countries are markedly low compared to elsewhere in Europe. In Ireland, the proportion of bloodstream isolates of *Staphylococcus aureus* that have been found to be methicillin resistant has been close to or over 40 per cent, compared to under 10 per cent in eight of the 28 states and 1 per cent or under in Scandinavia.[26]

The EARSS has reported a steady annual rise in many countries, including some countries with hitherto low overall resistance rates. Over the period 2000–2003, a significant increase in the proportions of MRSA was observed in Belgium, Germany, the Netherlands, Portugal and the United Kingdom. In Britain, the EARSS has reported that the 'relentless increase of MRSA proportions among bloodstream infections that occurred between 1992 and 2000 seems to have stabilised.' EARSS data showed no further increase in the UK in the three years from 2001 to 2003.[27] In Ireland, the proportion increased marginally over the first four years of data collection, from 38.8 per cent in 1999 to 42.7 per cent in 2002, but has decreased (again marginally) over the last two years to 41.8 per cent in 2004. These trends are not regarded as statistically significant.[28]

Programmes to control infection have proven effective in other states:

> In a Spanish study, three time periods were studied, i.e., pre-outbreak, during an outbreak of MRSA, and when a control programme was instituted; the authors estimated that the programme prevented 76 per cent of expected MRSA cases and 85 per cent of expected fatalities due to MRSA in the ICU. The

experience in Finland, where two successive MRSA outbreaks in the early 1990s were successfully managed and where there is now no endemic MRSA, suggests that it is possible in the non-endemic situation to control the spread of MRSA and eradicate it.[29]

Measures to control infection

The Minister for Health has launched national guidelines on hygiene and the control of MRSA, with a particular emphasis on hospital cleanliness and hand washing by staff and visitors. The HSE has conducted a hygiene audit of Irish hospitals. There is published evidence that staff hygiene needs to improve. A study of ICU staff by Síle Creedon, a lecturer in nursing at University College, Cork, found that only 51 per cent of hospital staff followed hand-washing guidelines before a hygiene campaign. Hand washing improved by an average of 32 per cent after a six-week hygiene programme, from 51 per cent to 83 per cent. Doctors showed the lowest compliance levels and the smallest improvement, rising from 31 per cent before the campaign to 55 per cent after it. Nurses' compliance increased from 50 per cent to 89 per cent and compliance by other health care staff, such as physiotherapists and care assistants, rose from 66 per cent to 96 per cent.[30]

The national guidelines for the control and prevention of MRSA were produced by an expert Infection Control Sub-committee[31] and published by the Health Protection Surveillance Centre (formerly the National Disease Surveillance Centre and now subsumed into the HSE). While the guidelines emphasised hand hygiene before and after each patient contact, this was only one of many recommendations. The experts made clear that other issues that needed to be addressed were hospital over-crowding, the provision of single rooms for infection control and the recruitment of more specialist personnel. They recommended that new hospitals or units should have at least 50 per cent of their beds in single rooms, with appropriate facilities for patient isolation, and that there should be at least 2.9 metres between the centre of adjacent beds in multi-bedded wards. They observed that when more patients are added to a defined area, infection is likely to increase, and that increased patient/staff ratios and increased staffing by temporary or locum nursing staff are also associated with increased transmission rates.

The expert subcommittee made it quite clear that hand washing alone would not solve the problem of hospital infection and that additional investment in health service capacity and staffing was essential:

> Improvements in controlling MRSA are possible. However current resources (specialist personnel, hospital facilities etc) in Ireland are inadequate to achieve this…Current resources for the control of infection in hospitals and in community units are inadequate and additional investment such as the appointment of more microbiologists, infection control nurses and laboratory scientists, together with the provision of appropriate physical infrastructure, is required. This is likely to assist in the implementation of these guidelines, help contain hospital- and other healthcare-associated infection, and contribute to the more efficient utilisation of healthcare resources. [32]

The chief executives of the major Dublin teaching hospitals share this assessment. In a submission to the Minister for Health, they have argued that bed occupancy rates are significantly lower in countries where MRSA control has been achieved, and that inadequate ward infrastructure and high bed occupancy rates in their hospitals were contributing to the level of infection.[33] The president of the Irish Association of Emergency Medicine, Anthony Martin, has pointed out that the risk of cross-infection is similar if not greater in an overcrowded A&E than on a ward: 'Why should ward patients need to be separated by 2.5 metres for infection control purposes, while it is deemed suitable for A&E department patients to be jammed together within centimetres of one another?'[34]

Discrimination against public patients in public hospitals
Bed designation
Since 1991, all Irish citizens have had the right to free accommodation and treatment, including consultant care, in public

hospitals, apart from a limited overnight charge (€55 per night up to a 10-night per annum maximum in 2005). However, under the provisions of the Health (Amendment) Act 1991, hospitals must designate a proportion of their beds as public and a proportion as private, subject to the Minister's approval. This means that patients who pay private fees, whether covered by insurance or out of pocket, gain fast-track access to public hospitals.

The 1991 Act stipulated no explicit ratio of public to private beds. The proportion of designated private inpatient beds rose from 19 per cent in 1991 to 20 per cent in 1993 and remained at that level in 2002. The proportion of designated day beds rose from 27 per cent nationally in 1991 to 33 per cent in 2002, having apparently evaded the 80/20 split from the start. In 2002 in Limerick Regional Hospital, 50 per cent of day beds were private. In Cork Regional Hospital, 40 per cent of day beds were private.

Although the so-called '80/20 split' was introduced as a policy tool to protect public patients' access to public hospitals, as a Department of Health working group reported in 2001, the 80/20 public/private bed designation 'has not held to that level of mix in some key areas affecting equity of access'. The 2001 National Health Strategy observed that in the case of elective admissions, the area where waiting lists arise, the ratio was 'less than satisfactory'. The Strategy's promised 3,000 additional beds were therefore to be designated public.

However, despite the increase in the number of acute inpatient beds since 2002, the Department of Health has not changed its bed designations, which it says are 'under review'. In the absence of up-to-date bed designation figures from the Department, it is not possible to say what direction, if any, hospitals have been given on how their additional bed stock should be deployed.

In public hospitals in 2004, private patients accounted for 33.4 per cent of patients discharged after elective inpatient treatment, 24 per cent of patients discharged after day treatment and 23.6 per cent of patients discharged after emergency treatment. Private patients accounted for 25.6 per cent of total cases in public hospitals in 2004.[35]

While day beds are a small proportion of all acute beds, day activity has come to dominate elective treatment, and, as discussed above, many treatments do not require beds at all. By 2004 there were 424,000 day cases, representing 43 per cent of all hospital activity and 71 per cent of all elective activity. An internal analysis following the Department's February 2003 bed count concluded that 'it is clear from the exercise that the designation process alone is not sufficient to control the amount of private activity occurring in hospitals.'

The same review commented on one hospital where there were no designated private day beds, 'yet the public private mix in day case work is 72/28.' It observed that in some hospitals private patients were admitted for minor day procedures, where they did not need the use of 'any form of "bed"'. A patient who underwent laser surgery had complained to the Ombudsman that she had been charged a private day charge 'where she did not occupy a day bed, recliner, trolley or couch'.[36]

In 2003, the Department wrote to health boards and voluntary hospitals asking them 'to review arrangements for the monitoring of the public/private mix in order to ensure that private practice within public hospitals is not at the expense of fair access for public patients.' The Department concluded from the responses it received that 'there is little evidence that formal arrangements are in place with consultants regarding the management of their private practice.'[37] The CEO of the Southern Health Board had responded that only 20 per cent of beds in Cork University Hospital (CUH) were private and 'the emphasis should be on revising this upwards consistent with trends in activity.' He wrote that 40 per cent of the population had private health insurance, adding 'CUH has a strong and sustained focus on income generation for quite some time, and this needs to be protected.'[38]

The chief executive of St John's Hospital, Limerick, where the day care unit had 'a nominal 10 beds with a 6 public and a 4 non-public approved bed designation', acknowledged that 'activity levels in the day care unit are skewed in favour of private patients relative to this designation and we are in on-going discussion with a number of our consultant staff with a view to remedying this situation.' He observed that 'while we have lengthy public waiting lists for other [non-gynaecological] day case procedures, current contracted scheduled sessional commitments do not allow for the ready adjustment of activity to cater for these imbalances.'[39] The chief executive was responding to data for 2001, when 51 per cent of St John's day cases were private. This had dropped to 41 per cent by 2004.

Utilisation, access and waiting lists

It might be argued that since the privately insured have now grown to 52 per cent of the adult population,[40] hospitals might be expected to treat growing numbers of private patients and that private patients' medical need might legitimately require their prior allocation of more than 20 per cent of public hospitals' resources. The evidence suggests, however, that it is not greater medical need which secures private patients their growing access to public hospitals.

A telephone survey of 2,620 people conducted by the ESRI in 1999 found that of those on waiting lists for inpatient surgery, not one insured person had waited for more than a year, whereas 22 per cent of the uninsured had done so.[41] A further survey of 1,250 people in 2000 found that whereas 56 per cent of the insured had experienced no wait for day treatment, not one uninsured person had been admitted for day surgery without a wait.[42] Confirmation that private patients' faster access is not just a consequence of the availability of private hospitals but reflects their privileged access to public hospitals as well was provided in a 2002 Eastern Regional Health Authority survey, which disclosed that the average waiting time for private patients in public hospitals in the East was 3.4 months, whereas the average waiting time for public patients was 6.7 months.[43]

A survey conducted by the CSO in 2001, using a much larger sample of 39,000 households, surveyed waiting times for hospital outpatient appointments, inpatient procedures and day procedures or investigations for people aged 18 and over.

As Table 7.7 illustrates, experiences of waiting differed markedly according to whether the patient had private health insurance, Medical Card cover or neither. For day procedures, now the majority of elective procedures, fully a quarter of

Medical Card patients waited over six months, compared to 8 per cent of the privately insured. Even more strikingly, whereas a quarter of the privately insured waited over six months for inpatient treatment, this rose to 46 per cent for Medical Card holders and to 60 per cent for those people with neither Medical Cards nor private health insurance. Of this latter group, 39 per cent waited over one year for inpatient treatment.

Table 7.7: Waiting times according to method of payment, 2001

	Outpatient				Inpatient				Day			
	Less than 1 month	1 to less than 6 months	6 months to 1 year	Over 1 year	Less than 1 month	1 to less than 6 months	6 months to 1 year	Over 1 year	Less than 1 month	1 to less than 6 months	6 months to 1 year	Over 1 year
Medical Card holders	26	50	16	8	14	40	21	25	29	47	15	10
Private health insurance	44	46	5	5	35	39	13	13	50	43	5	3
Both	42	49	9		40	32*	28**		33	67		
Neither	31	48	13	8	17	24	21	39	27	47	15	12

*Source: CSO Quarterly National Household Survey, Third Quarter 2001. *1 to less than 3 months **Over 3 months*

Of particular significance is the finding for waits for outpatient appointments, since until a patient secures an initial outpatient appointment with a hospital consultant, he will not go on an official waiting list. A quarter of Medical Card holders waited over six months for outpatient appointments, compared to 10 per cent of the privately insured. Regrettably, the survey did not ask how much longer than a year patients had waited for procedures or appointments. However, the authors have heard GPs report that public outpatient waits can be so long that they may not refer their patients onwards for specialist treatment, since they consider it to be a pointless exercise. In 2005 the National Treatment Purchase Fund (NTPF) initiated pilot projects in co-operation with 14 public hospitals to provide outpatient appointments for up to 5,000 public patients. The Minister for Health announced in May 2005 that 'people waiting longest in a number of specialties will receive consultations at outpatient level in private hospitals. If it is decided that any of the patients involved in the pilot projects require surgery then, of course, the Fund will make these arrangements.'[44]

The CSO's 2001 survey discovered that among the population aged 18 or over in 2001, 46.3 per cent had private health insurance only, 25.9 per cent had Medical Cards only, 2.1 per cent had both and 25.6 per cent had neither. Whereas this survey put the percentage of the adult population with private insurance at 48.4 per cent, subsequent surveys based on smaller samples for the HIA found private insurance coverage to be 47 per cent of the population in 2002, rising to 52 per cent in 2005.[45] This most recent survey also recorded that 26 per cent of the sample had Medical Cards and 3 per cent had both private health insurance and Medical Cards, leaving 25 per cent with neither.

A further perspective on inequity in access to care in Ireland was provided in a study analysing 1996 data for 14 OECD countries, which discovered that Ireland, along with Portugal, had a notably greater pro-rich distribution of medical specialist care than other European countries. This paper concluded that the lack of private insurance coverage 'does seem to act as some access barrier to specialist care for lower income groups, in spite of their entitlement to free specialist care.'[46]

A recent study of equity in the utilisation of health care in Ireland surprisingly concluded that hospital services are distributed equally in relation to need across the income distribution. However, the data available to this study were so highly aggregated that this conclusion must be questioned. The data did not distinguish between day procedures and outpatient visits, so that, for instance, it implicitly equated a public patient's repeat outpatient visits, to be informed that he remains on the waiting list for treatment, with the same number of day visits by a sequence of patients, who benefit from day case procedures. Equally, the study treated inpatient nights as of equal value as a measure of 'service utilisation'. But this fails to capture the difference between the very large number of inpatient bed nights which may be 'utilised' by patients who are due for discharge but for whom no long-stay place has yet been found, a typical experience of poorer, older patients, and the much more effective utilisation of hospital care, which the same number of bed nights represents, when they are attributable to a sequence of patients experiencing short stays for treatment.[47]

There have been other studies which support the perception of two-tier access to hospital care in Ireland. An analysis of liver transplants found significant inequity in transplant allocation in Ireland. In this study, published in 2004, the possession of private health insurance appeared to increase the chances of receiving a liver transplant. Patients without private health insurance living distant from the liver transplant unit appeared particularly disadvantaged. Surveying the experience of 202 patients who were admitted to the national liver transplant unit between 1 April 2000 and 31 March 2002, this study discovered that 43 patients received liver transplants (21.3 per cent). Of patients with private health insurance, 17 of 50 (34 per cent) were transplanted, compared with 26 of 152 (17 per cent) without private health insurance. For residents of the East (close to the liver transplant unit), patients with private health insurance were no more likely to be transplanted, whereas for residents of other areas, patients with private insurance were three times more likely to receive a transplant than those without health insurance. Patients living outside the Eastern region without private health insurance were only half as likely as all other patient types combined to receive a transplant.[48]

A study in 2001 of the diagnostic care of patients with coronary heart disease from one general practice provided evidence of the differing care received by public and private patients. The study of 30 private and 40 public patients found that 77 per cent of private patients and 25 per cent of public patients had had angiograms; all but one of the private patients had had an exercise electrocardiogram, whereas 15 of the public patients were not offered this test.[49]

This study provided confirmation that public patients may not only have greater difficulties accessing care, but that they may also have differing experiences of care. Under the terms of the consultants' contract, consultants may delegate care to their juniors. Whereas consultants will see private patients in their private rooms and private patients will expect and, in general, receive personal care from their consultant, public patients may well see more junior doctors when they go for outpatient appointments and may ultimately be treated by more junior doctors. A survey in 2002 disclosed that almost a quarter of patients said they rarely or never saw their consultant.[50] The medical staffing of public hospitals quite simply does not provide for public patients to have the kind of personal relationship with their consultants that private patients expect.

Private patients are on average younger, healthier and higher earners than public patients. Poor health makes one less rather than more likely to have insurance. Although the most recent survey evidence is that by 2005, 52 per cent of over-18-year-olds had taken out private health insurance, this was a self-selecting group. While approximately 60 per cent of 45- to 64-year-olds were insured, this dropped to 48 per cent for people aged 65 and older. Whereas 85 per cent of the richest social group (AB) were insured, this dropped to 18 per cent of the lowest income group (DE). On middle incomes it is apparent that paying for insurance is a struggle. The highest proportion of formerly insured people (6 per cent) was in social group C2.

The probability of having poor health rises with age and is greater the lower one's income. The privately insured are therefore on average less likely as a group to require care than the rest of the population. Survey evidence has shown that when admitted to hospital, the privately insured generally stay there for less time than Medical Card patients.[51] On the other hand, even before the extension of Medical Cards to everyone aged 70 and over, Medical Card patients were as a group older and sicker than the rest of the population and stayed in hospital on average 25 per cent longer than non-Medical-Card patients. It is against this backdrop that the bed designations need to be seen.

The privately insured have unimpeded access to the beds in private hospitals. There is no competition for these beds from emergency admissions and scheduled surgery goes ahead as planned. In addition, private patients are admitted for elective surgery to the designated private beds in public hospitals in advance of public patients in greater need. No matter what the length of the public waiting list is and no matter how much sicker the people on that list may be, private patients may take up beds in public hospitals. Even if privately designated beds are not formally available, there is sufficient latitude in the definition of day places and laxity in how bed designations are policed to ensure that private patients whom consultants have listed for treatment receive their treatment much faster than public waiting list patients. In the words of an internal Department of Health working group on the public/private mix, which reported in 2001, 'the system involved separate waiting lists for public and private beds'.[52]

How many patients are now waiting for care and how long have they been waiting?

The establishment of the National Treatment Purchase Fund (NTPF) has unquestionably reduced waiting times for public patients by concentrating on purchasing care for long waiters, in private or public hospitals, at home or abroad. The NTPF has reported that whereas in January 2003, 39 per cent of public patients on lists waited over 12 months for surgical treatment and 16 per cent of patients over 24 months, by January 2004, 20 per cent of patients waited over 12 months and 2.5 per cent had waited over 24 months.[53]

Highly desirable though it is to ensure that patients are treated speedily, the establishment and operation of the NTPF has created a strange circularity in the Irish public health care system. While private patients continue to receive preferential access to public hospitals, the public patients whom they displace may in turn be treated in private hospitals. The private sector gains – in private fees to public hospital consultants for private treatments in the public hospital, and in private fees to private or more probably public consultants, who treat public patients in the private hospitals. This circularity is neither a good use of public money nor an equitable way to treat patients. In addition, given the absence in private hospitals of multi-disciplinary care, it would appear that public patients who undergo NTPF-funded procedures in private hospitals may be denied the free follow-up care, like physiotherapy, which they would have received had they been treated in the public hospital where they first presented.

The unfortunate decision by former Minister for Health, Micheál Martin, that the Department should cease collecting national waiting list data and that this function should be assumed by the NTPF has made it impossible to assess the achievements of this new agency. In the new administrative system, in which the Department and HIQA are intended to act as checks and balances for the HSE, this is not a logical or sensible allocation of functions. The NTPF should be subsumed by the HSE. The Department should have the role of judging its achievements. HIQA has responsibility for the collection of information and maintaining standards. The authors recommend that responsibility for maintaining, verifying and publishing waiting list data should be given to HIQA, which would give the Department – and the public – an objective standard by which to judge the performance of the NTPF within the HSE.

When the NTPF assumed responsibility for collecting national waiting list data in May 2004, it informed the Department of Health that in the region of 4,500 patients should be removed from the list of 27,318 patients whom health agencies had reported to the Department as waiting for treatment at the end of 2003. The NTPF reported that these patients were variously not available for treatment, not medically suitable to undergo treatment, no longer required treatment or had postponed treatment at their own request. Given that upon its establishment the NTPF discovered patients who had waited as long as 10 years for treatment, it is plausible that significant numbers of patients on official waiting lists may have died, chosen to pay privately for treatment or decided against treatment. However, there remains the possibility that patients whom the NTPF has offered treatment might not wish to be treated privately by a doctor other than their original consultant, possibly outside their own hometown, and might therefore not have chosen to avail of the treatment offered. While the authors have heard only anecdotal evidence of such possibilities, we recommend that an agency other than the NTPF, probably HIQA, should examine the reasons why patients might decline its offer of treatment.

Although the NTPF has legitimately argued that the former waiting list data contained inconsistencies in agencies' recording, definitions and reporting of patient data, and its development of an accessible Patient Treatment Register (PTR) is welcome, the authors believe the original waiting list data series should have continued to be published until the NTPF's new data were available. Indeed, there should have been a period of overlap between the two systems in order to afford continuity for analysis and transparency in judging the work of the NTPF.

The NTPF launched its new PTR on 9 September 2005, following over a year in which there had been no published national waiting list data. Described as 'phase 1', this version of the PTR records waiting lists for only seven hospitals, which formerly accounted for 40 per cent of patients waiting nationally. The NTPF said it would extend the PTR to the whole country in 2006. The PTR continues to define as being on a waiting list only patients who have waited over three months for an inpatient or day surgical or medical procedure. Patients with a scheduled date for a procedure within three months are described as 'pre-scheduled'. Waiting times are measured from the date a patient is placed on a list for treatment.

In August 2005, the seven 'phase 1' hospitals had 4,944 patients waiting for surgical procedures and 2,103 for medical procedures, a total of 7,047 patients waiting. In total, 2,134, or 29 per cent, of waiting list patients in these hospitals had waited for over a year – 24.4 per cent of surgical patients and 39 per cent of medical patients. A further 1,020 patients were on a list for pre-scheduled surgical procedures.[54]

The former waiting list series published by the Department of Health recorded that in December 2003 these seven hospitals had 12,189 patients waiting, of whom 4,745, or 39 per cent, had waited over a year. There therefore seems to have been a significant overall reduction in both the absolute number of patients waiting and in the numbers waiting over a year in these hospitals. Although the authors do not know how many patients were removed from these lists because of treatment and how many were removed as part of a validation process, the NTPF has reported that 544 surgical patients of these hospitals are currently suspended because they are 'not currently ready (for clinical reasons) or not available (social or personal reasons) for their procedure.'

Both in 2003 and in 2005, hospitals' waiting lists show great variance. In 2003, over 45 per cent of patients were recorded as waiting over a year in St Vincent's and in Tallaght, whereas none waited over a year in St James's, a hospital which was notably co-operative with the NTPF from its inception. The latest NTPF figures continue to show great variance between hospitals. Beaumont has increased its waiting lists in absolute terms from 1,842 patients in 2003 to 2,564 patients in 2005, of whom 1,162, or 45 per cent, have been waiting over a year. The authors cannot say how much of this deterioration is to do with the change in counting methods, but it contrasts with the progress made by most of the other hospitals.

In 2004, the NTPF had a budget of €44 million and arranged for the treatment of 13,627 'cases'. While its internal accounting does not assign administrative costs when calculating the average cost per procedure, we would consider that appropriate. Average cost per procedure in 2004 was therefore €3,273, of which €188 paid for administration. The NTPF's annual report is sparing in the financial and activity details it supplies. The authors would consider it appropriate for this state-funded agency to publish precise details of how many procedures have taken place respectively in public and private hospitals, in Ireland and abroad, and of the cost per procedure in each of these hospitals.

In the first published scrutiny of the operations of the NTPF, the Comptroller and Auditor General (C&AG)[55] has answered some of these questions. His report raises other disturbing questions about the operations of the NTPF which have yet to be answered. Centrally, the C&AG disclosed that 36 per cent of the NTPF cases examined by him were carried out in the same public hospital from which the case had been referred. Furthermore, the NTPF did not systematically record information relating to the referring consultant and the consultant carrying out the surgical procedure to enable it to guard against the risk of excessive self-referral. There exists, then, considerable scope for public consultants to earn private fees for the treatment within their hospital of their own public waiting list patients. Nearly half the NTPF treatments examined (44 per cent) took place in public hospitals. This raises the related question of whether it would have been a better use of state funds to permit these public hospitals to work at full capacity, and their salaried staff to perform to their full potential, rather than for the state to pay again through the NTPF for the use of public capacity and the work of public staff. The report states that some of this public work was undertaken outside core hours and on staff overtime, but how many cases this represents is not quantified.

The Minister for Health introduced a policy in 2005 that no more than 10 per cent of NTPF work might take place in public hospitals. While the authors believe it is preferable for the state to fund public hospitals directly to work to their full capacity, in the absence of such funding this decision will deny public hospitals with excess capacity the opportunity to compete with private hospitals to undertake NTPF work. Since NTPF funding has become an important source of income for public hospitals, there is a risk that some public hospitals will have to reduce activity and staffing as a consequence of the Minister's decision. To say the least, it is a strange manner of funding public health care to afford private hospitals the right to compete to supply the publicly funded treatment of public patients and to deny this right to public hospitals.

The C&AG uncovered wide variations in the rates paid by the NTPF for the same procedures. The highest rates for some procedures were twice or three times the lowest rates. The C&AG said he had acceded to a request from the Department of Health 'not to disclose the prices paid for procedures by the NTPF on the basis that the publication of commercially sensitive information would affect NTPF's negotiating position and as a result its capacity to deliver a value for money service.'

However, there is the implication that the NTPF is regularly paying higher rates to private than to public hospitals, since the report states that the NTPF argued that prices might need to take into account the 'capital costs and depreciation considerations which arise for private hospitals in some instances.'

For a state body to pay higher prices to private hospitals when public hospitals systematically subsidise their operation would be an indefensible use of state funds. Whereas public hospitals must pay the pensions and indemnity costs of the consultants on their staffs, private hospitals do not have to do so. Private hospitals overwhelmingly use the services of publicly salaried and pensioned consultants.

The focus of public attention on conditions in A&E, and the suppression for over a year of information on waiting lists, has temporarily obscured the issue of public patients' waits for elective operations and treatments. Yet public patients continue to wait much longer than private patients for care, hence many Irish people buy private health insurance, not because they have chosen private care but because they recognise that this is the only way they can be sure of public treatment when they need it.

Conclusion

This initial discussion of Irish acute hospitals has disclosed that there remains a crisis of inadequate acute bed capacity, that the 2001 Health Strategy's targets for expanding capacity have not been met and that a growing and ageing population is going to make this crisis ever more severe, particularly in the East, unless the government responds with a planned and serious programme of investment. We recommend that the HSE should produce a plan for expanded hospital capacity. This should begin with a transparent bed count, validated by HIQA. It should include an assessment of the actual ratio of beds to population in each region, and it should be reconciled with the regional reorganisation of acute hospital services. Investment in extra acute beds should take place against a backdrop of explicit identification of which hospitals should grow, which should change function and of changes in how hospitals are staffed, managed and financed. If the government, the HSE or official policy-makers are no longer convinced of the merit of the assessment of capacity needs in the Acute Hospital Bed Capacity Review, we recommend that the government should initiate a further review as a matter of urgency. This review should take into account the considerable increase in population and population growth forecasts since the 2001 Review.

The capacity crisis makes it very difficult to counter hospital-acquired infections. The Irish rate of MRSA infection is higher than in many other countries. This growing problem reinforces the case for greater investment in hospitals in order to increase capacity, the number of single rooms and the space around beds in wards, as well as to modernise outdated facilities. The authors endorse the Infection Control Sub-committee's strategy for the control and prevention of MRSA, and point out that while improved hygiene has an important role to play, the sub-committee was clear that present staffing and hospital facilities are inadequate to control MRSA.

Although the NTPF has reduced patient waiting time, the two-tier system remains a reality. Hospital patients are treated on the basis of income, not need. Patients without private insurance wait longer for care, receive inferior care and may be denied care altogether. We recommend that there should be a common waiting list for patients in public hospitals, but with care to be provided promptly so that few patients appear on waiting lists and none stays long. We recommend that if public hospitals offer patients who choose to pay for them enhanced, private rooms, they must provide them with the same care as all other patients. There should not be any private and public patients in public hospitals.

Public hospitals with unused capacity should be funded to treat more patients within the public system, not via the NTPF. The NTPF's annual report should contain precise details of how many procedures have taken place respectively in public and private hospitals, in Ireland and abroad, and of the cost per procedure in each of these hospitals. It is the authors' view that until such time as there is a common waiting list in public hospitals, public hospitals with excess capacity should be permitted to compete to supply NTPF-funded treatments on the same footing as private hospitals.

Subsequent chapters will develop our discussion of Irish acute hospitals, firstly by examining the A&E crisis and the relationship between hospitals and others sectors of health and social care.

8

THE ACCIDENT AND EMERGENCY CRISIS: SOLUTIONS WITHIN AND OUTSIDE HOSPITALS

Introduction

Accident and emergency (A&E) departments are the primary route of entry to Irish hospital care. Even when an experienced general practitioner (GP) has decided that a patient needs admission to hospital and has referred that patient to the local hospital, the patient may then spend long hours waiting to be seen by a hospital doctor, who is quite likely to be relatively junior and still in training.[1] This may then be followed by many days and nights on a trolley in A&E, although a hospital doctor has concurred that the patient's condition requires him to be admitted as an inpatient. While A&E sees some patients who should have been treated at primary care level, the problem of patients on trolleys is not caused by patients inappropriately attending A&E who should be in their GP's surgery. Patients on trolleys are patients who have been medically judged to require admittance for treatment and/or the advanced assessment which acute hospitals can offer. They remain on trolleys in A&E departments quite simply because this treatment or assessment takes place in inpatient wards and, for a complex combination of reasons, hospitals have no free beds into which to admit them.

An examination of the A&E crisis reveals that it is only the tip of an iceberg. The indignities which patients suffer result from a long chain of causation, which includes recent cutbacks in community and public long-stay care; low capital investment in health and social services over many decades; the political system's continued failure to address how Irish society should access and pay for long-stay care in old age; failure to reform the system of hospital medical staffing; failures of internal management within hospitals; and the perennial problem of lack of integration between primary, acute and community care.

Just as the reasons for the A&E crisis are multiple, so are its solutions: increased investment in capacity in long-stay, community and palliative care; increased capacity in acute hospitals; better admissions procedures and units; better discharge planning; reform in how hospital doctors work and greater flexibility from all staff; initiatives led from the top to encourage greater integration between the arms of the health service; and, critically, political leadership to win community support for a new system of funding and access to long-stay care.

Who comes through A&E?

Although the popular view of an acute hospital is as a place where patients go for surgery, in reality, the majority of patients who stay overnight in Irish hospitals require medical, not surgical, treatment. In 2003, 76 per cent of inpatients in acute hospitals nationally were medical and 24 per cent were surgical patients. Most hospital inpatients come to hospital as emergency, not elective, cases. Almost 70 per cent of all inpatient admissions to Irish acute hospitals are admitted as emergencies, and most emergency admissions are for medical, not surgical, care. In 2003, 84 per cent of all medical inpatients were admitted as emergencies, compared to 39 per cent of surgical inpatients. The majority of surgical patients are treated electively – by arrangement – and of those, the majority are day, not inpatient, cases.[2] A typical A&E admission would be an older person who has had a stroke and whose treatment will require the skills of a multi-disciplinary team, in which nursing care, speech therapy, physiotherapy and the assistance of a social worker in ensuring that the patient returns home with proper supports will be every bit as important as, if not more important than, medical care.

How bad is the A&E crisis?

Public perception of the health service has suffered because of the public's awareness of the conditions in A&E. It could hardly be otherwise. As Figure 8.1 recounts, it is commonplace for people of advanced age to spend up to five days on trolleys. Hospitals regularly cancel elective or emergency admissions because of A&E overcrowding. Numbers waiting on trolleys nationwide regularly run to over 200 or even 300. In 2005, they peaked at 422 in January, according to a count by Irish Nurses Organisation (INO) members. They hit that level again in January 2006. In March 2005, the Health Service Executive (HSE) began an official count of people 'waiting on trolleys in A&E for admission following assessment by a consultant.' This count was taken in the afternoons on weekdays. In 2005, it recorded a peak of 294 people on trolleys in the first week of April. On the same day the INO, who assemble figures from local union representatives at about 9.00 a.m. each weekday morning, counted 362 patients on trolleys. The worst-affected hospital is frequently Tallaght in West Dublin, which can have over 60 patients on trolleys.

In the autumn of 2005, the HSE pointed out that the numbers on trolleys declined on average in May and had remained down to September, and attributed this to a programme to reduce delayed discharge of patients from hospital, which we discuss below. The real test of its success had yet to come in the winter of 2005–2006. At the time of writing at end-January 2006, numbers on trolleys had climbed steeply (see Figure 8.2). The January average count by the INO exceeded the January 2005 average. It might be argued that these figures were not comparable, since the INO did not yet have a complete nationwide count in January 2005. However, at an average of 336 people on trolleys nationwide each weekday morning in January 2006, the HSE was clearly facing an intractable problem.

On 17 January 2006, the INO counted 422 people on trolleys in the morning and the HSE counted 363 in the afternoon. Tallaght, the hospital with the busiest A&E, was typically worst affected, with 50 people on trolleys in the morning and 39 still on trolleys in the afternoon; the Mater had 25 in the morning,

15 in the afternoon; Beaumont had 23 in the morning, 27 in the afternoon; St Vincent's had 19 in the morning, 17 in the afternoon; and Naas in County Kildare had 36 in the morning, 15 in the afternoon. While the most persistent problem of patients waiting for beds on A&E trolleys occurs in and near Dublin, the problem has been manifest all over the country. On the morning of 17 January 2006, the worst affected hospitals outside the Dublin region were the Mid-Western Regional Hospital, Limerick (32), Our Lady of Lourdes Hospital, Drogheda (22) and Wexford General Hospital (21).[3]

There is evidence – but no one has attempted to quantify it – that people are leaving A&E departments without medical attention. A nurse has described to the authors the experience of triaging (assessing) a patient as urgent, who, after six hours of waiting to be seen by a doctor, left the hospital and died within minutes in its car park. Emergency department crowding (EDC) has been reported in other countries. EDC is defined as a 'situation in which the demand for emergency services exceeds the ability of a department to provide quality care within an acceptable time frame.' A 2002 study by the US Joint Commission on Accreditation of Healthcare Organizations cited EDC as the cause of a significant number of patient deaths.[4]

DEATH IN A HOSPITAL CAR PARK

'I have specialised in A&E nursing, triage. There has been a huge increase in waiting times. Patients have died as a result of this. There are five triage categories. Category I gets seen immediately – for example, cardiac arrest. Category II should wait no more than 10 minutes – for example, someone whose ECG is showing changes. Category III should wait no more than an hour – they probably wait six hours now. Category IV should be seen within two hours – they wait six to 12 hours. Category V should have been seen within four to five hours. They shouldn't bother coming to A&E.

'A man came in with chest pain. I triaged him. He didn't show ECG changes but I was concerned about him. I called him an urgent Category III. He should have seen a doctor in one hour. He waited six hours. Then he left. He arrested in his car outside and died.'

– *A&E nurse in conversation with the authors, July 2005*

Figure 8.1: Tales from A&E	
2004: October	All elective admissions cancelled at University College Hospital Galway because 16 patients are on A&E trolleys awaiting beds.
	Kathleen Byrne (72) spends five days on a trolley in Dublin's Mater hospital following a series of strokes. She contracts the winter vomiting bug and bedsores.
	Her daughter, Janette Byrne, co-founds Patients Together, a group of relatives and health professionals protesting about A&E conditions.
	An 84-year-old woman spends five days on a trolley in Dublin's Mater hospital A&E.
	In Cavan General Hospital 18 patients wait on trolleys in the X-ray department, outpatient department and corridors. One patient spends five days on a trolley.
2004: November	In Limerick a 74-year-old woman spends 33 hours on a trolley beside an entrance door. Another patient takes her trolley when she goes to the toilet. The health board apologises.
	Minister for Health, Mary Harney, announces a 70 million 10-point plan to improve A&E services.
2005: January	'I remain extremely hopeful that by the autumn of 2005 we will see measurable results.' Minister for Health, Mary Harney, on A&E crisis.
	There are a record 422 patients on trolleys, says INO.
	Kevin Kelly, interim CEO of HSE, says A&E overcrowding 'unacceptable'.
	Mater hospital goes off call due to A&E overcrowding.
2005: February	INO begins campaign of protest about A&E conditions. 239 patients on trolleys, says INO.
2005: March	73-year-old woman spends five days on trolley in Mater.
	Cork University Hospital closes A&E department to all except ambulance patients.
	335 patients on trolleys, says INO.
2005: April	Dublin fire brigade sends personnel to Tallaght hospital after member of public says that fire exits are blocked in A&E department, where there are over 60 patients on trolleys.
	HSE begins its 'official' trolley count each afternoon.
	The INO counts in the morning. 350 patients on trolleys nationwide, says INO.
2006: January	On Tuesday, 17 January, INO counts 422 patients on trolleys. INO average count for the month is 336, HSE average count is 269.

What has made the A&E crisis so bad?

There are many pressures on acute hospitals – and they have been mounting. In 2004, Comhairle na nOspidéal, the body with responsibility for consultant appointments, listed these factors:

- 'heightened public expectation and demand for prompt and high quality healthcare and hospital treatment;

- increased public expectation that the acute care of emergency admissions should have direct consultant input;
- a preponderance of medical emergencies being older people, often with multiple medical conditions in addition to the acute illness for which they have presented;
- the acknowledged bed capacity deficit within acute hospitals in Ireland;
- occupancy of acute hospital medical beds by patients who no longer require acute treatment, but who are not discharged forprolonged periods because of a lack of appropriate alternative facilities and infrastructure outside the hospital to receive and support them.[5]

Figure 8.2: Monthly average of patients on trolleys awaiting admission, January 2005–January 2006

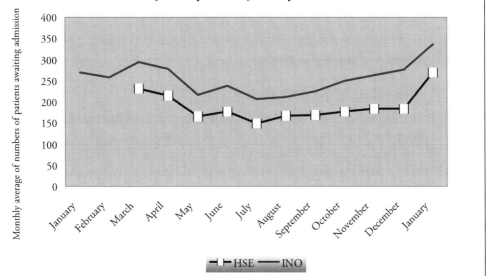

Source: HSE, INO. Counts taken on weekdays only. HSE an afternoon count of patients on trolleys awaiting admission, who have been seen by a consultant. INO a morning count. HSE count began in March 2005. INO January 2005 count did not cover all hospitals.

These factors, combined with the needs of a rising and ageing population and the treatment of more conditions because of medical advances, caused:

severe pressure on acute hospitals, their beds, their staff and other resources, by virtue of the sheer volume of patients presenting with acute medical illnesses. Some of the greatest effects of this pressure can be seen in the regular disruption and frequent cancellation of elective work, both medical and surgical and the persistence of waiting lists nationwide despite a series of initiatives to address this problem. Additionally, there is an increasing practice of acute patients being referred to A&E who should be more appropriately admitted directly to a medical or surgical bed. Furthermore, an increasing number of patients, for whom an elective admission to hospital would be more appropriate, choose to access inpatient care via attendance at the A&E department, as this route may offer the only prospect of being admitted expeditiously.[6]

Irish hospitals can be 'chaotic'. Managers and consultants told Comhairle that 'In a number of hospitals…, management and consultant staff described the current medical assessment, admission and discharge pathway as being "chaotic". The most serious issues cited concerned resource utilisation, the impact of delays on patients' health and well-being and ultimately the public's perceptions of the health service.'

Responding to the A&E crisis

In November 2004 the Tánaiste and Minister for Health, Mary Harney, announced '10 actions to improve Accident and Emergency services'. These would be funded by €70 million in new current expenditure. The actions addressed three distinct issues: enhanced GP services, the internal working of acute hospitals and the provision of post-acute care outside acute hospitals. The Minister also announced that 300 new beds would be available in 2005 in public hospitals, in addition to some in acute medical units (AMUs).[7]

We discussed earlier the considerable potential for improving health care and health in Ireland by modernising GP services and widening access to care. The Minister's proposals in this regard – ensuring out-of-hour services in North Dublin and increasing access of GPs to diagnostic services – might reduce pressures on hospitals in Dublin to some degree. When set against the potential of the disregarded Primary Care Strategy, however, they were very modest. In this chapter, we will examine the two other dimensions of the A&E crisis – how hospitals might change their admissions and other internal processes and the huge relevance of long-stay and community care to the acute hospital sector.

Improving the internal processes of acute hospitals

There are measures that are within the control of managers and staff which hospitals can employ to help ameliorate the problems of A&E. Some hospitals have already reduced pressures on A&E by changing how they admit and assess medical patients, through dedicated medical admissions units. All hospitals would benefit from greater flexibility in the use of their beds and other facilities and in the hours that employees work. A&E staff recount how they have admitted victims of domestic violence over weekends who do not need acute care but do need the services of a social worker, who does not work weekends. Nurse bed managers recount how patients remain longer than they should, occupying valuable inpatient beds, because hospital consultants conduct too few bed rounds. The INO has sought the appointment of senior nurses to A&E departments who could diagnose, treat and discharge patients with minor injuries.[8]

A recent investigation of the problems of A&E heard from one hospital that it was not uncommon for an acute medical patient to spend four or five days in hospital before appropriate treatment began. These delays could include waiting in the A&E department, waiting for an inpatient bed, waiting to be seen by the relevant consultant and his/her team, waiting for tests and their results and waiting for a diagnosis.[9]

Greater flexibility and creativity in the use of employees' time and skills will require negotiated change in their terms of employment and teamwork between professionals in the interest of patients. Providing cover out of hours will require increased staffing in some areas. Evolving such solutions will require leadership from the HSE and hospital managers. Solving the problems of A&E will demand a partnership approach.

In 2005, the HSE completed an assessment of clinical and organisational processes in 10 hospitals. The Minister's plan included commitments to providing or expanding minor injury units, chest pain clinics, respiratory clinics and acute medical units (AMUs). The AMUs were to be provided in three major Dublin hospitals – Tallaght, St Vincent's and Beaumont, which would also receive a second MRI. The nationwide development of AMUs was endorsed by Comhairle na nOspidéal in a report in 2004, which stated:

> while essential, the putting in place of additional beds in the public hospital system will not on its own address all the current difficulties being faced by acute hospitals in the state. Rather, additional measures and steps need to be taken in order to ensure that current and additional capacity is used more effectively and efficiently and existing processes changed in order to guarantee that patients have access to the right care, at the right time, in the right place, delivered by the right people.[10]

Comhairle recommended the development of AMUs in all acute general hospitals receiving acutely ill medical patients. Its report defined AMUs (also sometimes referred to as medical assessment units, or MAUs) as providing 'a short stay area for assessing medical patients who need further investigations before a decision on the most appropriate care can be made.'

These units would effectively fast track medical patients' access to assessment and treatment. By accepting patients directly referred by GPs, they would save the patient from unnecessary waits in A&E and the hospital from unnecessarily double checking an experienced GP's diagnosis prior to admitting the patient to specialist care. The AMU would accept patients referred by their GP, the A&E department or the hospital's outpatient clinics. Patients would be either acutely medically ill and needing immediate assessment and treatment, or might potentially be acutely ill but because of 'clinical uncertainty' would require further assessment and treatment. The unit would be staffed by a multi-disciplinary team led by a consultant physician. AMU patients might be treated in the unit and discharged directly home, they might receive continuing care in the unit if their stay was expected to be short, or they might be transferred to a ward or referred to an outpatient clinic. The AMU would have priority access to hospital investigative facilities and inpatient beds.

The Irish College of General Practitioners (ICGP) told Comhairle that 'GPs do not always require admission in cases of clinical uncertainty, but they often require particular investigation or assessment, to clarify a diagnosis. The absence of an assessment option may result in unnecessary admission, even for a short period.'

Advocating that such units should accept direct GP referrals, eliminating the need for such patients inappropriately attending A&E departments, the ICGP said that:

> the failure to recognise and maximise the potential of General Practice results in duplication, time delay, and is an inefficient use of scarce resources and expertise in our healthcare system. Lack of proper communication structures between the two sectors in effect ensures that the capacity of General Practice to reduce demand on A&E departments and hospital services, especially at times of crises, is underutilised.

The Irish Association of Emergency Medicine (IAEM), which represents emergency consultants, agreed that:

> the use of emergency departments as admission units for all general practice referrals to hospital is inappropriate. A vast amount of resources in A&E departments are taken up dealing with patients who have already been assessed by GPs and other doctors who think that the patient requires assessment by a specialist or admission to hospital. It is unreasonable to expect A&E department staff to reassess these patients basically to check out the opinion of the referring doctor before they are passed on. We would envisage these patients bypassing the A&E department direct to an admission/assessment area for the attention of the specialist team.

It should be noted that Comhairle did not think AMUs could function effectively without other changes and investment. While some hospitals could provide such units by redesignating existing beds, in others additional beds would have to be provided. Rehabilitation and community service beds would also need to be taken into account, since 'a shortage of community-based beds can present a serious exit block in hospitals, and will impact negatively upon the effective functioning of the AMU.'

Staffing might also have to increase. Comhairle reported that existing medical units which had the greatest positive impact on patients and their well-being were those that had the dedicated on-site services of allied health professionals, including occupational therapists and physiotherapists, and had direct access to community services.

Comhairle reviewed the operation of existing and discontinued units, which had varying success. At St Luke's Hospital, Kilkenny, 95 per cent of AMU patients were referred by GPs and 23 per cent of them were discharged on the same day. This reduced potential admissions by almost a quarter because prior to the introduction of the AMU, all GP medical referrals were admitted to the hospital.

Kilkenny is a small hospital and, when Comhairle reported, its AMU had six beds, but other hospitals face greater challenges. The large and highly pressurised Mater hospital in Dublin introduced a 24-hour medical emergency department (MED) in 2001, with 162 beds in three operation areas for cardiology, geriatric (including stroke) and other acute medical care. Medical patients were referred to the unit from A&E. The unit began discharge planning for the patient at the time of admission, so that the facilities the patient required would, in so far as possible, be in place at the time of discharge. The Mater said the MED project had helped to reduce the average length of stay of medical emergencies from 13.6 days to 6.1 days and the average length of stay of chest pain patients from 13 to 6.2 days. However, the MED had problems discharging patients who needed access to long-term care and rehabilitation beds. By only accepting patients from A&E, the Mater's MED has not solved the problem of access to specialist care for patients referred by GPs. As Figure 8.1 recounts, notwithstanding this facility, patients in the Mater's A&E have experienced some of the worst trolley waits.

Other hospitals with AMUs also reported problems. University College Hospital Galway's unit and St James's hospital in Dublin had trouble transferring patients into the main hospital wards because of insufficient beds. At St James's, which opened its unit in 2003, between 80 and 100 acute medical beds in the hospital were considered inappropriately occupied at any given time. However, St James's reported that it had managed to eliminate duplication of assessment of patients, resulting in a decline in waiting time in the emergency department and a significant reduction in length of stay for acute medical admissions. In Waterford, where the unit opened in 2000, the number of complaints, particularly about the treatment of elderly patients, had decreased considerably. A senior clinical decision maker would see patients at an earlier stage than under the traditional system.

Over a year after the announcement of the 10-point plan, progress had been slow in developing AMUs. At the beginning of 2006, the HSE had not reported any progress in developing units at three Dublin hospitals – Tallaght, St Vincent's and Beaumont – which were announced in November 2004. The authors note that a significant advantage in AMUs is the availability of senior clinicians to ensure rapid diagnosis. The limited availability of senior clinical decision-makers in A&E departments remains a serious issue of concern, which cannot be addressed comprehensively without following the recommendations of the Hanly Report on hospital medical staffing, which is discussed in Chapter 10.

A crisis behind a crisis: long-stay and community care

Irish society has belatedly begun to wake up to a very serious crisis of inadequate care provision for older people. In 2005 the government appointed a high-level working group of officials from a number of departments, including the Department of Health, to examine options for a financially sustainable system of long-stay care. The National Economic and Social Forum was working on a report on community care for older people. The Minister for Health's responses to the A&E crisis were heavily biased towards finding ways to speed older patients, whose discharge had been delayed, onwards and out of the acute system.

We have discussed above the growing need for more acute inpatient beds. There is also ample evidence that many hospitals could put the beds they have to better use. Many inpatient beds – as many as 10 per cent in some of the major hospitals in Dublin[11] – could be freed for incoming patients were there sufficient beds appropriate to their needs in long-stay or extended care institutions, and sufficient community care facilities and supports for patients who should be helped to return home. Increasing the capacity of Irish hospitals, long-stay and extended care institutions and strengthening community care will require increased government investment.

This care crisis should come as no surprise to the government. In 2001, management consultants Deloitte & Touche forecast that the level of investment in facilities for the elderly was 'likely to be of a very significant magnitude' and 'the historically low investment and service base' during the 1980s and well into the 1990s 'makes this challenge more difficult'.[12]

The 2001 Health Strategy identified inadequacies in existing services for older people:

- *In the community*: Paramedic services, community nursing services, health promotion, home help service, day care.
- *In acute hospitals*: Assessment and rehabilitation beds, day hospital facilities.
- *In long-stay places*: Community nursing units.

It promised 'a programme of investment to increase capacity':

- 800 additional extended care/community nursing unit places 'per annum over the next 7 years' (this would cumulatively add 5,600 beds);
- 600 additional day hospital beds;
- 1,370 additional assessment and rehabilitation beds;
- 7,000 day centre places;
- recruitment of multi-disciplinary staff to support domiciliary care, i.e. care at home, and day and respite services;
- improved staffing levels in extended care units.[13]

Progress on achieving these objectives can be judged from the Department of Health's annual reports on long-stay activity and facilities, which analyse public and private provision; limited-stay and long-stay facilities; care for older people and for younger people with chronic illness; and facilities for rehabilitation, convalescence, palliative and respite care. Since the publication of the Health Strategy, in the three years from end-2001 to end-2004 (the latest data available), the overall number of extended care

Table 8.1: Extended care beds, 2001–2004

Health Board area	Extended care beds in 2001	Extended care beds in 2004	Increase/ decrease 2001–2004	Increase/ decrease public and voluntary beds	Increase/ decrease private nursing home beds	Percentage of beds in private nursing homes 2001	Percentage of beds in private nursing homes 2004	Extended care beds per 1,000 population * 65 years or over	Public and voluntary beds per 1,000 aged 65+
ERHA	5,753	6,445	692	43	649	42	48	47.3	24.7
Midland	1,801	1,883	82	58	24	40	40	71.9	43.5
Mid-Western	2,428	2,107	-321	30	-351	46	37	53.4	33.7
North-Eastern	2,113	2,373	260	-20	280	52	58	65.1	27.4
North-Western	1,499	1,808	309	52	257	28	37	62.1	38.9
South-Eastern	2,507	2,379	-128	181	-309	48	37	47.8	30.0
Southern	2,939	3,497	558	156	402	41	46	50.4	27.4
Western	2,909	3,280	371	7	364	52	57	66.6	28.6
Total	21,949	23,772	1,823	507	1,316	44	46	54.5	29.3

*Source: Derived from Long-Stay Activity Statistics 2001 and 2004 (Department of Health, 2002 and 2005). *Population data from Census of Population, 2002.*

beds increased by 1,823, or 8 per cent, according to the Department's count (see Table 8.1). Of the increase, 72 per cent of additional beds came in private nursing homes, a sector which has benefited from tax incentives. The public and voluntary sectors contributed a minority of beds, 21 and 17 per cent, respectively. In the East, where demands on acute hospitals are most severe, the number of public extended care beds increased by 149, voluntary sector beds were reduced by 106 and there were an additional 649 private nursing home beds.

In 2004, the East and the South-East had the fewest extended care beds in relation to population aged 65 and over, as Table 8.1 illustrates. The East had fewer public and voluntary beds in proportion to its population of 65-and-overs than any other region. This has significance for the problems of the acute hospitals because private nursing homes do not offer the same range of supports for patients with high dependency and care needs as public institutions, so they may not be able or prepared to accept many post-acute patients. Furthermore, the location of private nursing homes is unplanned and may not meet the needs of discharged patients to be within affordable or practical reach of their families or spouses.

The then Minister for Health, Micheál Martin, announced plans in 2002 for the development of community nursing units for older people by public-private partnership (PPP). It was anticipated that 17 new 50-bedded community nursing units would provide 850 new beds in the East and the South, which the Minister described as the areas of most acute need. Services offered in the units were to include 'assessment/rehabilitation, respite, extended care, elderly mentally infirm and convalescent.' Day centres for the elderly were to be combined with the community nursing units in each site 'to help promote the dignity and independence of older people and to support them in living at home.'

The Minister said that 'the provision of the additional beds to be provided under the Pilot PPP Programme will free up acute hospital beds where older people may be inappropriately placed and provide a higher quality of care for those people who require the various services provided by Community Nursing Units.'[14]

For reasons which have not yet been publicly explained, the

Department of Finance did not sanction this development. The authors have heard from managers and health service professionals working in the East that this has been a great disappointment to providers of services. Had the 450 community nursing beds envisaged in this development for the East been provided in the three years to 2005, the problems of the acute hospitals could have been greatly alleviated. The PPP model proposed by the Minister was one in which the private partner would design, build, finance and operate the facility.[15] The state would own the facility, which would be run on a not-for-profit basis. It would be a public sector institution, with publicly salaried clinical and managerial staff, although facility maintenance staff would be supplied by the private sector operator. Such units would offer more complex care than the private, for-profit nursing homes which the government has effectively chosen to substitute for them. Development of these facilities would have required the Department of Finance to sanction an increase in public health service employment, which has been subject to a cap since 2002. The cap does not apply to growth in employment in private sector nursing homes, although these are subsidised by the Exchequer. We discuss the cap and its effects in Chapter 11.

The shortage of appropriate facilities for post-acute care predictably remains a major problem, particularly in the East. Comhairle na nOspidéal reported in 2004 that:

> One of the major difficulties experienced by patients and hospitals…is the shortage of alternative facilities and services such as rehabilitation, community care support and long term nursing care, for patients no longer in need of acute medical care. One Dublin hospital informed the committee that, at any one time, the hospital would have in the region of 60–70 patients awaiting placement in long term care. Delays in accessing long stay beds for these patients can range from six months up to three years. Twenty per cent of these patients are in the younger/middle-age group. The committee was informed of similar situations in other hospitals throughout Ireland.[16]

Pat McLoughlin, then chief executive of the National Hospitals Office (NHO), told the Joint Oireachtas Committee on Health and Children in April 2005 that:

> It is clear that the accident and emergency service is heavily dependent on the quality of services in the community for elderly patients. It is a medical admissions issue for the elderly. I have visited accident and emergency departments and they have confirmed that. At any one time, up to 400 beds are blocked, particularly in the Eastern region, with patients who could be cared for elsewhere. These include patients who are awaiting nursing home assessments, people awaiting long-term care, young chronic sick patients, those awaiting palliative care and patients who are awaiting adaptations to their home, for example, after a stroke. A variety of people make up that 400.[17]

The state-incentivised private provision in the period since 2001 and the measures for post-acute care announced by the current Minister for Health in 2004 as part of the 10-point plan will not provide either the amount or mix of care places which the Health Strategy envisaged. In extended care, as in acute care, the government has apparently abandoned the strategy's assessment of need without making this explicit or offering an alternative. Instead, as in acute care, the government continues to turn to private provision.

Over a year, the funding for the Minister's plan enabled the HSE to find places in private nursing homes for 48 patients with high-dependency needs. The Minister wanted the HSE to move 100 such patients to private nursing homes, but the private sector could not offer sufficient places with the more high-tech care, e.g. intravenous drips and oxygen, that these patients needed. As an alternative, the HSE began moving low-dependency patients out of public long-stay institutions and into private nursing homes to enable the public institutions to offer more high-dependency places. To achieve this without forcing the relocated patients to pay a proportion of private nursing homes' fees, the HSE contracted beds from private nursing homes, in effect adding them to the public bed stock. The cost efficiency of this method of providing public long-stay places has yet to be scrutinised. The HSE also turned to the private sector to locate places for intermediate care patients, who would return home after six weeks or so. This recourse to the private sector could have been partially obviated even in the short term because at least 65 long-stay beds had been closed in a number of public Dublin institutions, with the cap on public sector employment having contributed to their closure.

Palliative care is another area of post-acute care with considerable unmet needs. There can be as many as 14 patients in St Vincent's Hospital in Dublin at any one time who are terminally ill and in need of palliative rather than acute care. The *Report of the National Advisory Committee on Palliative Care* in 2001 recommended a specialist inpatient unit in every health board region to act as the hub of a hospital and community service and between eight to 10 inpatient hospice beds per 100,000 population. A study published in October 2005 reported that many of the 2001 report's recommendations had not been implemented. Only seven of the country's 35 acute General Hospitals with over 150 beds had full palliative care teams, and 11 hospitals had no service or depended on external support from community-based teams.

To provide 10 inpatient hospice beds per 100,000 population would require 390 beds. The current number of beds was 135. At December 2004 there were five specialist inpatient units which provided day care services for 538 patients (accounting for 5,961 attendees) in the year. There were no specialist inpatient units in the Midlands, North-East and South-East regions and in consequence no day care services in those regions.[18]

Community care

The Minister for Health stated in 2005 that as many as 5,000 older people who were in nursing homes could be cared for in their own homes with appropriate support and that she intended to increase supports for older people in the home.[19] In the 2006 Budget, she announced €150 million of additional funding for care of the elderly, largely in the form of enhanced community care, including additional funding for palliative care. The authors welcome this development but caution that such is the evidence of unmet need in care provision for older people that these extra supports for people at home should complement but not substitute for the expansion of extended care facilities planned in the

Health Strategy.

An OECD study published in 2005 showed that whereas 5 per cent of Irish people aged 65 or over were receiving home care benefits, this compared with over 20 per cent in the UK, nearly 15 per cent in Australia and Austria and 9 per cent in Sweden.[20] In 2005, the Institute of Public Health published a study which found that 7 per cent of people aged 65 and over in the Republic of Ireland had received home help services in the preceding 12 months compared to 17 per cent in Northern Ireland.[21] An evaluation of existing Irish home care grant schemes undertaken for the Eastern Regional Health Authority (ERHA) in 2004 observed that inadequacy of funding was resulting in a build-up of unmet need. Public health nurses and social workers interviewed for this evaluative study reported a 'high level of unmet care needs among older people in their areas.' They were concerned that 'a lot of older people are returning after a hospital stay to their homes to live in circumstances which are not always as safe as they should be.' They also observed that many families would qualify for home care grants 'if they knew about the system and if they were given access to it, but the lack of funding prevents this.'[22]

Whereas a publicly provided home help service has been a feature – albeit an erratic and under-funded one – of Irish community care for some time, giving direct home care grants to older people to purchase home supports privately is a new development, partially driven by the inadequacy of public community care. Dr Virpi Timonen, author of the 2004 evaluation of home care grant schemes for the ERHA, observed:

> Inadequacy of basic home help services, due to funding constraints, recruitment difficulties and lack of adequate structures, is causing a problem in that large numbers of older people in need of help are experiencing problems in accessing services. Lack of adequate day care and respite care services, and the uneven distribution of these services across the country, also poses a problem…One of the main motives behind the introduction of homecare grants was responding to the unmet care needs resulting from the absence or inadequacy of other services.

It emerges that in the community as in institutional care for

older people, the government has preferred to fund private provision rather than expand public provision. This new policy of
direct grants raises many issues. Dr Timonen recommended that
there should be more careful monitoring of the quality and adequacy of services purchased with the grants, and that there should
be mechanisms to ensure that the grants were adequate (since
over 50 per cent of those surveyed did not find them sufficient).[23]
The grants have since been increased by the HSE. The authors
would recommend that they should be up to the level of private
nursing home subvention offered by the government, since it is
medically and socially desirable to encourage older people to
remain in their own homes for as long as they can.

The expansion of care represented by the home care packages
may have been more apparent than real because it seems to have
coincided with a significant cutback in public home help provision. The Department of Health's personnel census no longer
includes home helps and it was never comprehensive, since in
some parts of the country the state funds home help services
through voluntary agencies and does not count numbers
employed. However, the Department has a count for most of the
state, apart from the East. This shows a 19 per cent drop in the
number of home helps employed (wholetime equivalent basis)
from a peak of 2,694 in 2001 to 2,180 by March 2005.[24]

The 2006 Budget expansion in funding for the elderly contained additional allocations for both home care packages and
home helps. This simultaneous expansion of both services should
result in an expansion of community care. However, taken
overall, the government's preference for private provision and its
abandonment of the Health Strategy's goals was once more evident in this package. The Minister announced no planned
expansion in public long-stay places for the elderly. The package
instead included €8 million 'to cover the cost of 250 extra
nursing home beds which the HSE is already in the process of
sourcing from private nursing homes.'

Dr Timonen reported that there were no national standards
for any form of home care service, including home help services
provided by health boards.[25] The issue of consistent inspection
and standard setting also arises in institutional care. The 2001

Health Strategy stated that the remit of the Social Services Inspectorate would be extended to include residential care for older people and that national standards for community and long-term residential care of older people would be prepared. Neither has happened. The existing position is untenable. The HSE, a provider and purchaser of care, is responsible for policing providers' standards. In our discussion of health administration in Chapter 12, we recommend that as an independent institution, HIQA should be statutorily empowered to require externally validated standards in Ireland's health care system, including public and private long-stay care facilities. HIQA should have statutory powers to inspect extended care facilities and police these standards.

The 2005 OECD study observed that 'examples of inadequate care in institutional and community settings are numerous' internationally. Bringing quality up to expectations would require 'increasing public spending and initiatives in better regulation of long-term care services, such as by establishing quality assessment and monitoring outcomes.'

The OECD advised that better quality care would require improved staffing levels and improved pay and working conditions for staff in long-stay care to make sure qualified jobs in the sector remained competitive with alternative acute health care jobs. Staff shortages and staff qualifications were the number one concern of long-term care policy-makers in OECD countries.[26]

Paying for post-acute and community care

Remedying the deficiencies in post-acute care will require investment in facilities and staff. As Deloitte & Touche observed, services must be built up from a historically low base. However, there is encouragement to be taken from the OECD study, which reported that 'even in countries with relatively comprehensive coverage, spending on long-term care is currently only 10 to 20 per cent of total spending on health and long-term care together. In addition there is no evidence that long-term care expenditure has grown faster than spending on acute health care – at least after an initial period of introduction of long-term care programmes.'[27]

A study by Mercer in 2003 on the future financing of long-term care in Ireland noted the survey evidence that the Irish public was strongly in favour of public coverage of long-term care. It concluded that the case for the state to take the lead in care 'seems compelling, having regard to the uncertainty and to the distribution of the risk of needing long-term care.' Mercer argued for a universal approach to financing long-term care. This should include statutory entitlement to home care benefits to promote the policy of maintaining people in the community as far as possible. Mercer advocated financing through the social insurance (PRSI) system: 'The strong entitlement to benefit that social insurance financing would confer, along with earmarking of the contributions to pay for the benefit, would, we believe engender good public support.'[28]

After the enactment in 2005 of new legislation to give a statutory footing for charges in public long-stay institutions, and the introduction of measures to reimburse patients who had been charged without legal basis, and given the continued controversy about charges faced by patients in private long-stay institutions who cannot be accommodated in public care,[29] it is evident that Irish society needs to address this issue in an honest and coherent manner. If it is indeed the consensus or majority view that long-stay care, like acute care, should be available universally to all who need it, then a manner of sharing the cost must be found, and the Mercer proposal has considerable merit. We recommend that the state should take responsibility for providing a secure, well-funded and high-quality system of long-term care for frail elderly, severely disabled and others unable to care for themselves, to be provided by or funded by the state, either from taxation or social insurance, or with a co-payment element, which is proportionate to the income and assets of the beneficiary but is neither an unpredictable private charge, nor an effective confiscation of the income of pensioners, as is currently the case.

Mental health services

Mental health services are another area of care where under-resourcing of services in the community affects the functioning of acute hospitals. For the last four decades the national policy on mental health care has been to move from large centralised institutions towards a community-based approach.[30] In keeping with this policy, mental health units have been developed in general hospitals, supported by a network of community-based facilities. But the provision of community-based residences since de-institutionalisation has not been adequate, particularly in the East, leading to a situation where a 1999 study of mental health services in the East found that 45 per cent of acute psychiatric beds were occupied by those who no longer required acute care but for whom alternative community-based facilities were unavailable. One-third of these people were homeless.[31] Agencies for the homeless have estimated that 40 to 50 per cent of homeless people suffer from mental illness.[32] It has been reported that one in four inmates in Irish prisons was homeless when sent to prison and more than 80 per cent of these were using heroin and/or cocaine on committal. Of the 25 per cent of the 3,200 prison population who were homeless on committal, one in three had been previously diagnosed with a mental illness and two in three had spent time in a psychiatric hospital.[33]

Among those who present at A&E departments are people who become acutely psychotic, or those who have engaged in deliberate self-harm, estimated by the National Parasuicide Registry at more than 11,000 cases in 2003. These people ought to be assessed by the mental health services, yet as we noted in Chapter 1, mental health services are under-resourced. Many general hospitals do not have liaison psychiatry services that should properly undertake this work.

The World Health Organization (WHO) acknowledges the enormous burden of disability caused by mental illness, and suggests that approximately 20 per cent of total health-related disability falls in the domain of mental ill health.[34] This high level of disability has not been reflected in resource allocation or service development. Public spending on mental health has declined from 10.7 per cent of the total health spend in 1990 to 6.7 per cent in 2004, and is forecast at 6.6 per cent in 2005. The equivalent spend in Northern Ireland is 9.2 per cent, and in

England and Wales, 11.6 per cent. There appears to be no governmental recognition of the need to develop and deliver a quality and comprehensive mental health service.[35]

There has been a considerable increase in spending on disability programmes, from 9.6 per cent of current health spending in 1990 to 12.4 per cent in 2004 and a forecasted 12.5 per cent in 2005. It might be argued that increased spending on disability should result in reduced demands on psychiatric institutions, which had traditionally and inappropriately housed many people with disabilities. However, current spending on both programmes combined was in 2004 (and remained in 2005) a smaller proportion of the health care budget than in 1990 – 19.1 per cent compared to 20.3 per cent. It is evident from the notoriously outmoded facilities of some Irish long-stay public psychiatric institutions that this sector requires much greater capital investment. The sale of some of the valuable land on which many of these institutions are located could provide capital for service modernisation and development.

The *Report of the Inspector of Mental Health Services 2004* presents a picture of:

- Deficiencies in acute care, well illustrated by the serious failure to develop a range of specialty services, and the long-recognised lack of availability of inpatient units for adolescents.
- Deficiencies in community care, evidenced by the movement of people from long-stay wards to community residences which, in the absence of dedicated rehabilitative input, has for some done little to change the social isolation and loss of independence associated with life in institutional care. Such residences have become little better than long-stay wards in a community setting.
- Considerable variation in indices of service development, resource and activity, reflecting the absence of a national minimum standard of care and modern mental health strategy.

In January 2006, the *Report of the Expert Group on Mental Health Policy* was published. The Minister for Health said its 'values and principles would guide both Government and service providers'.[36] The report was radical in scope. It recommended that 'steps be taken to bring about the closure of all psychiatric hospitals and to re-invest the resources released by these closures in the mental health service.' It envisioned 'an active, flexible and community-based mental health service where the need for hospital admission will be greatly reduced.'

The authors welcome the report but caution that it is critical that closures should be *preceded* by the provision of adequate alternative community facilities if the history of recent decades is not to be repeated and the population of homeless mentally ill greatly expanded. This implies that for some time institutional and community facilities should operate in parallel, which will require considerably increased funding for mental health services. The Expert Group recognises that implementing its recommendations will require substantial funding but points out that 'there is considerable equity in buildings and lands within the current mental health system, which could be realised to fund this plan.' While this is true, there is a substantial risk that this equity might be unlocked by closing outmoded institutions prior to the establishment of alternative community facilities, and that, as in recent history, the alternatives would prove insufficient to meet need. In mental health, as in care of the elderly, services need to be planned, expanded and funded in response to analysis of unmet need, not as stop-gap measures to reduce pressures on acute hospitals.

How far have we gone to resolving the A&E crisis?

How does one measure progress in resolving the A&E crisis? Since the problems of A&E reflect problems in so many other aspects of the health service, unless there is progress in resolving problems elsewhere, improving the experience of patients in A&E may only be achieved at a cost to patients with other competing demands on the health service. Medical patients may gain faster admittance to hospital beds, but elective operations may be cancelled, eventually leading to longer public waiting lists. Inpatient wards may accept additional patients on extra beds or trolleys, but the cost may be borne in increased infection due to greater overcrowding. Patients in need of long-stay care may be discharged from hospital more rapidly, but if community care services are inadequate to their needs, or the standard of care in long-stay institutions is poor, then they may pay a price in poor health or premature death, or may simply reappear in A&E. The homeless mentally ill may be discharged to the streets.

The HSE stated at end-September 2005 that its priority in implementing the 10-point plan was to maximise patient safety and comfort, and to make A&E and hospitals as efficient as possible, so that patients could move through the department and hospital 'in the most appropriate and efficient manner': 'In a scenario where people have been awaiting admission on trolleys in an Accident and Emergency Department, it is clearly safer and more appropriate to, where possible, have one ward absorb one extra bed for a short period.'

The HSE pointed out prematurely in September 2005 that since the introduction of the plan, the number of people waiting for admission from A&E departments had decreased. The rise in numbers on trolleys in subsequent months suggests that this reduction had been caused by seasonal factors like reduced illness and hospital attendance, and did not represent a sustained improvement.

The government's approach to addressing the A&E problem could unwittingly exacerbate it, for if it takes admission to hospital to secure supports for living at home or accelerated access to long-stay care, then older patients and their doctors may be encouraged to seek hospital admission. The HSE is not unaware of this potential 'pull factor' through hospitals. This potential problem demonstrates that provision for long-stay and community care should be planned, funded and delivered in response to an objective assessment of need in the community, not turned on and off in the form of short-term purchases from the private sector and in response to a hospital trolley count.

The number of patients with delayed discharge from Dublin hospitals tended to fluctuate between 350 and 375 in the autumn and winter of 2005 to 2006. There was still a very real sense that any big increase in illness, or worse still, a serious epidemic like avian flu, could plunge hospitals and their A&E departments into even deeper crisis.

What measures could help? The authors recommend that any

existing public long-stay capacity should be reopened immediately. In the short term, public purchases of private nursing home care, flexibility in working practices and better hospital team-working can play a role in easing A&E pressures. But the real solutions will take longer and require investment in public long-stay, community and acute care. Acute medical units should be developed in all acute hospitals. The AMUs for Tallaght, Beaumont and St Vincent's should be fast-tracked by government.

As a matter of urgency, the government should develop public community nursing units for older people, as envisaged in the Health Strategy. The units should offer services and facilities for assessment/rehabilitation, respite, extended care, care of the elderly mentally infirm and convalescence. Day centres for the elderly should be combined with the community nursing units. The first of these units should be developed without delay in Dublin, where inadequate extended care facilities place the greatest pressure on acute hospitals. Community care supports for people at home should complement, but not substitute for, the expansion of extended care facilities planned in the Health Strategy. Lastly, the state should take responsibility for providing a secure, well-funded and high-quality system of long-term care for people who are unable to care for themselves.

9

SPECIALIST CARE IN THE ACUTE HOSPITAL SETTING

Medical practitioners

In Ireland, medical practitioners fall into two main groups: specialists, providing care in, or based in, acute hospitals, as discussed in this chapter; and general practitioners (GPs), providing primary care in the community, as discussed in Chapter 6. Specialists in turn fall into two main groups: consultants and non-consultant hospital doctors (NCHDs). In general, most specialists are salaried employees, though as we have discussed earlier (see Chapters 4 and 5), some have private practices as well, making them self-employed practitioners to that extent. In general, GPs are self-employed.

About 78 per cent of Irish doctors are Irish or EU nationals; the non-nationals are found predominantly among NCHDs.[1]

Specialist care

Specialist care in an acute hospital setting is provided by specialist consultants and by medical graduates in sub-consultant, mainly training, posts collectively known as non-consultant hospital doctors (NCHDs).

Consultants are fully trained, skilled physicians deemed ready to assume full responsibility for patient care. NCHDs are junior physicians who have not yet completed their post-graduate specialist training. In order of ascending skill and seniority, NCHDs are interns (in their first post-graduate training year); house officers; registrars; and senior and specialist registrars.

On 1 January 2005, there were 1,947 approved permanent consultant posts and 4,170 approved NCHD positions salaried in the public sector in Ireland. Because NCHDs outnumber consultants, and, moreover, presumably work longer hours,[2] it is they who provide the majority of specialist care in an acute hospital setting in Ireland. They do so under the (sometimes nominal) supervision of consultants. For this reason, the Irish system of specialist care has been described as a 'consultant-led' service, as distinct from a 'consultant-provided' service. A consultant-led service is defined[3] as 'a service supervised by consultants who lead and advise teams of doctors in training and other staff in the delivery of care to their patients', while a consultant-provided service is one 'delivered by teams of consultants, where the consultants have a substantial and direct involvement in the diagnosis, delivery of care and overall management of patients.'

The Hanly Report[4] has called for a shift to a consultant-provided service, a proposal endorsed by the authors. Such a change, if achieved, would effect a major transformation in the character of specialist care in Ireland. It would require a substantial increase in the numbers of consultants, approximately doubling the present number of posts.

Under the present consultant-led service, most specialist care is provided by under-trained and over-worked junior physicians. There are three important further negatives in the current arrangement:

- It exacerbates the two-tier system of acute care. It would not be false to say that care of private patients in public hospitals is already a consultant-provided service, while care of public patients is a deficient consultant-led service. Care for private patients in public hospitals is provided by consultants, who, while they receive salaries for treatment of public patients, also receive fees for treatment of private patients, treatment sometimes provided during the hours for which their public salary is paid. That means that there is less consultant time available either for care of public patients or even for leadership of care.

- NCHDs often work without benefit of supervision by consultants, especially in smaller hospitals.
- Many NCHD posts provide no real training. The Hanly Report (discussed further in Chapter 10) proposed top-to-bottom reform of the training system, with training provided only in settings with senior supervision, free time for training and a statutory post-graduate training authority to co-ordinate, manage, regulate and inspect teaching hospitals. The Buttimer Report, released in early 2006, proposed phasing out NCHD posts with limited training value, a recommendation accepted by the government.[5]

Shortage of specialist doctors

It is acknowledged that Ireland has a consultant shortage and a specialist shortage. The Hanly Report proposed more than doubling consultant numbers, from 1,731 to 3,600, by the year 2013. Even when NCHDs are counted, Ireland has a specialist shortage. In 2005 Ireland had 0.5 consultants (public and private) per 1,000 population. If NCHDs are also counted, Ireland had 1.55 specialist doctors per 1,000 population compared to an EU15 average of between 1.8 and 1.9.[6] To meet the EU average for the current population, Ireland would require 7,641 specialist doctors, an additional 1,230 doctors.

After one completes medical school, one must serve at least eight years as an NCHD in training positions. Training consists of the first or intern year, after which the graduate is eligible for listing in the General Medical Register, as discussed below; at least two years as senior house officer; and then five or six years as senior or specialist registrar. The NCHD category has been the most rapidly growing in Ireland in recent years, in effect compensating for the shortfall in numbers of consultants. There are insufficient numbers of Irish (or other EU) medical graduates to fill the NCHD positions, which have therefore been filled with large numbers of non-Irish (and non-EU) nationals.

One reason for the shortfall in Irish nationals among NCHDs is that there has been a cap on the number of Irish (or EU) nationals enrolled in Irish medical schools of 305 per year. A taskforce, the Medical Education and Working Group (or the Fottrell Working Group), which released its report early in 2006, recommended an increase in the cap from 305 to 725 per year, a proposal accepted by the government.[7] One reason for the cap was that non-EU students pay full fees and medical schools have come to depend on high numbers of them as a source of revenue. If that revenue were not to be lost, the total number of places in Irish medical schools would have to increase. An additional €4 million will be provided in the Education Vote in 2006 to allow for an additional 70 EU places in undergraduate medicine in the autumn of 2006.

The authors support the increase in the cap, an increase in the overall number of places in Irish medical schools and an increase in state funding of medical education.

Students go from Leaving Certificate to medical school. As an alternative track, the Fottrell Working Group has proposed enrolment in medical school as a post-graduate subject, as in the US, a recommendation which has been accepted by the government. The authors support this proposal as well.

These changes will also help address the GP shortage, discussed in Chapter 6.

Consultants' contract

In Chapter 4 we outlined some reasons why the consultants' common contract is one of the most problematic and controversial issues in the Irish medical care system. It is widely criticised because it permits consultants to receive a salary for being present in public hospitals but to delegate public patient care and earn fees for treating private patients during their salaried hours. Consultants are not accountable to anyone, either administratively or clinically. A significant minority of publicly-salaried consultants and a majority in Dublin hold contracts which permit them to conduct private practice in private hospitals.

The Value for Money (VFM) audit of the Irish health care system by the consulting firm Deloitte & Touche[8] expressed concern about the management implications of consultants' extraordinary degree of autonomy[9]:

Consultants are not subject to effective management from a non-clinical perspective...There are issues in relation to: scheduling time inputs; managing cover; provision of locums; managing rest days etc. This is further exacerbated by the degree of delegation to NCHDs.

Senior level clinical decision-making is not available within our system at all key times...A significant level of frontline services at Accident & Emergency are provided by NCHDs which has a consequential impact on requirements for additional tests, referrals to other NCHDs, and waiting times...

Deloitte & Touche were concerned with the management consequences of excessive delegation to NCHDs. Were they concerned with medical consequences, they might have mentioned the harmful effects excessive delegation has on quality of care, and hence necessarily on medical outcomes, patient health and even mortality.

The VFM report continued:

There is no question as to the consultants' rights in terms of clinical independence. However, the independent nature of consultants does provide other difficulties. A consultant must decide on what the balance in his practice will be between emergency and elective clinical work and between teaching, research, or other work. The employing authority has little control over what that balance should be. In addition the preferences of a consultant for a particular type of work within his specialty can over time dictate what gets referred to him. This profile of work may not necessarily match the overall needs and priorities of the Employing Authority.

The Brennan Commission Report, *Commission on Financial Management and Control Systems in the Health System*,[10] which was particularly critical of the consultants' contract, recommended that *new* consultants be signed to contracts which deny them private practices, requiring that they work exclusively in the public sector. The report also recommended that consultants be unambiguously accountable, both financially and clinically, for their work. The Brennan Commission accepted that existing consultants could not be brought under these terms, but recommended revisions in their contracts to make them less ambiguous and 'more transparent' and to underline consultant accountability. The authors endorse these recommendations.

In the interviews and consultations conducted by the authors in preparation for the present study, we found fundamentally no change in the picture as painted by the Brennan Commission and by Deloitte & Touche.

The authors regard the system described here to be wholly unacceptable. Clinical freedom must be preserved, but clinical freedom cannot mean an absence of clinical accountability (clinical accountability is discussed later in this chapter). Clinical freedom also cannot be interpreted as meaning an absence of administrative accountability. The job of a hospital CEO is an impossible nightmare when the key personnel are not obliged to accommodate to the needs of the hospital, region and health care system in which they work as salaried employees.

Clinical freedom and Catholic ethos

A number of voluntary hospitals, including the Mater and St Vincent's in Dublin, as well as the private hospitals the Blackrock Clinic and its sister institution, the Galway Clinic, profess a Catholic ethos. An issue arose in October 2005 showing that hospital management's interpretation of Catholic ethos may conflict sharply with hospital consultants' clinical freedom and with patient care.

As the issue arose in the Mater, Catholic teaching regarding birth control meant that a widely used cancer drug could not be used for patient care. As reported by Eithne Donnellan in *The Irish Times*:[11]

> The issue of religious influence on hospitals and how it can influence what services a hospital provides resurfaced in the past week, following a decision by the Mater hospital to defer giving approval for clinical trials of Tarceva, a cancer drug. The Mater was concerned that information in a leaflet drawn up for patients participating in the trials ran counter to the hospital's Catholic ethos.
>
> It was said initially this was because artificial contraception had to be used by women taking part, though it later emerged abstinence was also acceptable. Pregnancy had to be avoided

by women on the new drug as it could damage an unborn child.

The net result of the decision by the Mater is that patients at five hospitals across the State may, if they are suitable, be able to avail of a drug which can prolong life in people with advanced lung cancer, but patients at the Mater cannot. A clearly frustrated Dr John McCaffrey, a cancer specialist at the hospital, was quoted as saying doctors needed to be able to offer patients the best treatments available. 'We can't do that at the moment and it's a disaster,' he said.

Maurice Neligan, a heart surgeon at the Mater hospital for many years, said he was surprised in this day and age that something like this should happen.

'This is a Catholic hospital, but at the same time the sick are the sick, and we are meant to be a non-sectarian State,' he says. 'I would have thought anybody going into hospital would be entitled to receive the treatment they needed, or that the hospital would arrange for them to go somewhere else.'

Following adverse publicity, the Mater's board subsequently reversed the hospital's earlier decision and the hospital announced that the clinical trial would proceed.[12] The Mater campus was about to benefit from a major state investment, funding the redevelopment of the hospital and the relocation there of a children's hospital. At a reported €500 million, the cost of the project over time was comparable to the state's entire annual investment in health and social care facilities.[13]

There is a fundamental conflict between the very considerable state support the Mater and other voluntary hospitals receive and its decision to deny any patient the best care as determined by a senior consultant. There are other alternatives which are consistent with the continuation of a Catholic ethos at these voluntary hospitals. One would be that these hospitals not offer care in areas likely to create conflicts between clinical freedom and patient care on the one hand and Catholic ethos on the other. In this instance, for example, if the Mater anticipated a conflict between Catholic ethos and cancer care, it should arrange to close its cancer service and the Health Service Executive (HSE) could transfer that service to a public hospital. A less drastic solution would be for the voluntary hospital to arrange to transfer to other facilities any patients whose best care, as determined by the consultant, conflicted with the hospital's guiding ethos, as interpreted by hospital management. What does seem inappropriate is that the patient continues to be treated in the voluntary hospital but not be given the best care.

Remuneration of consultants

One of the most justly criticised features of the Irish health care system is the two-tier system of care in Irish acute hospitals. The two-tier system manifests itself primarily in two ways. Public patients often have to wait months or years longer for care than private patients. There are, unnecessarily and inequitably, two separate waiting lists for acute care. Private patients are almost certain to be treated personally by the consultant, while public patients are likely to be treated by an NCHD.

As is discussed in detail in Chapter 5, methods of remuneration of consultants play a central role in producing the two-tier system of care.

Consultants are paid by salary for their work for public patients and by fee for private patients. This gives consultants an economic incentive to privilege private patients over public patients. If consultants were paid in the same way, at the same rate, for public and private patients, their motive to privilege private patients would disappear.

Physician competence assurance and contract fulfillment

In most countries, there is a peer-governed mechanism protecting the public through mandatory physician quality assurance, clinical audit and continuing medical education. Also in most countries there is an employer-governed method to assure that doctors fulfil their contracts.

Neither exists in Ireland. The Medical Council, an institution established for peer governance by Irish physicians, has signaled that it is ready for competence assurance but awaits overdue revision of the Medical Practitioners Act. There has been no movement toward assurance of contract fulfilment by the General Medical Service, which contracts with GPs, or the HSE, which contracts with specialist consultants.

The Drogheda scandal

In 1998, it came to light that a County Louth consultant obstetrician practising in Our Lady of Lourdes Hospital in Drogheda had performed what ultimately proved to be over a hundred hysterectomies on women undergoing caesarean sections over a period of more than 20 years. Approximately 130 women have identified themselves as possible victims of operations unnecessarily removing their wombs. The Medical Council, whose role in the Irish health care system is described in more detail below, struck the physician off the register of physicians in 2003, a power vested in them under law, performed through their Fitness to Practice Committee.

Our purpose in raising this case, which made headlines for years, is not to review the scandal of one doctor's shockingly inappropriate care. Further, we will not comment on the legal actions which have been brought and may still be brought. Instead, what cries out for debate and action is the system under which this physician's practices, which were far from secret and which occurred in a major Irish hospital, failed to come to light for years, even decades.

The alarm was finally raised by two nurses in the Drogheda hospital, not by the doctor's fellow consultant obstetricians, not by his senior registrar obstetrician colleagues, not by the anaesthetists and pathologists who were necessarily involved in these surgeries and not by the London-based Royal College of Obstetricians and Gynaecologists, which provides limited clinical oversight for the Drogheda obstetricians.

Mr Finbar Lennon, a consultant general surgeon in Our Lady of Lourdes Hospital, Drogheda, and at the time medical adviser to the North Eastern Health Board, commented on how such events could be for so long unnoticed:

> The explanation that we, his fellow professionals, did not know or appreciate what was happening is a sad indictment of our medical system and how it is regulated. His failure was our failure. We did not recognise his faultline, correct it and assist him. The events in Drogheda represent both individual and collective professional failures as well as corporate and institutional failures. The latter may well be the more significant.[14]

The reason it did not come to light is that there are no formal peer review requirements for practising consultants or GPs in Ireland and no mandatory system of clinical audit. Though the doctor's unusual proclivity for caesarean-hysterectomies seemingly escaped the notice of many potential protectors of the public interest, in fact none of them had either the responsibility or the authority to intervene, and under Irish law and the consultants' common contract, he was not clinically accountable to any of them, or in fact to anyone, with the exception of the Medical Council, an accountability dependent on a formal complaint being lodged.

This means that, even today, there could be other, similar cases which have yet to come to light, or which, in fact, may never come to light.

That may not be the biggest problem. Even if there may be no physicians quietly endangering patients with scandalously inappropriate patterns of care, it is almost certain that across Ireland there are widely varying standards, methods and qualities of consultant – and GP – care, resulting in insufficient, excessive or inappropriate care, harmful or dangerous to patients and costly in economic terms. Modern health care around the world, with the exception of Ireland, increasingly includes mandatory peer review, clinical audit and a set of techniques known as quality assurance (QA) and quality improvement (QI).

QA and QI are typically periodic mandatory inter-disciplinary processes, governed and led by physician peers but including other clinicians and even lay persons, designed to maintain adequate standards and to raise standards of the delivery of preventative, diagnostic, therapeutic and rehabilitative measures. In many countries, QA and QI are part of standard procedures in hospitals. They are less well developed in out-of-hospital primary care.

The Medical Council

The Medical Council,[15] a statutory regulatory body for Irish doctors, regulates the medical profession in Ireland, as provided for in the Medical Practitioners Act 1978. It has a duty of care on behalf of the state to supervise undergraduate medical education and post-graduate training of specialists, in both general practice and consultancy streams. The Medical Council registers doctors on their General Medical Register when they become eligible to practise. To practise, Irish doctors must appear on this register.[16] The Council also maintains a Register of Medical Specialists for physicians who have successfully completed specialist training, in either a general practice or a consultancy stream. There is no legislation requiring practising GPs or consultants to be listed on the specialist register. However, to be a publicly salaried consultant, a doctor must be eligible for the Specialist Register and must have obtained membership (by showing competence) in the relevant self-governing specialty college, e.g. Royal College of Physicians in Ireland.[17]

Through its Fitness to Practice Committee, the Medical Council also considers complaints (its own or those brought by others) against registered doctors. It has the power[18] to strike doctors from the General Medical Register on two grounds: their professional misconduct or mental or physical disabilities which adversely affect their ability to practise. It also has available a range of other sanctions which it can employ.

Hence, it will be seen that in the exercise of this power, the Medical Council primarily plays a disciplinary role. However, the Medical Council is prepared to expand its role. In 2003, the Council initiated a process which it calls competence assurance, under a system which it calls Competence Assurance Structures (CAS).

Competence Assurance Structures

The Medical Council lacks the legislative authority to make CAS mandatory. Doctors can participate on a voluntary basis, and the structure is ready for legislative changes which are needed for mandatory participation. Obviously, a voluntary mechanism does not go very far to protect patients. Physicians who would not meet the standards will simply decline to participate. Not every physician who does not participate can be assumed to fail to meet the CAS standards, of course.

According to the Council, 'The purpose of CAS is to ensure that doctors maintain the necessary knowledge and skills to function as effective practitioners throughout their working lives. In this way, CAS aims to enhance the standard of care provided by all doctors and to protect the public from those who are performing poorly.'[19]

There are two separate components of CAS. The first is a set of quality assurance processes the Medical Council refers to as Clinical Quality Assurance (CQA). The second consists of performance appraisal processes to identify and work with doctors who may be performing poorly.

Clinical Quality Assurance

CQA in turn is comprised of three programmes: continuing medical education (CME), clinical audit and peer review.

The CME component is in place. Doctors acquire CME credits in a variety of ways to keep their knowledge fresh and current with advances in medical knowledge. CME is wholly voluntary and not all doctors participate. In particular, GPs generally do not participate.

While CME has been introduced on a voluntary basis, clinical audit and peer review procedures do not exist on any basis. The Council states:

> The Medical Council recognises that Clinical Audit and Peer Review cannot be introduced until the necessary statutory and financial supports are in place. Among other things, this will necessitate a revision of the 1978 Medical Practitioners Act. In anticipation of legal reform and resolution of funding issues, the Medical Council is now actively planning for the introduction of Clinical Audit and Peer Review.[20]

The Medical Council is not ready to present its clinical audit and peer review programmes. It has funded eight pilot projects in clinical audit and peer review and states that it expect that the pilot projects will yield appropriate models of clinical audit and peer review.

The introduction of clinical audit and peer review is waiting on legislation. It is hard to imagine a more important regulatory reform for the Irish health care system. The authors strongly call for the needed legislation to be enacted without further delay.

Performance appraisal

The Medical Council is also establishing procedures to identify and work with doctors whose performance is poor, though they may not be guilty of professional misconduct.

The Royal Colleges

In each specialty, the appropriate Royal College provides a limited peer oversight mechanism. By establishing standards for membership, they define their respective specialist disciplines. They supervise the post-graduate training of specialists in hospitals. They do not provide a true clinical audit or peer review process.

Contract fulfilment

As has been seen, the consultants' contract is anomalous in many respects and can be regarded as among the most serious structural problems in the Irish health care system. It would not be a stretch to say that the central problem of the consultants' contract can be viewed as one of contract fulfilment.

Consultants are paid public salaries for being present in public hospitals for at least 33 hours each week, but they need not care for public patients during all (or any) of that time, though if and to the extent that they do not it is clear that they are not earning their salaries. Further, they need not account for their time. They are permitted private practices in public hospitals, and time spent treating private patients for fees can count toward the 33 hours obligated. It would be hard to imagine an employee contract as devoid of accountability.

Without accountability of key employees for their job performance, it is impossible to have an efficient organisation which achieves even adequate productivity. Nothing is more basic in any organisation than that salaried employees are accountable for fulfilment of their contracts.

The authors believe that consultants must be made legally accountable for care of public patients (or for other public work for which they do not receive a fee).

Malpractice

From time to time Irish medical practitioners are sued in court for medically negligent injuries to patients. Because court awards may be substantial, Irish doctors protect themselves with clinical indemnity, a form of insurance cover.

Employed medical practitioners are required by law to be indemnified against claims for negligence. In turn, the state pays for the largest share of the costs through a system called enterprise liability, through the Clinical Indemnity Scheme adopted in 2004.[21]

Does the medical malpractice system in Ireland provide another, additional method of competence assurance, along with or in place of clinical audit or peer review? This is an important question, but the answer is not known. There seems to be no published research on medical malpractice in Ireland. In the US, whose legal system differs in important respects from Ireland's, the medical malpractice system does not seem to serve such a function. In the US, research has shown that the majority of patients who are victims of medically negligent in-hospital injuries do not collect from the medical malpractice system, while the majority of those who do collect do not actually suffer from medically negligent injuries.[22]

Need for reform

The area of specialist care in acute hospital settings in Ireland is desperately in need of sweeping and radical reform. Effective management of hospitals, care equity, quality of care and patient life and health are all at stake.

There is a need for more consultant numbers and for a consultant-provided service in the public sector, as proposed in the Hanly Report. There is a need for more places in Irish medical education, as well as a need for structural changes in Irish medical education, as called for by the Fottrell Working Group. The Medical Practitioners Act must be revised immediately, with appropriate legislation providing a statutory basis for clinical audit and peer review.

The more difficult reforms are in consultant remuneration and the consultant contract itself. Reforming the consultant contract is extraordinarily challenging. In 2006 the Department of Health and the HSE were entering talks with the Irish Medical Organisation and the Irish Hospital Consultants Association concerning new terms for the contract. It is important that clinical and administrative accountability should be provided for in the new contract. It is no longer tolerable that salaried medical practitioners be answerable to no one for their care of patients and their use of time.

Should consultants with public appointments and substantial public paychecks be permitted to continue to have fee-paying private practices within their own hospitals, as provided for in Category I contracts, or in private hospitals, as provided for in Category II contracts? From the standpoint of public patients, permitting salaried consultants to have private practices is a failed experiment, with enormous costs. It is hard to disagree with the Brennan Commission's recommendation that henceforth, all new consultants be signed to contracts which deny them private practices, requiring that they work exclusively in the public sector. The authors have recommended the introduction of a common waiting list for patients in public hospitals (see Chapter 7), so that every patient has access to timely care based on need. To achieve this, the consultants' contract must be reformed. It is central to inequity in access to hospital care and is an obstacle to rational management in Irish hospitals. The authors appreciate that revising the contract will be a difficult and time-consuming process. A reformed contract should provide for clinical and administrative accountability; should require all consultants to treat patients according to need, drawn from a common waiting list; and should require all consultants to work as rostered members of teams, answerable to a head of department or clinical director, who is in turn answerable to the hospital/hospital group's CEO.

Part of the solution of the two-tier system of care will be to change the method of consultant remuneration. Ideally, as discussed in Chapter 4, consultants should be paid on behalf of both public and private patients under the same hybrid system. Consultants should continue to be paid a salary, to which private health insurance carriers would contribute in relation to covered private patients, and also fees in relation to all patients, public or private. Such a change does not require universal health insurance (UHI), but UHI obviously facilitates it.

If they are not pleased with the idea of a hybrid remuneration system common to both public and private patients, consultants might be asked what solutions they might offer which would achieve a common waiting list and a consultant-provided service for both public and private patients.

10

THE ORGANISATION OF ACUTE
HOSPITAL CARE

Introduction

In this chapter we address the related themes of how hospitals are medically staffed, where they are located and how they should be managed. There can hardly be an adult in Ireland who has not heard of the Hanly Report and who is unaware of the strong feelings it has provoked. Yet there has been little informed debate about it and scant effort by the government, which commissioned and published the report, to convince the public of the value of its recommendations and approach. The authors are convinced of the fundamental value of the Hanly argument for reform in medical staffing in order to achieve consultant-delivered care and for change in how hospitals work together to deliver care within a region in order to ensure patients are treated by highly skilled and practiced teams of physicians. But the authors also recognise the genuine fears felt by people who see services leaving their locality and who have little faith in their replacement. We believe those fears should be respected and that this has important implications for the context in which the implementation of the Hanly Report should take place.

Although Ireland has adopted a centralised model of health administration, we nonetheless see an opportunity for decentralisation within the hospital care system by giving greater power and autonomy to regional hospital networks. In this chapter, we explore how those hospital groups should be managed and governed, with boards reflecting the interests of their locality and major stakeholders. We advocate a system of funding which will incentivise hospitals yet protect them from unmitigated market forces. We suggest a governance structure for the regional centres of excellence, which should grow from well-resourced and well-thought-through implementation of the Hanly reforms.

What the Hanly Report said

In October 2003 the Minister for Health, Micheál Martin, published the *Report of the National Task Force on Medical Staffing* (popularly referred to as the Hanly Report because the taskforce was chaired by David Hanly).[1] This Report recommended a fundamental reorganisation of the Irish public hospital network.

The taskforce had been established by the Minister with the brief 'to devise an implementation plan for reducing substantially the average working hours of non-consultant hospital doctors (NCHDs) to meet the requirements of the European Working Time Directive (EWTD), to plan for the implementation of a consultant-provided service, and to address the medical education and training needs associated with the EWTD and the move to a consultant-provided service.' The taskforce's terms of reference gave it the task of 'devising, costing and promoting implementation of a new model of hospital service delivery based on appropriately trained doctors providing patients with the highest quality service, using available resources as equitably, efficiently and effectively as possible.'[2]

The EWTD required that by August 2004, NCHDs should not work for more than an average of 58 hours per week on the hospital site. By August 2007, they could not be required to work more than an average of 56 hours per week on-site, and by August 2009 this must decrease to an average of 48 hours. When the taskforce reported, there were 3,943 NCHDs, delivering frontline services in more than 40 public acute hospitals and many other health agencies. They worked an average of 75 hours per week on-site, 'often for continuous periods of more than 30 hours, with minimal rest'.

As the phased working limits took effect, the ability of NCHDs to provide medical cover for long periods of time would diminish significantly, the Report observed. In 2003 there were

1,731 hospital-approved consultant posts in public hospitals. Consultants were already covered by the EWTD and could not therefore work for more than an average of 48 hours per week.

The taskforce recommended more than doubling the number of consultants to 3,600 and almost halving the number of NCHDs to 2,200 in the 10 years to 2013. This would achieve a change from a ratio of one consultant post to every 2.3 NCHD posts, to a ratio of 1.6 consultants for each NCHD. It would mean a change from a 'consultant-led' service, in which much hospital care is delegated to junior doctors, to a 'consultant-delivered' service. The Report explained:

> This is in line with the recommendations of a number of reports on hospital medical staffing over the past two decades. It is also the only solution that simultaneously addresses the need to improve patient care, reform medical education and training and support the continued provision of safe, high quality acute hospital care 24 hours a day, 7 days a week. It contrasts with the present reliance on large numbers of NCHDs who work excessively long hours and have limited access to formal training.

Implementing this solution implied radical change to the organisation of hospitals, many of which had hitherto largely depended on NCHDs to provide care. The taskforce concluded that all hospitals providing emergency care must have acute medicine, surgery and anaesthesia on-site, which meant that 'an irreducible minimum' of 21 consultants, seven in each of medicine, surgery and anaesthesia, would be needed to provide basic on-site medical cover within a 48-hour working week. 'Comprehensive acute care' would require a minimum of 45 to 50 consultants.

As an illustration, the taskforce examined in detail what this would mean for two pilot areas: the mid-west or area surrounding Limerick, and on the east coast from north Wicklow to south Dublin. It recommended principles for how hospital networks should be organised nationally, without applying them in practice to the rest of the country. This was to be the work of a second report. However, due to the non-participation of consultants because of their dispute with the government over arrangements for professional indemnity cover, and perhaps also because of the political storm created by the publication of the first report, in 2005 the Minister for Health, Mary Harney, abandoned plans for a second report.

The Hanly recommendations for hospital networks

The Hanly recommendations for how hospital networks should be organised are as follows.

- *Major Hospital*: Ideally should have a catchment population of 350,000 to 500,000. Provides acute, consultant-provided care around the clock, seven days a week. Requires a minimum of seven consultant staff in each specialty and sufficient specialties to provide a spectrum of care. Implies a minimum of 45 to 50 consultants. The actual envisaged team of consultants is much larger, since consultants based at the Major Hospital will also work at the Local Hospitals (see below). The Major Hospital is the major trauma-receiving hospital for the region, responsible for regional emergency services and taking complex cases referred from other hospitals. Emergency cases are treated here and en route by ambulance staff trained as emergency medical technicians.
- *Local Hospital:* Here the consultant teams from the Major Hospital perform elective day surgery and medical procedures and attend outpatient clinics. Local general practitioners (GPs) might admit their patients here. Overnight patients would be long-stay and rehabilitative patients, with overnight nursing care but ultimately no overnight on-site medical presence. These hospitals would not offer a traditional accident and emergency (A&E) department. Instead, nurse-led minor injury units would handle less urgent cases, which currently constitute the majority of A&E cases. All major traumas and medical emergencies would go directly to the Major Hospital.
- *General Hospital*: In areas with widely dispersed populations, for many of whom it would be difficult to reach the Major Hospital in an emergency, this intermediate hospital would offer emergency care, but its range of services would not be as wide as in the Major Hospital.

- *National and supra-regional specialties*: National specialties like liver transplant to be offered at only one site. Supra-regional specialties like neurosurgery continue to be offered at only a few Major Hospitals.
- *Single specialty hospitals*: Maternity, orthopaedic or other specialised hospitals should ideally move to the site of the Major Hospital.

Discussion of the Hanly Report

The Hanly Report has raised a great many issues for local communities, for the staff of hospitals, for people working in primary and community care and for health service planners. None of these has been resolved because of the uncertain status of the Report's recommendations. In Chapter 12 we review the policy-operational divide between the Minister for Health and the new Health Service Executive (HSE). We argue that the location of hospital services is quintessentially a policy issue on which the Minister must give clear direction. To achieve that, she will need the clear support of the government.

The issue of the location of hospital services and of health and social services generally is also the essential stuff of democratic politics, which the Dáil should debate and in which the regional forums provided under the HSE legislation could play an important role in ensuring that communities and stakeholders have a voice about the kind of health and social services they would like to see develop.

The Hanly Report is readily available through the Department of Health or on its website, so we will not exhaustively reproduce its reasoning here. However, we wish to highlight a number of issues which arise from it.

Patient safety: the strongest argument in favour of Hanly

Tired doctors make mistakes. If those tired doctors are also relatively young and inexperienced, not in formal training programmes and not working under the direct supervision of fully trained superiors, then mistakes are even more likely. This is the sub-text to the Hanly Report, which tends not to be debated, because not even the Report's supporters – in the government or the Department of Health – want to tell the Irish public that Irish hospitals are not safe. The Hanly Report can be read to state this implicitly, as have earlier reports.[3] Notwithstanding this, a large number of Irish hospital doctors are relatively young, relatively inexperienced, work for too many hours and in many cases with inadequate training or senior supervision. For the Irish public, this is a strong argument in favour of adopting the direction proposed in Hanly, i.e. reducing the hours worked by NCHDs, ensuring that they have adequate training and supervision and changing hospital staffing so that consultants either treat most patients directly or very closely supervise their treatment.

Irish patient safety is further compromised by the very small size of many acute hospitals, where even the most senior doctors may see too few patients to enable them to maintain their skills in certain specialised areas. There are many procedures, especially in surgery, but in other specialties too, where doctors who do not perform a sufficient volume of them cannot maintain their expertise. The Report argued that 'there is convincing evidence that the best results in treatment are achieved when patients are treated by staff working as part of a multi-disciplinary specialist team and that better clinical outcomes are achieved in units with appropriate numbers of specialist staff with relevant skills and experience, high volumes of activity and access to appropriate diagnostic and treatment facilities.'[4]

For the Irish public, this is a further strong argument in favour of adopting the direction proposed in Hanly, i.e. concentrating acute services in major regional hospitals, which are well staffed and well resourced, so that patients receive the best possible care. There has been debate as to whether acute medical, i.e. non-surgical, care needs to be regionally centralised to the same degree as acute surgical care. This argument should be revisited in light of the needs and configuration of services in each region.

But hospital reorganisation must not be viewed in isolation

While in the authors' view these arguments for better care are compelling, we also consider it imperative that the reorganisation of hospital services should not be viewed in isolation from the many other factors which affect patients' access to and experience of care. These include primary care, community care, ambulance services, the capacity and quality of existing regional hospitals, travel distances to hospitals and the quality of roads, the quality and availability of public transport, population projections, spatial planning and the commitment of investment.

Proposals for the development of primary care have been discussed above. We believe that communities in many parts of Ireland depend on their local hospitals for the provision of services which they should rightly receive from well-resourced primary care networks. They consequently very much fear the loss of their local hospital emergency treatment room, even though patients with acute trauma may already bypass it to go to the regional hospital.

Every existing local hospital should also be the location for a 24-hour primary care centre, on the model proposed in the Primary Care Strategy. If care at such a centre were free at the point of access, and if experienced GPs were available to triage patients and access a local ambulance service for patients who need to go the regional hospital, patients would have achieved better access to higher-quality care than they often currently receive in local hospitals, largely staffed by unsupervised NCHDs. Investment in the ambulance service is also an essential prerequisite to hospital reorganisation.

It is axiomatic that patients should not receive inferior care or access to care because of hospital reorganisation. To ensure that is the case, the sequence in which reorganisation takes place is critical. It should only take place against a backdrop of investment in primary care, i.e. the convincing roll-out of the Primary Care Strategy; of investment and significant improvement in the ambulance service, both the vehicles themselves and the level of expertise of their staff; and of investment in and expanded capacity in regional hospitals. It follows, therefore, that there will have to be a period in which there is some duplication of services in which a new regional service gets up and running before the functions of a local hospital change. If this is not the case, patients will experience reduced access to care and may substitute long waits on trolleys in a regional hospital for the care of inexperienced NCHDs in a local hospital. This has already been the experience of some patients. That is medically unacceptable. It is also a sure path to preventing the convincing Hanly agenda for reorganised networks from ever acquiring popular and political understanding and support. The authors strongly advise that when hospital networks are reorganised, no service should be withdrawn before the substitution of a convincingly better service within the region.

When the National Hospitals Office (NHO) comes to planning regional networks, it must do so with an informed understanding of local transport routes and public transport services. In research for this study, the authors variously heard of a woman in her eighties with a fractured wrist who was obliged to take two buses and a six-hour round trip when orthopaedic clinics were centralised in her area, and of a young woman, injured because of domestic violence, who was taken by ambulance to a regional A&E department, was seen and treated there, and then found herself in the middle of the night many miles from her hometown, without money or any means of returning. No civilised health and social service should be planned or staffed in a manner which allows such treatment of patients.

In some former health board areas provision exists for transport supplied by the health board, e.g. local buses which take patients to outpatient clinics in Dublin hospitals. Local transport to and from regional hospitals must be planned for, costed and funded. In a number of border counties, there is obvious potential for cross-border co-operation in the provision of acute care. Residents of County Donegal could benefit from their proximity to Altnagelvin Hospital in County Derry and residents of County Monaghan from their proximity to Craigavon Hospital in County Armagh. We recommend the active pursuit of such potential for linkages.

Planning for population growth is a huge issue which affects much more than the health services. The population living and working in Ireland is growing rapidly. New towns are springing up around former villages without planning for schools, child care or public transport. As outlined in the earlier discussion of the government's failure to advance the increased bed targets of the 2001 Health Strategy, planning for additional health service capacity is effectively in stasis. This cannot continue. Reorganised hospital networks must be planned against the backdrop of up-to-date analysis of patterns of population growth and of local authorities' plans for accommodating future growth. If the HSE attempts hospital reorganisation without detailed and convincing plans for hospitals and other health services for a growing population, on which there is political sign-off and a commitment to multi-annual funding, it will almost certainly fail. Local opposition will grow and political support will dissipate. The losers will be the Irish people, who will continue to receive poor care in under-funded hospitals.

Hospital management, organisation and budgeting

As we have seen, the Hanly Report proposed a series of regional hospital networks, consisting of Major Hospitals staffed with 24-hour, seven-day consultant coverage, with full emergency services and serving catchments areas ranging from 350,000 to 500,000 populations, and a number of Local Hospitals with more limited services. Some regions with more dispersed populations might have intermediate General Hospitals providing emergency care. Some Major Hospitals might offer either national or supra-regional specialties.

The authors advocate the creation of a governing board, with significant local and regional representation, for each hospital network. The authors also advocate gradually increasing hospital autonomy, matched by increasing power, responsibility and accountability for the governing board. The Major Hospital and affiliated Local (and General) Hospitals in a region would constitute an organisational entity. They would have a single budget, would be led by a single CEO and would share consultant staff, some of whom would rotate among the hospitals to provide care.

The HSE initially announced 10 hospital networks and in June 2005 announced the appointment of seven permanent and three acting CEOs. But in October of that year, HSE CEO Brendan Drumm revealed plans to reduce the number of networks to four.[5] The authors have not seen Professor Drumm's plans in any detail, so it would be premature to judge his idea.

However, they are concerned that the Drumm plan may involve excessive centralisation and too few Major Hospitals.

The Hanly Report advocates a 'clinical directorate' model of internal management within hospital networks. In that model, seemingly based largely on the system in place at St James's Hospital, related specialties are grouped into units which are analogous to small business firms. Each directorate has responsibility and accountability for a defined group of patients. It is to have its own budget and will have considerable autonomy within the hospital. Each directorate has a clinical director, a nurse manager and a business manager. A purpose is to bring senior clinicians into management roles in hospitals,[6] and thereby to enable enhanced clinical and administrative accountability.

There are advantages and disadvantages in the clinical directorate model. It facilitates the kind of team care advocated by the Hanly Report. 'It improves accountability and responsiveness through a stronger link between the delivery of services and the use of resources.'[7] These are desperately needed values for Irish hospitals.

The main disadvantage of the clinical directorate model is that it weakens the already weak hospital CEO. While it brings rationality and accountability to sub-units within the hospital, it actually works against the integrity of the hospital, or hospital network, as an entity. The Hanly Report argues, 'The chief executive retains overall responsibility for the hospital, but delegates a wide range of important operational and planning functions to each clinical directorate.'[8] This euphemistic statement is actually false. 'Delegation' implies that the delegator has the authority and voluntarily relinquishes it to subordinates. In the Hanly model of clinical directorates, the hospital CEO *cedes* authority to the clinical directorates. The authors advocate a modified version of the clinical directorate in which budget and planning powers are retained by CEOs, who then can truly 'delegate' them to clinical directors.

The authors believe that clinical directors should be chosen by hospital CEOs, or at the very least with the concurrence of hospital CEOs.

From bureaucracy to decentralisation

As we described in Chapter 5, many European countries have moved to decentralise their health care systems, providing increased autonomy to important sub-units. The Irish system, particularly in relation to acute hospitals, retains the older, less flexible, more bureaucratic system of state control and micro-management. The creation of regional hospital networks, as contemplated in the Hanly Report, especially if each network is headed by a governing board with true authority and by a CEO with enhanced powers, facilitates a move toward flexibility and autonomy in the governance of Irish hospitals.

Neither the Hanly Report nor the newly structured HSE con-templates significant changes in the budget process, except that, as described, hospital budgets will go to regional networks of hos-pitals and, within them, clinical directorates. The authors advocate a gradual, step-by-step move toward decentralisation and autonomy.

Hospital budgeting

It is important to reform the way Irish hospitals get their budgets. The current method was discussed in Chapter 4.

There are three components in the budgets received by most Irish hospitals: budget allocation, casemix and revenues.

Budget allocation: Irish public hospitals receive an annual budgetary allocation which is primarily incremental. This method locks in historic inefficiencies and inequities and results in inter-regional inequities. There is an administrative discretion component, primarily to deal with changes in services or equip-ment from the prior year. This method is also inconsistent with hospital autonomy and it does not include any incentives for effi-cient behaviour.

Casemix: A small but growing proportion of budget amounts are based on casemix measurement. Under casemix, as discussed in Chapter 4, a hospital whose casemix was average in costliness has no adjustment. Hospitals with less complex or severe, and less costly, casemixes experience a reduction. Those with more costly casemixes receive an increment.

Under casemix, hospitals receive payments based in effect on the average national cost of treating a particular condition; those able to treat it at less cost than that gain financially, and those who do so at greater cost lose. Thus, hospitals share financially from any cost saving they are able to achieve. Casemix-adjusted budgets are consistent with increased hospital autonomy.

Revenue: The third component of Irish hospital budgets consists of revenues for patient care. These consist of charges imposed on private patients, nominal revenues from public patients who do not hold Medical Cards and payments from the National Treatment Purchase Fund (NTPF).

The present method of incremental budgeting should be replaced with a more flexible, more transparent and more equitable system. Further, hospitals should be paid in the same ways for public and private patients to remove any incentives for hospitals to differentiate between them in ways that favour private patients.

The authors advocate that hospital budgets should be set in large part on the basis of their case loads – the numbers of their patients, the conditions with which they are diagnosed, their severity and their treatments. This principle could be achieved through a combination of insurance-covered charges to patients, reflecting true economic costs of care, and casemix-based allocations from the state. Both charges and casemix-based payments result in the desired state in which 'money follows the patient'.

However, the authors believe that hospital budgets should not be based wholly on case loads. There should continue to be a significant component in the budgets of Irish hospitals which is set in a discretionary manner by the HSE. This component will permit budgets to reflect individual circumstances that vary from hospital to hospital and allow adjustments for added/closed services or equipment. They also might be thought of as providing a continuing payment to hospitals to reflect the service that hospitals provide to their communities through their mere existence and availability, apart from actual patient care. And non-case-load-based payments can act as a buffer between hospitals and their bottom lines, assuring that no hospitals need to automatically close or reduce services when demand for care declines.

Hospital autonomy

The casemix method of determining hospital budget allocations can be viewed as a move toward a purchaser-provider model. The budget reforms discussed above can be viewed as steps toward hospital autonomy, in place of the present bureaucratic command model. Ultimately hospitals – meaning in all cases major/local networks of hospital buildings – should make major capital investment, networking, service plan and personnel decisions.

The authors believe that every hospital network should have a governing board, which will act, as the HSE Executive Board does, as an interface between the HSE and the hospital. The governing board, which should represent a variety of interests – the state (the Department of Health, the HSE), local and regional economic interests, the trade union movement, non-governmental organisations (NGOs) and patients – should eventually have the power and responsibility to appoint the CEO, approve budgets and capital plans, hear audit reports and otherwise function as a governing board functions.

Thus, the system advocated here is one of regional networks of hospitals offering integrated, team-based, consultant-provided care; governed by strong CEOs working through clinical directorates and answerable to governing boards; with the boards in turn answerable to the HSE but reflecting the views and interests of localities and major stakeholders.

Conclusion

The authors recommend that hospital services should be reorganised to ensure a consultant-delivered service for all patients, to ensure supervised and genuine training for all NCHDs and above all, to ensure that patients, wherever they live, receive high and consistent standards of treatment and care. To achieve these objectives will inevitably require some smaller hospitals to cease offering A&E and acute surgery services. They will have to become satellite hospitals to larger regional centres. Every region should develop a genuine centre of excellence.

However, we caution that reorganisation of hospital services should not be viewed in isolation from the many other factors which affect patients' access to and experience of care. Smaller hospitals should not discontinue services until extra capacity and staffing have been provided in the regional centre to meet their needs.

We recommend a system of governance, funding and management which will foster strong, autonomous hospital groups, well connected with their communities and well aware of their needs. Such hospital groups should be in a position to plan integrated care with primary care networks and providers of continuing care in a region.

11

HEALTH SERVICE STAFFING

Introduction

A skilled labour force is central to the delivery of health and social care, thus planning to meet skill needs is critically important in health care. In Ireland, such planning has been notably deficient. Cutbacks in nurse training places in the 1990s contributed to shortages of nurses by the end of that decade. The subsequent expansion of training places has now increased numbers of graduating nurses, some of whom may not find employment in the public health sector because of an employment cap introduced in 2002. A cap on medical training places has given rise to serious shortages of domestically qualified doctors. In this chapter we examine trends in health sector employment; we analyse the effect of the cap, which, in combination with other policies, has substituted private for public health and social employment; we look at how Irish health employment and skills compare internationally; and we examine some recent analysis of Irish health care staffing needs.

Health and social services are highly labour intensive. Delivering more services generally requires more people: physiotherapists, psychologists, social workers, home helps, child care workers, receptionists and payroll clerks, as well as doctors and nurses. So when critics of increased health allocations say that all or most of the money has gone toward pay, this does not tell us whether it covers an increased payroll for additional employees delivering extra services, or an increased pay budget because of sectoral and national pay increases for existing employees delivering the same volume of services. In the recent past in Ireland, increased health spending has funded both.

The cap on health service employment

The Department of Health conducts an annual census of public health and social service employment, including employment in the publicly funded voluntary sector, such as the voluntary hospitals. Numbers employed rose rapidly in the years from 1997 to 2001, when there was a steep increase in health and social care budgets. In the years from 2001 to 2005, the increase was much less sharp, even though the 2001 Health Strategy had envisaged considerable further increases in health sector employment (see Table 11.1 below).

This slowing in the growth of health sector employment was a direct consequence of a government decision to cap employee numbers throughout the public service. The government took this decision in December 2002, when the international and national economic outlook was poor.[1] Public service employee numbers were to be capped at their existing authorised level and reduced by 5,000 across all sectors by the end of 2005. The government had been influenced by a report commissioned by the Department of Finance, which showed that numbers employed in the public service had increased by 19 per cent over four years, from 222,000 in 1997 to 265,000 in 2001, and that health had recorded a bigger increase than any other sector at 37 per cent. The *Report of the Independent Estimates Review Committee* observed that:

> Control of health service employment was devolved by the Department of Health and Children to health boards at end-2000. The Department's 2001 Health Service Census discloses that total employment was nearly 4,000 above the employment ceiling which had been approved by the Department of Finance. Centralised control of health service employment needs to be re-established by the Department of Health and Children as a matter of urgency.

Having rejected an embargo on public sector recruitment as 'too crude a policy instrument', the committee recommended:

In present circumstances overall employment in the public service (i.e. civil service, education sector, health sector, local authorities, security services and non-commercial State bodies) should be capped at existing levels and reduced where practicable. In each sector the emphasis should be on an appropriate skills mix policy aimed at maintaining the quality of service provided by front line delivery staff.[2]

Table 11.1: Numbers employed in public and voluntary health and social services, wholetime equivalents (WTE)

Health sector	Management /admin	Medical/ dental	Nursing*	Health and social care professionals	Support and other staff	Total
1997	8,844	4,976	25,611	5,969	20,705	66,105
2001	14,714	6,285	31,429	9,228	28,645	90,301
Increase 97–01	5,870	1,309	5,818	3,259	7,940	24,196
% increase 97–01	66	26	23	55	38	37
2002	15,690	6,775	33,395	12,577	27,242	95,679
2003	15,766	6,792	33,766	12,692	27,485	96,501
2004	16,157	7,013	34,313	12,830	28,410	98,723
March 2005	16,260	7,102	34,693	13,350	28,324	99,729
Increase 01–05	1,546	817	3,264	4,122	-321	9,428
% increase 01–05	11	13	10	45	-1	10

*Source: Department of Health Personnel Census. Wholetime equivalents. The census totals have been adjusted by the Department to exclude student nurses and home helps. *There were 1,735 student nurses in 1997. The exclusion of home helps inflates employment growth between 2001 and 2005 by 514, the amount by which home help wholetime equivalent numbers fell.*

When the government took this advice at the end of 2002, the consequences were immediately apparent in health and social services. Hospitals reduced staffing and closed wards during 2003, community care services suffered and the health boards cut their home help services.[3] The number of home helps retained by those health boards, who make such returns to the Department, fell from 8,709 in 2002 to 6,929 in 2003, a drop in wholetime equivalent numbers from 2,534 to 2,281.[4] Paradoxically, the employment cap increased health expenditure in some areas. In order to maintain services while reducing employee numbers, health boards employed agency nurses at a higher cost than permanent staff.[5] In a year when the population increased by 1.6 per cent, jobs in public health and social services increased by 0.8 per cent. Including the recorded fall in home help numbers, excluded recently from the Department of Health's count of public health sector personnel, lowers the increase to 0.6 per cent.

As well as capping employment, the Department of Finance required spending departments to operate on an 'existing level of service' (ELS) basis. Consequently, in 2004 it emerged that new health care facilities, funded at a cost of some €400 million under the National Development Plan, could not open because health authorities were not permitted to recruit employees to staff them. In September 2004 the Minister for Health, Micheál Martin, announced that the Department of Finance had permitted the hiring of 1,200 additional staff to run these units.[6]

The contrast between the 66 per cent increase in the number of 'management and administration' staff in the years from 1997 to 2001 and the 26 per cent increase in the number of doctors and 23 per cent rise in nurse numbers[7] had caused considerable adverse criticism. In its examination of financial management and control systems in the health service published in 2003, the Brennan Commission did not agree that the health service had recruited too many administrators.[8] The Department of Health census points out that this category includes 'staff who are of direct service to the public', such as consultants' secretaries, outpatient departmental personnel, medical records personnel and telephonists and non-frontline staff in areas like payroll, human resources (including training), IT and communications. This category of staff increased proportionately less in the years from 2001 to 2004.

The government decision to cap health sector employment had come just one year after the 2001 Health Strategy recommended substantially *increased* employment over the 10 years to 2011. It was a weakness of the strategy that these increases were unspecified. An exception was the primary care element of the strategy, which calculated that an additional 500 general practitioners (GPs) and 2,000 nurses and midwives would be required to achieve two-thirds implementation of the strategy over 10 years. It observed that similar large increases would be required among professional therapists, administrators, home helps and health care assistants.[9] In general, the Health Strategy envisaged that 'substantial further numbers of staff will be employed over the next five to seven years, including consultants, nurses, allied and paramedical, and support grades.'[10] Subsequently, the Hanly Report recommended an increase in consultant numbers and a reduction in non-consultant hospital doctor (NCHD) numbers over the 10 years from 2003 to 2013. This recommendation was designed to substitute consultant for NCHD care, but the Hanly taskforce did not calculate the increase in medical staffing which would be required to meet the needs of a growing population.

Substitution of private health employment for public health employment

While the employment cap has applied in the public health sector, it has not applied to private health and social services, even though these are frequently substantially funded by the Exchequer. After the introduction of the public employment cap in 2002, private developments subsidised by the state included:

- employment of private agency nurses by public hospitals in place of staff nurses;
- establishment of tax-subsidised private hospitals;
- NTPF funding of public patient care in private hospitals in Ireland and abroad;
- payment of private fees to public hospital consultants for the treatment of public patients;

- tax-subsidised expansion of the private nursing home sector, in which patients who cannot be accommodated in public institutions receive state subventions for care;
- state payment of home care packages to people requiring care in the community so that they can source private care.

Each of these developments has come at a cost to the state. Each has been driven by deficiencies in public care, and at a time of constrained employment in public health and social care. In light of these developments, the cap on public health employment is a questionable policy instrument. Employment in health and social care can be expected to increase both in absolute terms and as a percentage of total employment in a country with a growing and ageing population, with rising incomes and with rising expectations for higher-quality care. The Department of Finance cap is not stemming this inevitable growth in employment. What it is achieving is the diversion of health employment growth from the public into the private sector, and into institutions and arrangements where, in many cases, quality of care is more poorly supervised and assured than in the public sector. In the process, this policy is providing opportunities for private profit in a significantly state-funded sector.

Overall numbers employed in health and social care, as measured by the Central Statistics Office (CSO), increased by 25 per cent from 2001 to the first quarter of 2005. Over that period the Department of Health's personnel census recorded a 14 per cent increase in numbers employed. Comparison of the growth of these two measures must be treated with caution since, although they are both head counts of numbers employed, they remain different counts, employing different methodologies. Under health and social employment, the CSO includes categories like veterinary services and, more significantly, employment in crèches, clearly a growth area. Unfortunately, the CSO cannot disaggregate these components from its count. It is nonetheless of interest that the number of people employed in the broadly defined non-public health and social service sector increased by 46 per cent over the years from 2001 to the beginning of 2005. Of the 37,100 additional people employed in the sector, as broadly defined, between 2001 and 2005, fewer than 15,000 were employed in the public sector and 22,000 in the private sector. Whereas public health employment had been 68 per cent of total health employment in 2001 and 2002, in 2005 it had dropped to 62 per cent. It might be conjectured that this reflects the rapid growth in the private nursing home sector, the switch from public home helps to private agency services funded through home care grants and the replacement of staff nurses with agency nurses, as well as any growth in private hospital capacity.

The proportion of total employment accounted for by health is lower in Ireland than in other countries with more developed health care systems. In Germany and Norway in 2003, over 10 per cent of employees and over 8 per cent in wholetime equivalent terms worked in the health sector, according to *OECD Health Data*. Comparisons must be treated with some caution because countries' compliance with the OECD definition of health care varies. Ireland has reported to the OECD that 7 per cent of employees and 5.7 per cent of wholetime equivalents were employed in health care in 2003. These data are not comparable because they include employment in social care programmes and exclude private health care employees.[11] There is no official Irish count of employees in health care as defined by the OECD.

The other available source is the CSO's Quarterly National Household Survey, which has shown a sharp rise in health and social employment as a proportion of total employment, from 7.8 per cent in 1999 to 9.7 per cent in 2005 (see Table 11.2).[12] As noted above, the CSO counts private sector health employees but also includes people involved in social care. Since social programmes are highly labour intensive and have many part-time workers, it can be concluded that the purely health share of employment in Ireland, as defined by the OECD, is still some percentage points behind countries such as Germany and Norway with more developed health care systems. The increase in health sector employment, which so alarmed the Independent Estimates Review Committee, can be expected to continue because the international evidence is that as national income rises, so too does employment in health and social care.

There has been some evidence of cabinet disagreement about the acceptability of raising taxes to pay for expanded health and social services.[13] The decision to constrain public employment may have forestalled tax increases to pay for increased public health and social care, but it has not reduced the burden on Irish society of paying for health care. Privately purchased care has substituted for publicly purchased care. In contrast to tax or social insurance, which can be levied on the entire community, thus avoiding too high a burden on any individual, the incidence of private payment for care, particularly nursing home care, falls on the individual at a time when he or she is by definition unwell, older and likely to be on a fixed income.

Table 11.2: Numbers employed in public and private health and social services									
Head count of numbers employed									
	1998	1999	2000	2001	2002	2003	2004	2005	% increase 01–05
	thousands								
Total health**	115.9	127.9	140.1	150.9	163.2	175.8	182.5	188	25
Public health*	78.9	82.3	89.9	102.0	110.8	115.4	115.9	116.7	14
Private health	37	46	50	49	52	60	67	71	46
Public as % total health	68	64	64	68	68	66	64	62	
Total in all employment	1,547.1	1,647.4	1,712.6	1,759.9	1,782.3	1,828.9	1,894.1	1,929.2	10
Health as % total employment	7.5	7.8	8.2	8.6	9.2	9.6	9.6	9.7	

Source: CSO for total health employment and total employment, from quarterly national household survey. Department of Health personnel census for public health employment. All figures head counts, not wholetime equivalents. *End-December total, except 2005, which is end-March. ** Sept.-Nov. total, except 2005, which is March-May quarter. See text for qualifications about comparability.

Health skill needs

The lack of specificity in the 2001 Health Strategy about the staffing implications of its plans for expanding health and social services led to the commissioning of a report on health care skill needs, which was published in October 2005. The FÁS *Healthcare Skills Monitoring Report* attempted to forecast demand

and supply for 29 health care occupations in the years to 2015.[14] It identified considerable current and future skills shortages and recommended an expansion of training places to address present and/or future shortages of doctors (consultants, interns and GPs), dentists, children's nurses, dieticians, chiropodists, radiographers and radiation therapists.

In other occupations, the report concluded that expanded training places might not be necessary if measures were effective to adjust the skills mix, improve retention rates, promote immigration and increase productivity. The report recommended that the effect of current policies should be monitored before increasing training places in the occupations of registered general nurses, health care assistants, physiotherapists, social workers, dental hygienists, optometrists, dispensing opticians and clinical psychologists.

FÁS identified a third category of occupations with either no major gap between domestic supply and demand, or for which mandatory qualifications did not apply so that 'supply can be taken from the general population'. The occupations which FÁS judged did not currently need expanded training places included dental technicians, dental nurses, intellectual disability nurses, psychiatric nurses, public health nurses, midwives, occupational therapists, speech and language therapists and pharmacists.

Among the factors FÁS took into account in analysing future demand for health care workers were the needs identified in the government's strategies, current vacancies (although it observed that these were constrained by the cap on public employment), population growth forecasts and the discrepancy between Irish and international ratios of health care staff to population. The report observed that 'unfortunately, official forecasts are not available for many of the government's healthcare strategy plans.' FÁS employed a relatively conservative population growth forecast, equivalent to the lowest of the CSO's range.[15]

There is a dichotomy between the future health skills market forecast by FÁS and the present reality of constrained public health service employment. The FÁS report is predicated on assumptions that the government will expand health service employment to meet the health care demands of a rising population and will implement the Health Strategy and Hanly reforms. FÁS therefore implicitly assumes that the government will end its cap on public sector employment. FÁS has stated that the Department of Health is 'in broad agreement' with its analysis and recommendations.[16]

However, the FÁS analysis is hampered by the existence of the cap. It is difficult to assess skill shortages when vacancies do not arise because employers are not permitted to expand services to meet need. The FÁS analysis recognises shortages in occupations such as radiation therapy, on which there have been recent expert reports. But it is arguably too sanguine about the improbability of shortages arising for occupations like social work, for which there has been no recent comprehensive analysis of need. The public employment cap can give the false impression that need for services has been met, when this is not the case.

In health professions where training places have been increased, the combined effect of the employment ceiling and the Department of Finance's ELS requirement have led to new graduates encountering difficulty in finding employment or going into the private sector when their skills are badly needed to address public sector waiting lists. Most controversially, starting from the premise that Ireland has more nurses in proportion to population than many other states, a statement which we examine in detail below, the FÁS report advocates a policy of reducing the proportion of nurses in the health workforce. The discussion that follows reviews some but not all of the occupations analysed by FÁS.

Doctors

FÁS stated that there are approximately 9,200 medical practitioners in the public and private sector, including 2,000 consultants, 4,000 NCHDs, 2,500 GPs and 650 doctors working in other areas. With the second lowest doctor per 1,000 population ratio in the EU15, FÁS calculated that for Ireland to meet the EU15 weighted average of 3.26 doctors per 1,000 people for the current population, the number of doctors employed would have to increase to 12,955, a 41 per cent increase.

To meet the less ambitious target of increasing the number of doctors in line with population and implementing the reforms recommended in the Hanly Report, the number of doctors required by 2015 would rise to 12,200, a 33 per cent increase, FÁS calculated. It concluded that there would be a 3,958 shortfall, which could only be met by increased immigration, unless training places increased significantly. Already in 2004, 34 per cent of doctors fully or temporarily registered by the Medical Council had qualified outside Ireland. FÁS concluded:

> There is an urgent need for policymakers to address the shortage of places in undergraduate medical training. The number of funded undergraduate places available for Irish students has not been increased since the quota set in 1981. At that time there were approximately 5,000 medical practitioners. In the current environment, with over 9,000 medical practitioners employed, this number of places is no longer sufficient. If the supply from domestic sources is not increased, the analysis shows that a further substantial increase in immigration will be required to meet demand.

In Chapter 6 on primary care and Chapter 9 on specialist care in hospitals, we have already endorsed the recommendations of the Fottrell Report for an increase in Irish medical training places and in funding for medical education.

Other occupations for which FÁS recommends increased training places

FÁS accepted that a shortage in children's nurses was evident from the use of temporary and agency staff and the existence of 100 wholetime equivalent (WTE) vacancies in 2004. It recommended that to meet future demand over and above population growth, the number of training places would have to increase from 133 places to approximately 200 annually. FÁS also accepted that the number of training places available for dieticians was too low and should more than double from 21 to 50 places annually; that training places for diagnostic radiographers should increase further, although the annual intake of students doubled from 20 to 40 in 2003; and that student places for radiation therapists should increase by 10 to 15, although they had increased from 10 to 25 annually in 2001. The Hollywood Report on *The Development of Radiation Oncology Services in Ireland* (2003) identified a profound deficit in radiation oncology services and a shortfall in the number of qualified radiation therapists.

Occupations in which FÁS concluded extra training places might not be necessary

General nurses

FÁS observed that 'the Irish ratio of nurses to the population is much higher than the ratio found in other developed countries. The average ratio of nurses per 1,000 population in the OECD is 8.1, while the average for the EU is 8.5. The ratio in Ireland is 12.2 nurses per thousand population.' It further stated that 'comparisons with the other member states of the EU show that the level of nursing employment in Ireland is the highest in the entire EU.'

Based on this observation, FÁS adopted an optimistic view that an otherwise large gap between the supply and demand for nurses could be avoided if 'certain changes are made' which 'should bring the health service in Ireland into line with those in other OECD countries.' Chief among the changes advocated by FÁS was the 'widespread introduction of healthcare assistants': 'It is current government policy that the skills mix in nursing needs to be addressed with the expansion of the role of health care assistants. This should moderate demand for nurses in the medium term.'

There was unquestionably going to be a shortage of new Irish nurses in 2005 because the move to a degree-length course in nursing meant there would be no graduates that year. Ireland would require many more immigrant nurses to fill vacancies. Immigration had been the main source of supply of general nurses for the last five years. FÁS forecast that the domestic supply of general nurses would decrease slightly from 30,485 in 2003 to approximately 27,312 by 2015, 'as new entrants from education sources are not sufficient to replace the numbers lost through attrition and further specialisation each year.'

FÁS concluded that if demand for general nurses rose as it had done in the past, approximately 48,000 would be needed in 2015 against a domestic supply of 27,312 nurses. It then made two brave assumptions. The first was that nurse immigration would rise from 3,015 in 2003 to 5,900 in 2015. The second was that health care assistants would take over many tasks formerly performed by nurses.

FÁS summarised:

There will be a large gap between supply and demand unless certain changes are made. These include improving retention and changing the skills mix between this occupation and others. These changes should bring the health service in Ireland into line with those in other OECD countries. If these reforms are successful, supply and demand of general nurses will be more balanced in the future.

FÁS argued:

If for example nurses spend 25 per cent of their time on non-nursing work and this was freed up by health care assistants, then by 2015, 36,000 general nurses would be able to do the work of 48,000 general nurses based on current work practices. Supply, both domestic and foreign, should be able to match this level of demand especially if retention issues are solved.

This argument could have profound consequences for the future staffing and organisation of Irish health care, so it deserves to be examined closely in each of its steps.

Firstly, is the Irish ratio of nurses to population much higher than the ratio found in other developed countries and the highest in the entire EU? The available international data do not support this statement. The data are poor. The OECD compares head counts of nurses in relation to population and acknowledges that the comparability of its data on nurses is limited. The primary limitation is that head counts are not the same thing as whole-time equivalents. There is a great deal of part-time working in Irish nursing. While there were approximately 40,700 nurses employed in the Irish public sector in December 2004, because of part-time working these nurses filled fewer than 34,300 whole-time equivalent posts.[17]

FÁS calculated an Irish ratio of 12.2 nurses per 1,000 population on the basis of the CSO's Quarterly National Household Survey count of 48,600 nurses employed in the public and private sectors in 2003. It then compared this Irish ratio with international averages. The averages of 8.1 nurses per 1,000 population in the OECD and 8.5 for the EU are averages derived from head counts of nurses in countries where working patterns and rates of part-time working may differ greatly. The Irish count includes midwives, which the OECD comparison requires countries to exclude. Some countries, like Austria, only return numbers for nurses working in hospitals; others, like Italy, only include nurses working in the National Health Service. Iceland recorded 13.7 nurses per 1,000 in 2003. The latest data for the Netherlands was 12.8 per 1,000 in 2001. According to the OECD, Australia, Canada, Denmark, Germany, Luxembourg, Norway, Sweden and the UK all have a head count of close to or over 10 nurses per 1,000 population (see Table 11.3).

Therefore, the Irish ratio of nurses to population is not much higher than the ratio found in every other developed country. In so far as one can compare from the available data, Ireland appears to have fewer nurses proportionally than the Netherlands or Iceland. However, the Netherlands' numbers are probably overstated since they include nurses who may not be actively working in health care. While it could be the case that Ireland has the highest level of nursing employment in the EU, in the absence of comparable wholetime equivalent data for nursing employment in the EU, this statement cannot be made with certitude. Irish nurses may on average work fewer hours than nurses in other countries. To discover what the true difference is between numbers of nurses, the hours they work and the roles they play, it would be necessary to examine in detail the work practices in different states, a study which has not been done in relation to Irish nursing.

Can one assume, as FÁS appears to, that the widespread introduction of health care assistants would bring the health service in Ireland into line with those in other OECD countries? A recent OECD study of nurses in advanced roles in the health service observed that 'most of the policy attention on using skill-mix

Table 11.3: International employment of doctors and nurses (head counts)					
As percentage of total health employment			Numbers per 1,000 population		
	2002 % doctors	2002 % nurses	2002 % doctors and nurses	2003 Doctors	2003 Nurses	Doctors and nurses
Australia	n.a	n.a	n.a	2.5	10.2	12.7
Canada	n.a	n.a	n.a	2.1	9.8	11.9
Denmark	10.6	37.4	48	2.9	10.3	13.2
Finland	8.5	29	37.5	2.6	9.3	11.9
France	10.8	23.2	34	3.4	7.3	10.7
Germany	7.3	21	28.3	3.4	9.7	13.1
Iceland	n.a	n.a	n.a	3.6	13.7	17.3
Ireland	**7.8**	**49.4**	**57.2**	**2.6**	**12.2**	**14.8**
Italy	21.9	27.1	49	4.1	5.4	9.5
Luxembourg	n.a	n.a	n.a	2.7	10.6	13.3
Netherlands	10	n.a	n.a	3.1	12.8	15.9
Norway	n.a	n.a	n.a	3.1	10.4	13.5
Portugal	23.9	29.6	53.5	3.3	4.2	7.5
Spain	16.9	42	58.9	2.9	7.5	10.4
Sweden	n.a	n.a	n.a	3.3	10.2	13.5
United Kingdom	6.6	29.6	36.2	2.2	9.7	11.9
Average	12.4	32	45	3	10	13
Ire as % average	63	154	128	87	127	118

Source: OECD Health Data 2005, with the exception of Irish nurse:1,000 pop.ratio, which follows the FÁS method. Not all data for 2002 and 2003, some for latest year available, none before 2001. See text for discussion of limitations to comparability of data.

changes to improve health system performance has been on the mix between physicians and nurses.'[18] This study found large differences in reported physician/nurse ratios across OECD countries and evidence of significant changes in the ratio over time in some countries (see Table 11.4). Whereas Ireland had 159 doctors to every 1,000 nurses in 2000,[19] the average across 23 OECD countries was 426 doctors per 1,000 nurses. The ratio ranged from 1,121 doctors per 1,000 nurses in Greece in 1999 to 113:1,000 in Norway. The OECD study noted that in Australia, the ratio of doctors to nurses had risen from 183:1,000 in 1980 to 233 in 2001, whereas in France it had fallen from 557:1,000 in 1990 to 477 in 2001.

It is apparent, then, that to bring the Irish health service 'into line with other OECD countries' is not possible because there is no OECD norm in staffing relationships. What is apparent is that Ireland has fewer doctors relative to population and relative to the number of nurses. When doctors and nurses are combined to find the ratio of both professional groups to 1,000 population, at 14.8 Ireland is above the average of the range of developed countries in Table 11.3.[20] Once again, the absence of wholetime equivalent data makes this comparison of limited usefulness. In Ireland, there is a significant amount of part-time working among both doctors and nurses. There is a ratio of 1.16 doctors and dentists for each WTE in the public sector, while there is a ratio of 1.18 nurses for every WTE.[21]

Ireland is now following other states by extending to nurses the power to prescribe, a measure taken elsewhere to reduce the ratio of doctors to nurses. Even without such measures, nurses in Ireland have for many years informally filled roles which doctors fill in other states. The authors have been told by a hospital consultant with responsibility for an area of highly specialised care that he has arranged for a senior nurse to oversee his clinics because she offers greater expertise and continuity of care than the alternative NCHDs on short training rotations.

To entertain the argument for a reduction in the proportion of nurses in the health workforce based on international comparison requires acceptance of an accompanying argument for an increase to international averages in the number of fully trained

Table 11.4: Practising doctors per 1,000 practising nurses	
	2000
Australia	228
Austria	651
Belgium	336
Canada	211
Denmark	359
France	488
Germany	339
Greece	1,121
Ireland	**159**
Italy	808
Japan	242
Korea	431
Mexico	581
Netherlands	128
New Zealand	233
Norway	113
Portugal	867
Slovak Republic	493
Spain	883
Sweden	344
Switzerland	327
United Kingdom	228
United States	289
Average	429

Source: OECD Health Project from table in Buchan and Calman (OECD 2005). Data for Greece and Italy (1999), Japan (1998), Belgium (1996).

specialist doctors working in Irish health care. It also requires accepting an argument for enhancing numbers of other professionals to international levels. The authors have heard evidence that nurses also step in to fill the roles of social workers, also in short supply in Ireland (see below). The deficiency in the number of social workers requires nurses to become more involved in ensuring that patients are discharged to adequate care than they would be in states with more social workers and better community care. The assumption that increased numbers of health care assistants will significantly reduce the need for nurses in the Irish health workforce ignores the many other functions which nurses perform in Ireland.

The *Report of the Commission on Nursing* supported health care assistants taking on some tasks which are inappropriate to highly trained nurses. A national programme of training for health care assistants was introduced on a pilot basis in autumn 2001. The grade of Health Care Assistant was introduced in 2002. FÁS observed that 'it is not possible to carry out a supply and demand gap analysis for this occupation as currently it is not mandatory to hold the qualification to enter the occupation.' A range of grades carry out what broadly are assistant roles in Irish health and social care. In 2003 there were 8,465 people employed in these grades in the public health service (WTE).

The absence of mandatory training and standards for health care assistants and the lack of any analysis of future supply of candidates for this post raises fundamental questions about relying on the expansion of this occupation to fill a very large anticipated gap between the future demand for and supply of nurses. The authors recommend as a matter of urgency that the Department of Health should commission a health care specialist to conduct a study on the type of work which is typically undertaken by nurses in countries at a comparable level of development. From such a study it should be possible to develop a more considered interpretation of the statistical data, and of the degree to which expanding a lower-skilled occupation can reduce the need for Irish nurses. To conclude on the available evidence that training places for Irish nurses need not increase is unwarranted and premature.

The authors also recommend that health care assistants should have mandatory training and nurse supervision. There is evidence from the US, where care assistants are widely employed, that hospital patients receive better care and have better outcomes when they have a higher proportion of hours of nursing care provided by registered nurses and a greater number of hours of care by registered nurses per day. A study of 799 hospitals in 11 states found that a higher proportion of hours of care provided by registered nurses was associated with lower rates of pneumonia, shock or cardiac arrest and 'failure to rescue', which was defined as death from pneumonia, shock or cardiac arrest, upper gastrointestinal bleeding, sepsis or deep venous thrombosis. Among surgical patients, a higher proportion of care provided by registered nurses was associated with lower rates of urinary tract infections and a greater number of hours of care per day provided by registered nurses was associated with lower rates of 'failure to rescue'.[22]

Social workers

In the course of interviewing for this study, the authors heard from people working in hospitals, primary and community care that shortage of social workers is a significant problem. The demands that new child protection legislation has placed on social workers has led to a serious shortage of adult social workers in the community. FÁS has not published an assessment of the current demand for social workers and bases its projections of future demand on population growth and the past trends in social work employment. This approach fails to capture current deficiencies. At the time of writing, the National Social Work Qualifications Board (NSWQB) was surveying social work posts in Ireland. Its most recent survey in 2001 recorded that there were 983 social work posts in child and family care, fostering and adoption and 18 for older people.

International evidence supports the view that Ireland has too few social workers. While comparisons must have regard for the fact that social welfare and health systems differ, as do the social workers' qualifications and the roles they undertake, according to data compiled by the NSWQB, the ratio of social workers to 100,000 population was 90.2 in the UK in 2000, 129.1 in Sweden in 2001 and 52 in Ireland in 2001. [23]

FÁS observed that:

> Demand for this occupation is generally driven by government policy and its response to shifts in the social structure of society. This structure is changing rapidly especially in areas such as immigration, the disabled and older people. Government policy may change to reflect these changes and, as such, these changes will alter the demand for social workers in the future.

Its conclusion that the number of social workers available to work would grow faster than population growth was highly qualified: 'The situation should be monitored to ensure any rise in unmet demand is matched with increased places on social work courses.'

The authors recommend that as a matter of urgency the Department of Health undertake a survey which quantifies unmet need for the services of social workers in hospitals, primary and community care.

Physiotherapists

Approximately 1,700 physiotherapists were practising in Ireland at the beginning of 2004. Despite an increase in training places for physiotherapists, FÁS estimated that by 2015 domestic supply would be approximately 400 physiotherapists below the 2,600 needed, as estimated by the 2001 Bacon Report.[24] FÁS concluded that, depending on the rate of immigration of physiotherapists, it might be necessary to look at providing a new course (or expanding the numbers on existing courses) in the medium to long term. At 43.4 physiotherapists per 100,000 people in 2003, Ireland had fewer physiotherapists than most other EU states. The UK had 56:100,000, France 92.7, Germany 103 and Denmark 163.[25]

The Irish Society of Chartered Physiotherapists has calculated that implementing the Primary Care Strategy would require an additional 2,173 chartered physiotherapists working in primary and community care. This is in line with the envisaged 10-year target of 400–600 primary care teams. This group can identify considerable unmet need for physiotherapists in acute, rehabilitation, primary and community care throughout the country.

Occupations in which FÁS envisaged no major shortage emerging

Speech and language therapists

The 2001 Bacon Report found a large gap between supply and demand for speech and language therapists. Bacon recommended a substantial increase in the number of student places. Two new courses opened in 2003. Nonetheless, FÁS envisaged that domestic supply alone would not be able to meet the need foreseen by Bacon and 'a certain level of immigration will be needed to meet demand'. FÁS advised that it might be necessary to consider a new course (or expand the numbers on existing courses) in the medium to long term. However, the Irish Association of Speech and Language Therapists (IASLT) has expresssed fears that new graduates might not find jobs from 2005 onwards because of the cap on public sector employment.

Once again, the cap masks considerable unmet need. In 2005 the IASLT reported very long waiting lists for services. Children with intellectual disabilities who attended mainstream schools could wait three years for therapy. Service provision to adults was reported to be very sparse outside of the acute hospitals.[26]

> IASLT had a recent report of an adult recovering from a CVA (stroke) in an acute Dublin hospital who, from a general health point of view, was ready for discharge home, but who was kept as an inpatient by the hospital consultant because if he were to be discharged, he would not be able to access the necessary speech and language therapy services.

Limerick Regional Hospital had no speech and language therapy service, so that adults with neurological disabilities had no access to therapy in hospital. The IALTS reported that there were no diagnostic services for children who had swallowing disorders in the Health Service Executive (HSE) Western Area. There were not enough staff therapists available to provide clinical placements for expanded student numbers.

Conclusion

The most serious staffing issue facing the Irish health service is the shortage of domestically trained doctors. To meet need, develop primary care and move to consultant-delivered care in acute hospitals, it is necessary to increase training places for Irish students in medical schools. The authors therefore welcome the government's commitment to implement the Fottrell Report's recommended increase in Irish and EU medical student places. The persistence of a cap on Irish medical students from 1981 to 2006, notwithstanding population growth and developments in medicine and Irish society in that period, underscores the urgent need for a more planned approach to the staffing of the Irish health service. The arbitrary cap on employment in the health service is the latest instance of an unplanned approach to health staffing needs. It has been harmful and inefficient and the authors recommend that it should be lifted so that health staffing can grow to meet unmet needs. Planning for future staffing needs should become an integral part of the operations of the Department of Health and the HSE. Planning should be based on assessments of need across care areas and disciplines and should be informed by regular monitoring. Decisions on the number of educational and training places for health and social service staff should be based on evidence of need, analysis of the inter-relationships of health care staff and population growth projections. The Department of Health should undertake a survey which quantifies unmet need for the services of social workers in hospitals, primary and community care.

To conclude on the available evidence that an increase in training places for nurses in Ireland is not required, notwith-standing the probable emergence of a considerable nursing shortage within the next 10 years, is unwarranted and premature. The government's policy of relying on the employment of many more health care assistants to reduce the need for nurses requires rigorous and detailed evaluation in all its aspects. The authors recommend that the Department of Health should commission and publish a specialist study on the type of work typically undertaken by nurses in countries at a comparable level of development to Ireland in order to assess the feasibility, safety and efficiency of this policy. This should include an analysis of the role played by nurses in the Irish health care system, which has very much lower numbers of doctors and other allied professionals in proportion to population than in many comparable countries. However great or limited a role they play in the Irish health service, health care assistants should have mandatory training and nurse supervision.

12

ACCOUNTABILITY AND ADMINISTRATION IN HEALTH

Introduction

In preceding chapters we reviewed significant government strategies for investment in and reform of Irish health care – the 2001 Health Strategy, the Primary Care Strategy, the Hanly Report – all of which appear to have been shelved or abandoned. We have presented a case for reform in many aspects of Irish health care. It is striking that the one reform which the government has decisively advanced has been a reform of the system of health administration. This reform does not address two-tier access to care, the consultants' contract, the deficiencies of primary care, the inadequacy of acute care or the great needs in community and continuing care. What this reform does do, or purports to do, is reorganise the manner in which public health and social care is administered and relates to the body politic.

The government has embarked on this huge reform, among all the reforms of health care which it might have undertaken, in the apparent belief that it can thereby achieve enhanced results without greater expenditure, a questionable proposition. It has limited the scope of its own reform by failing to offer exit packages to those employees of the health boards who wish to leave. The reform has been and may continue to be enormously disruptive for the administration of Irish health services. It is a tribute to the employees of the former health boards that, so far, little of that disruption has been apparent to the general public. But unless the reform is implemented with much greater clarity, transparency and efficiency than heretofore, and unless there are some significant amendments to the legislation governing it, its disruptive consequences will have effects on the delivery of services.

The creation of the Health Service Executive (HSE) in 2005 and the prior abolition of the health boards in 2004 removed the last vestiges of local democracy in Irish health care. A unitary administrative structure has responsibility for the delivery of health services for the first time in the history of the state. In centralising the Irish health care system in an era when other states have sought to decentralise their systems (see Chapter 3), the government has sought to create a more efficient and responsive structure, which will put national and regional interests above local concerns. The HSE receives almost one-third of government current spending in its own direct Vote and must remain democratically accountable, yet the mechanisms by which it is accountable are far from clear.

The theory of the new structure is straightforward. The Minister for Health and her Department remain responsible for determining issues of health policy. The HSE is responsible for the management of the health service and associated social services. The Minister appoints the board of the HSE. The Minister appointed its first chief executive, on the recommendation of the board. Professor Brendan Drumm took up his position in August 2005. The board is responsible for appointing subsequent chief executives.

How this new structure will work in practice is untested at the time of writing. It is already apparent that some key issues relating to the functioning of the HSE and its democratic accountability require clarification and may require amending legislation. The legislation providing for the establishment of the HSE, the Health Act 2004, passed all stages in the Dáil in a guillotined debate in November and December 2004, without time for many provisions to be discussed and fully understood within or outside the Dáil, even by the government which promulgated them. There was no previous White Paper outlining the intent of the legislation. The policy-operations divide between Minister and CEO leaves great scope for confusion and blame.

The legislation is deficient in accountability because the Minister's discretion in the appointment of board members is too great. For the first year of its existence, the HSE operated without openness and in an effective vacuum of accountability because of the absence of ministerial regulations governing the answering of parliamentary questions and the appointment of regional health forums. Neither at national nor at local level was there an established pathway for the HSE to respond to the concerns of elected representatives. At the time of writing in early 2006, although these regulations had been made, their framing made it unlikely that they would allay concerns about accountability. The alienation of the community as a whole from the making and implementation of health policy was exacerbated because the Minister had not yet made an order to establish a national consultative forum, and the HSE had not yet established any local advisory panels.

The Health Act is unclear in its financial provisions, chiefly because of the assignment of a separate Vote to the HSE and of the role of Accounting Officer for that Vote to its CEO. Already, the Minister for Finance has made it clear in writing to the Tánaiste and Minister for Health that he intends to deal with her and her officials, not with the HSE, notwithstanding the responsibilities statutorily assigned to its CEO. The HSE is also operating without the intended checks and balances to protect the integrity and quality of the health care system. Legislation to establish and empower the Health Information and Quality Authority (HIQA) has yet to come before the Dáil.

There has been too great a delay in key components of the reform programme. It is not in the interests of the public, the HSE or its officials that the HSE should operate without adequate oversight and transparency.

History

The HSE replaced 11 health boards,[1] administrative structures answerable to representative boards, whose members were elected local councillors, representatives of health professionals and ministerial appointees. The health boards were established under the 1970 Health Act in a tradition of local democracy in health administration. They took over from county councils, which had been funded initially by local property taxes or rates.[2] With the phasing out of the health charge on the rates in the 1970s, the central Exchequer entirely funded public health services so that local health boards had power without fiscal responsibility.

In 1989, the government-appointed Commission on Health Funding concluded that the health board structure confused political and executive functions. It recommended that the Minister for Health should appoint a centralised Health Service Executive Authority to manage health and social services, leaving the Minister and Department free to formulate health policy. The government did not adopt the Commission's recommendations.

The 2001 Health Strategy also concluded that organisational reform was necessary 'to develop a single integrated system, rather than one which varies between the approaches taken in individual health board areas.'[3] Although the strategy stated that the health boards would remain, in June 2003, the government announced an Administrative Reform Programme, in which a Health Service Executive (HSE) would be established as 'the first ever body charged with managing and delivering the health service as a single national entity.' The reform programme drew on two reports: the *Commission on Financial Management and Control Systems in the Health Service* (the Brennan Commission, mentioned in earlier chapters) and the *Audit of Structures and Functions in the Health System* (Prospectus).[4] While these two reports concurred in recommending a centralised HSE, they differed in detail.

The Brennan Commission recommended retaining an unspecified number of regional health boards whose CEOs would report to the CEO of the HSE. Health board members would approve financial reports, monitor policy implementation and should be consulted on the regional service plan. This local accountability would complement the primary accountability of the Minister for Health, who would be 'the ultimate accountable person, accountable to the Dáil and Oireachtas for the performance of the health service.'[5]

The Prospectus report recommended abolition of the health boards, the transfer of their functions to the HSE and subsuming

27 other agencies into the HSE, a Health Information and Quality Authority (HIQA) and a restructured Department. The Prospectus report said that in the health board system, local area concerns had predominated over regional interests and objective need.[6]

The government adopted the organisational structure proposed by Prospectus. The HSE would have 'two service pillars': a National Hospitals Office (NHO) to oversee the acute sector and a Primary, Community and Continuing Care (PCCC) pillar to administer non-acute services through four regional offices. The regional offices would oversee the work of the existing community care structures, renamed as local health offices (LHOs). A National Shared Services Centre would rationalise the provision of corporate services across the system.

In November 2003 the Minister for Health, Micheál Martin, announced the appointment of a former banker, Kevin Kelly, as chairman of the interim HSE board. In September 2004 the Minister announced the HSE's four regions: Western, with headquarters in Galway; Southern, with a Cork HQ; Dublin/North-East with a HQ in Kells, County Meath; and Dublin/Mid-Leinster, with a HQ in Tullamore, County Offaly.

In June 2004 the Department of Health published a Composite Report on its website, summarising the views of departmental action committees on how to reconcile the Brennan, Prospectus and Hanly Reports. This was informally renamed the 'compost report', as the balance of power on shaping the HSE shifted from the Department to the interim organisation. The Composite Report recommended that the Minister and her Department should remain in clear control of health policy and health spending. The legislation establishing the HSE did not eventually have that clarity, particularly in relation to the role of the Department, as we will discuss further below. The Composite Report recommended that the Department should be responsible for holding the delivery system to account for its performance. The Minister and the Secretary General of the Department (as Accounting Officer) would be accountable to the Dáil for the spending of the Health Vote and for implementing legislation. But the role of Accounting Officer was eventually assigned to the CEO of the HSE, with unforeseen consequences, as we explain below.

The Composite Report observed: 'It is not possible to anticipate all scenarios in order to validate the proposed split of the policy and executive roles between the DOHC and the HSE...Potential blurring of roles and responsibilities is anticipated in a number of areas.'[7] The report provided an insight into unease within the Department about the transition to the HSE:

> The risks associated with the development of a programme of change of this scale are numerous. The Health Service Executive as the key new organisation in the newly structured system needs to take a strong leadership role early on to build confidence in the change programme; to generate momentum for change and to give a greater sense of certainty around key questions as yet unanswered.

The Report listed three specific risks: insufficient time to develop the system, the magnitude of the task involved and potential skills loss. In the following year, the HSE manifestly failed to take a 'strong leadership role', arguably a consequence of its failure to appoint a chief executive for a further 12 months, following the withdrawal of the first appointed candidate, Professor Aidan Halligan, deputy chief medical officer of the UK's National Health Service (NHS). The absence of confidence among staff in the change programme was apparent in threatened industrial action by IMPACT on the eve of the establishment of the HSE in 2005. The skills loss, which the Department feared, also occurred. Respected senior administrators retired from the system because they were assigned no role in the changeover to the HSE. The reform was probably not assisted by a changeover in Minister for Health at the end of September 2004 and by the subsequent changeover in Secretary General of the Department in April 2005.

The administrative staff employed by the former health boards and other organisations, which have been or will be subsumed into the HSE, have lived with great uncertainty since the government announced its reform programme. Most unfairly, in the view of the authors, the problems of the health care system have been painted as the fault of administrators per se rather than as the consequences of how the system has been constructed and has developed over time. The IMPACT deal of December 2004 has been criticised because competition for significant posts was restricted to existing staff. If the government and the interim HSE had taken more time and care in planning how to effect this organisational change and had not been driven by an arbitrary deadline for the HSE's establishment, the authors conjecture that this deal might have been done differently. While it is understandable for the staff represented by IMPACT to wish to secure jobs of equal or better value in the changeover, it would have been preferable for more posts to have been open to greater competition. Given the commitment of employers and unions in the current partnership agreement, *Sustaining Progress*, to reviewing the operation of the common recruitment pool, which restricts the filling of vacancies in health boards, it would seem probable that agreement could have been reached on more open competition. The authors endorse the recommendations of the Brennan Commission for key positions in health administration to be filled by open competition and for further review of the common recruitment pool. We further suggest, however, that the government should offer early retirement and voluntary redundancy packages to existing staff who do not wish to remain in the new organisation. Such a package would give staff options, and would allow the new top management of the HSE greater scope in the challenging reorganisation, which has yet to be effected in any real way.

The Health Act 2004

The Health Act 2004 passed all stages in the Dáil by 9 December 2004, just three weeks after the initial publication of the Health Bill, and following an acrimonious and guillotined debate, in which the Minister for Health introduced amendments up to the final stage. The most significant difference between the Act and the provisions recommended in the Composite Report was the designation of the CEO of the HSE as Accounting Officer for the HSE's Vote.[8] The Act requires the Dáil to vote funding directly to the HSE rather than to vote health funding to the Department of Health, and leave it the power to allocate a budget to the HSE, as it had to the health boards. This was a highly significant development, apparently motivated by a desire to empower the HSE and correspondingly disempower the Department of Health and its Secretary General. It would have considerable consequences for the operation of the new executive, which we discuss further below.

The Health Act makes it very clear that the government and Minister for Health determine health policy and that the HSE must comply with the wishes of the Minister.

The Act states that 'the object of the Executive is to use the resources available to it in the most beneficial, effective and efficient manner to improve, promote and protect the health and welfare of the public.' Further, 'in performing its functions, the Executive shall have regard to…the policies and objectives of the Government or any Minister of the Government to the extent that those policies and objectives may affect or relate to the functions of the Executive.'

The Minister appoints the members of the HSE board and may remove them. While the Act states that it is the board's responsibility to appoint the CEO, it says that the Minister should appoint the first CEO 'on the recommendation of the Board', an amendment to the original Bill, introduced by the Minister, Mary Harney, during the Committee Stage debate.[9]

The Minister may issue written directions to the Executive, with which the Executive is obliged to comply. The HSE must produce three-yearly corporate plans, which the Minister must approve and to which she may require amendments. The HSE must produce annual service plans, which must 'accord with the policies and objectives of the Minister and the Government' and which the Minister must approve and may require amended. The service plan must 'indicate the type and volume of health and personal social services to be provided', 'indicate any capital plans proposed by the Executive' and 'contain estimates of the number of employees of the Executive for the period and the services to which the plan relates.'

The HSE requires the Minister's prior written permission before committing to any major capital spending. The Minister, with the consent of the Minister for Finance, determines what constitutes major capital spending. The HSE is also circumscribed in its relations with its employees. Its power to determine their terms and conditions of employment is subject to 'the approval of the Minister given with the consent of the Minister for Finance.'

While the CEO can be required to appear before an Oireachtas Committee 'to give an account of the general administration of the Executive', when he does attend, he 'shall not question or express an opinion on the merits of any policy of the Government or a Minister of the Government or on the merits of the objectives of such a policy.'

The Act primarily provides for democratic oversight of the HSE by its accountability to the Minister for Health, who is in turn accountable to the government and through the government, to the Oireachtas. Under the Act, the further mechanism by which the HSE can be held accountable to the Dáil is the requirement that its CEO or other designated officers should attend Oireachtas Committees. The Act also states that the Minister may convene a National Health Consultative Forum to advise her. While this is optional, the Minister is required to establish no more than four 'regional health forums' whose function is described as 'to make such representations to the Executive as the forum considers appropriate on the range and operation of health and personal social services provided within its functional area.' Local councillors, but not Oireachtas members, will sit on these forums. The Minister must determine by regulation how many members they should have, how often they should meet and what their procedures should be. The Minister or the Executive may also set up community, provider or advisory panels.

The Act is succinct and has some striking omissions. There is no reference to the role of the Department of Health and its Secretary General. It did not give force to the Composite Report's recommendation 'that the relative roles and functions of the DoHC (Department of Health and Children) and the Executive and their relationship should be given explicit articulation in legislation.'

The Composite Report had also recommended that the HSE legislation should clarify eligibility for services, which the Health Act 2004 did not do. When opposition deputies raised this issue, the Tánaiste responded: 'This is purely about putting in place a new administrative management system for the health service, so I will not pretend it is about anything else…eligibility and entitlement will be dealt with in different legislation.'

She argued against adopting 'a rights based approach': 'I am advised it would effectively mean somebody could argue in court that instead of getting a by-pass, he or she should have got a transplant or whatever. It is not a route we can take for obvious reasons and it is not desirable that we remove autonomy from clinical independence to legal independence, as it were.'[10]

Absence of clarity on entitlement led to the 2005 legislation to legalise charging Medical Card holders for their nursing home care, and to acceptance by government that it must repay patients and their estates for charges levied without a legal basis. The Prospectus report had also earlier flagged this issue, observing:

> There is no statutory framework which sets out a citizen's right to access services within a stated timescale or to ensure consistency across the country in the interpretation of legislation or regulations…[W]ork is progressing with the DoHC on a package of legislation reforms covering both entitlements and complaints procedures…The early clarification of the statutory basis for health services would be a powerful force for integration and send a strong signal of the modernising intent behind the overall system reconstruction.[11]

Issues arising from the establishment of the HSE

In a review of international best practice in public sector governance, Prospectus observed that no single model applied across organisations, but public sector governance could be based on some core principles: openness, integrity and accountability; an integrated whole-of-government framework; and clarity in roles and responsibility of boards and ministers.[12] The following discussion of the issues arising from the establishment of the HSE takes these principles as a framework.

Role of the Minister

The Health Act 2004 is clear about the Minister's ultimate responsibility for the health services and associated social services.

The Tánaiste and Minister for Health, Mary Harney, was also clear when she announced the publication of the Health Bill:

- The key to the Health Bill is clarity: clarity of roles and clarity of responsibility.
- The Minister for Health and Children will retain clear political responsibility for our health services.
- The Health Service Executive will manage the operations of our health services, bringing together the current roles of the Health Boards/ERHA and many agencies.
- The Department of Health and Children will be responsible for supporting the Minister and the Government in all policy matters.
- Most of all, the people will have clarity now about who is in charge of policy and who is in charge of the management of health services.[13]

When the Commission on Health Funding advocated a centralised executive in 1989, it observed that 'the simple question "who is in charge?" cannot easily be answered for the Irish health services.'[14] The administrative reform was designed to achieve clarity about accountability and responsibility. If it does not do so, it will have been of questionable value. However, it is striking that despite the Minister's initial clarity and the provisions of the Act, there remains a great deal of public confusion about where responsibility rests in this new structure. In interviews conducted over the summer of 2005, six months after the passage of the Act and the establishment of the HSE, we found confusion to be widespread even among senior employees of the health service, senior administrators and politicians. Indeed, the absence of a shared understanding of roles and functions within the new structure seemed to presage future conflict. To a great degree, this uncertainty is the consequence of the speed with which the Act was debated and the amount of amendment which took place during its passage, leaving little time for public discussion and elaboration of the intent of this important legislation.

The uncertainty has been exacerbated by some of the Minister's statements, in particular in relation to the Hanly agenda. Since the Minister has responsibility for policy and is politically accountable for the health service, one might assume that the highly political question of where regional hospital services should be located is an issue for the Minister to determine with her officials and advisers and on which she might be expected to give direction to the HSE. However, this has not appeared to be the Minister's view. She has sidestepped this issue in public.

The Tánaiste informed the Joint Oireachtas Committee on Health and Children in February 2005 that: 'I agree we need hospital reform, regional autonomy, more consultant-led services and that hospitals be appropriately used. I will not say what should happen in one hospital or another as I am not an expert.'[15]

Interim HSE chairman, Kevin Kelly, told the committee in April 2005 that 'the current position as regards the Hanly Report is that the Tánaiste and Minister for Health and Children has asked the National Hospitals Office to take it on board.'[16]

Pat McLoughlin, chief executive of the NHO, elaborated to committee members: 'In the coming year, we will begin a consultation process with the profession and community on the issue of configuration. The principles are in place and, as a planning unit, we now need to examine how the report will impact on each individual area, which will differ from place to place.'

The Minister appears, then, to have delegated to the HSE responsibility for determining how to implement the Hanly principles, an issue which has already caused divisions at the highest political level between cabinet ministers, after the Hanly taskforce reported on two relatively uncontroversial areas. There are few, if any, more politically contentious issues in health than the location of hospital services. Arguably the elected health boards' reluctance to comply with ministers' and the Department's views on this was the primary reason for their dissolution. Now, despite the Minister's accountability to the Dáil for the HSE's actions, she has apparently judged this an operational issue on which she and her Department have no immediate responsibility for determining policy. This affords a striking illustration of how elusive clarity may prove to be about the policy-operational divide. The Minister's reticence on this topic contrasts with her clear, detailed and public policy direction to the HSE in July 2005 to facilitate the development of private facilities on public hospital sites.[17]

The Minister also made clear her control of the HSE's investment plans when in June 2005 she publicly announced that she had written to the HSE to give her 'approval to allow it to progress its capital programme.'[18]

The Minister's provision of detailed instruction to the HSE on private hospitals, a project which she favours, and the contrasting absence of detailed policy direction on hospital reconfiguration, a project with potential for serious political repercussions, provides the HSE and its officials with a very unclear mandate. Consequently, to paraphrase the Commission on Health Funding, the simple question 'who is in charge?' remains difficult to answer for the Irish health services.

The policy-operations boundary

International experience of government devolution of managerial responsibility to executive agencies reveals that distinguishing between policy and operational issues is perennially difficult. In the UK, where such agencies proliferated from the late 1980s, this issue came to a head in 1995 when the first Director General of the Prison Service, Derek Lewis, was relieved of his post after a critical report into prison escapes. Michael Howard, then Home Secretary, was subsequently criticised for scapegoating Lewis, who sued for wrongful dismissal and received substantial damages. The *Financial Times* observed in an editorial, 'ministers must resist the temptation to wash their hands of all difficult problems by classifying them as "operational".'[19]

Derek Lewis maintained that as chief executive he had been subjected to a great deal of interference from above and used to be summoned to the Home Office at least once a day to discuss operational issues. He commented: 'The attempt to distinguish between policy and operations was no more than a political figleaf – such a small figleaf that it was grossly indecent.'[20]

In evidence to the House of Commons Public Service Committee, he said he had been surprised by 'the quantity of briefing and the level of detail in which Ministers became involved' and 'their involvement in decisions as opposed to being provided with information and consulted on matters.' This involvement 'caused those within the service to be uncertain about who was actually calling the shots.'[21]

In the period prior to Brendan Drumm taking up his position as chief executive of the HSE, it was apparent that the Minister and her advisers were closely involved in the affairs of the HSE. The Minister's amendment of the HSE legislation to assume responsibility for the appointment of the first chief executive was a public manifestation of this. It significantly undermined the role of the HSE board, as envisaged, for instance, by the Brennan Commission, which had described the board's 'power of hiring and firing its CEO' as the 'ultimate test of accountability'.[22] At the time of writing, it is too early to judge whether this level of involvement with the everyday affairs of the HSE would continue after Professor Drumm's appointment.

The Lewis affair gave rise to a considerable debate in the UK about the feasibility of separating responsibility for policy and operational decisions. One writer had earlier presciently observed: 'The secretary (Minister), held accountable politically, will soon resume command, for few politicians will be willing to accept the burden of defending an embarrassing situation in Parliament while allowing an agency chief executive to make the key decisions.'[23]

Charles Polidano, an academic defender of the so-called 'Next Steps' executive agencies, argued that agencies could 'live quite well with a policy-operations "boundary" that is shadowy, permeable, and prone to shifting from time to time. This implies uncertainty; but administrators have lived with uncertainty since time immemorial in the complex world that is government.'[24] Nonetheless, Polidano conceded that bureaucrats with high personal visibility like Derek Lewis – or indeed, Brendan Drumm – are in particular danger of becoming political scapegoats. Their best defence is that their agency should have a framework document with defined targets, 'an objective test of performance to which he or she can point if his or her career appears under threat.' British executive agencies have such framework documents, but the HSE and its officials have no such defence against an unpredictable blame game.

Despite the British move towards executive agencies, it is noteworthy that since 2000, the role of chief executive of the

NHS has been combined with the job of permanent secretary of the Department of Health, which is the equivalent of the Secretary General of the Irish Department of Health being simultaneously chief executive of the HSE, an effective merger of policy and operational responsibility. Although the Minister for Health alluded to this combination of roles in the UK during Dáil debate on the Health Bill, she nonetheless maintained that the HSE's 'relationship to the Department will be very much like that between the National Health Service and the Department of Health in the United Kingdom.'[25]

Financial accountability

The HSE now has a separate Vote, for which the CEO is Accounting Officer. When voting on the annual Estimates (the process by which state spending is annually allocated), the Dáil now votes separately on the HSE's funding.

The government decision to make the HSE's CEO the Accounting Officer for a separate HSE Vote was a late development, sponsored by Mary Harney, who told the Dáil:

> This reflects the principle that the board is solely responsible for the management of the health services. This will mean that the CEO will be accountable, in the same way as a Secretary General of a Department, for the appropriation account and for the Vote of the executive. This is a very strong form of accountability for a public body and will give much greater clarity than before as to where responsibility for the management of public funds lies.[26]

An internal Department of Finance briefing subsequently described her rationale for this decision: 'This measure was seen by the Tánaiste as ensuring the desired clarity in lines of accountability by making the HSE fully accountable in its own right in relation to financial and operational matters. By way of precedent, the CEO of the Courts Service is already an Accounting Officer and a similar approach is planned for the Garda Commissioner.'[27]

The Brennan and Prospectus reports had presumed that the Secretary General of the Department of Health would remain in his role as Accounting Officer for the overall Health Vote. Had this remained the case, the Dáil would still allocate the overall Vote to the Department, which in turn would then allocate a budget to the HSE as it had formerly allocated budgets to the health boards (referred to as their 'determination' by the Minister). The Composite Report understood that 'as envisaged by government, the role of the Department in the new structure' would include 'negotiation of the annual Estimates' and 'allocation of HSE budget, setting out the type and quantity of services which it expects to be provided for that allocation.'[28]

A Department of Finance intervention: financial accountability in practice

Documents released to the authors under Freedom of Information (FOI) reveal that during its passage through the Dáil, these provisions of the Health Bill caused considerable debate between the Departments of Health and Finance. The Attorney General's advice was required to clarify the implications of the decision that the HSE would have a separate Vote and the CEO would be an Accounting Officer, and to draft consequent amendments to the Bill.

Department of Finance documents describe how differences emerged between the two departments on these issues. 'The areas where we diverge are of fundamental and central importance', an official of the Department of Finance commented in an internal briefing note in November 2004.[29]

This official outlined that Health took the view that it was no longer in a position to hold the HSE to account financially because the HSE's separate Vote meant that all reports would go directly to Finance and bypass Health. Finance countered that the Minister for Health should still hold the HSE to account. She should negotiate the estimates, approve the service plan, receive and evaluate reports from the HSE, report to the Minister for Finance and government and 'is advised in all this by the DoHC.'

While the Bill was before the Dáil, the Minister for Finance, Brian Cowen, wrote to the Tánaiste presenting the Finance view of how the Bill should be amended. He observed: 'I think it is critically important to get the relationships between the Dáil, the

HSE, the Minister for Health and Children, the Department of Health and Children and the Minister for Finance right. We need to be agreed on the precise legislative basis for this.'[30]

Ultimately, despite some Department of Finance reservations about the appropriateness of its communicating to the Department of Health how it should report to Finance, in December 2004 the Minister for Finance wrote to the Tánaiste, effectively instructing her on her role, the role of her Department and the role of the HSE. The authors have seen no record from either department that the Tánaiste questioned or disagreed with the contents of this letter from the Minister for Finance, Brian Cowen:

> You as Minister for Health, with the assistance of your Department, have the central role in managing the health system overall and holding the HSE to account for its performance – specifically in negotiating the estimates, approving the service plan, ensuring value for money and receiving and evaluating reports from the HSE, with onward reporting where necessary to me and/or the Government.
>
> Your Department will necessarily have a key role in the reporting process. It will be best placed to validate and evaluate reports from the HSE and my Department will be relying on their expertise in that regard. My Department is writing separately to the interim CEO of the HSE outlining the minimum reporting requirements which will attach to the issue of money from the HSE Vote...all such reports by the HSE are to be submitted to you as Minister for Health and Children. I would expect that they would be examined and evaluated as necessary by your Department on your behalf before being sent, with appropriate comments, to my Department.
>
> I would anticipate a similar process operating in relation to requests to sanction additional projects or new schemes and in relation to all aspects of the estimates process – i.e. that my Department would require such proposals to be considered by you as Minister with the assistance of your Department in the first instance and to receive a recommendation regarding each such proposal.
>
> In short, reflecting your position as the Minister directly responsible for the overall performance of the HSE and to

ensure that the best available expertise is utilised in decision making, I will, with my Department, operate through you as Minister and your Department when dealing with HSE matters...

Finally, and importantly, I would like to emphasise that it is critical that all necessary controls and arrangements are in place before an Establishment Order is made. It is of course a matter for you to decide that they are in place. The Board, management tiers and management controls for the HSE need to be fully operational before responsibility for more than €10 billion is handed over to the new organisation.

I have sent a copy of this letter and attachments to the Taoiseach.[31]

A further letter sent the same day to Health officials from David Doyle, Minister Cowen's Second Secretary General with responsibility for public expenditure, was even blunter: 'In short, our Minister's and this Department's day-to-day dealings with the health system will be through your Minister and your Department. We do not intend to maintain a direct line of contact with the HSE.'[32]

Although the Health Act 2004 had appeared to write the Department of Health out of the script, the Department of Finance's refusal to deal directly with the HSE effectively placed the Department of Health right back into the chain of command – and financial accountability. Finance appears to have justified this stance by reference to a memorandum for government of June 2003, when the reform programme was first announced, which stated that the Department of Health would conduct the estimates negotiations on behalf of the Minister.[33] This statement, however, pre-dated the subsequent government decision assigning a separate Vote to the HSE.

The apparent clarity in the Act had been muddied in practice yet again, in respect of financial accountability as in respect of the policy-operation divide, in this case even as the legislation was passing through the Dáil. Officials of the Department of Health reportedly lost no time in ensuring that the senior executives of the interim HSE were aware of the contents of Minister Cowen's letter to their Minister.

Consequences of assigning a separate Vote to the HSE and designating its CEO as Accounting Officer

In whatever manner the Department of Finance has interpreted the Health Act 2004, it remains the case that the HSE now has a separate Vote, for which the CEO is Accounting Officer. This has onerous consequences for the CEO, for the relationship between the CEO and the HSE board, for the financial management of the health service and for the operation of public hospitals.

The role of an Accounting Officer explained

The government decision to assign this role to the CEO of the HSE runs counter to custom and practice within the civil service, where Secretaries General take on the Accounting Officer role for their department's spend. A high-level Working Group on the Accountability of Secretaries General and Accounting Officers, chaired by former Secretary General of the Department of Finance, Paddy Mullarkey, reported in 2002. It observed that the Accounting Officer role of departmental secretaries had been inherited from the UK civil service, where:

> From the beginning it was considered that the best person to discharge the Accounting Officer function was the permanent head of the Department...It was considered that they were the only ones with sufficient authority within Departments to discharge the role...[I]t had also been recognised that finance was an essential element in all policy questions and that financial responsibility had wider implications for efficient management.[34]

The report defined the Accounting Officer for a Vote as 'the person appointed by the Minister for Finance...with responsibility for the preparation of the Appropriation Account(s) and for giving evidence before the PAC (Public Accounts Committee).' The key feature of the Accounting Officer role was the personal responsibility of the most senior official for the 'regularity and propriety of the transactions in the accounts for which s/he is answerable, the control of assets held by the Department, economy and efficiency in the use of the Department's resources and for systems, practices and procedures used to evaluate the effectiveness of its operations.'

Mullarkey observed that the Accounting Officer system was unusual because while the Secretary General was accountable to the Minister for managing the Department, as Accounting Officer he was personally answerable to the PAC. This differed from practice in the private sector, where responsibility would normally rest with the board. In appearing before the PAC, the Accounting Officer appeared in his own right rather than as a representative of the Minister. The duties of the Accounting Officer before the PAC were outside the normal system of civil service delegation where, in general, civil servants act in the name of the Minister. There are specific procedures governing a difference of opinion between the Accounting Officer and the Minister. While the Accounting Officer must comply with the Minister's wishes, he should also inform the Department of Finance and the Comptroller and Auditor General (C&AG) of the circumstances.[35]

Mullarkey identified 'significant overlaps' between the roles of Secretary General and Accounting Officer and concluded: 'The financial management responsibilities of Accounting Officers also necessarily constitute part of the general management responsibilities of Secretaries General under the Minister.'[36]

Effect of Accounting Officer decision on the role of the Secretary General of the Department of Health

Under the terms of the Health Act 2004, the Secretary General of the Department of Health and the CEO of the HSE now divide the roles which Mullarkey reviewed as being combined in the person of the Secretary General. Mullarkey said the Accounting Officer had a responsibility to ensure that financial considerations were taken into account in policy proposals with implications for income and expenditure.[37] This no longer applies in Health. The Secretary General, who has oversight of health policy, is no longer Accounting Officer for the consequent expenditure. Conversely, the CEO of the HSE, who is Accounting Officer for the expenditure, has no control over the policy proposals, which he must then implement.

Mullarkey identified 'important synergies' arising from the role of the Secretary General as Accounting Officer:

> The fact that the duties of Accounting Officer are vested in the most senior official in the organisation, who is personally answerable to the PAC, gives an important focus to managerial accountability for regularity, propriety and value for money in the operations of the Department. This, in turn, contributes to and underpins the exercise of the Secretary General function.
>
> The responsibility of the Accounting Officer gives him/her considerable authority within the organisation, particularly in relation to advice given to the Minister, without undermining the authority of the Minister who is in charge of the Department.

If one accepts this assessment, one can only conclude that the authority of the Secretary General of the Department of Health has been significantly diminished by his loss of the Accounting Officer role.

The Minister could have chosen an alternative route in the Health Act. Both the Brennan Commission's report and the Composite Report had recommended that while the Secretary General of the Department of Health should remain Accounting Officer for the Health Vote, the CEO of the HSE should also be made accountable for his budget. He would have been what the public service terms an 'Accountable Person', whose responsibility differs from that of the Accounting Officer, who has the duty of preparing the Appropriation Accounts of a Department.

The Composite Report said that the CEO should be 'designated an Accountable Person and should have statutory responsibility for giving evidence before the Public Accounts Committee (PAC) for regularity, propriety and Value For Money.'

> Giving evidence to the PAC, which reports to the Dáil, is a key element in the accountability framework for public funds. This will be a particularly important function in the HSE given the size of its budget. The detailed governance arrangements for the HSE, particularly the controls assurance framework, will need to take account of the responsibilities of the CEO as Accountable Person.[38]

It remains difficult to understand why the Minister did not take this recommended route, particularly in light of the Department of Finance's evident discomfort with the assignment of the Vote and Accounting Officer role to the HSE. The Finance refusal to engage directly with the HSE and its requirement that the Department of Health should oversee all aspects of the HSE's relationship with the estimates process has effectively restored to the Secretary General of the Department of Health much of the responsibility of the Accounting Officer without any of the accompanying statutory powers. There is clearly considerable scope for confusion between the roles of the CEO of the HSE, Brendan Drumm, and the new Secretary General at Health, Michael Scanlan.

Effect of Accounting Officer decision on relationship between CEO and HSE board

The CEO's Accounting Officer role has also considerably complicated his relations with the HSE board, weakening the board's control over the financial operations of the HSE and introducing the potential for conflict. Although the Health Act 2004 describes the board as the 'governing body' of the HSE, the CEO is personally responsible for the preparation of the Appropriation Accounts for the HSE's Vote. He signs off on them and reports on them to the Public Accounts Committee of the Dáil – not to his board. The HSE is obliged to prepare *two* sets of accounts: the Appropriation Accounts, which are the CEO's responsibility, and annual income and expenditure accounts, which the board signs off on and which the HSE must submit simultaneously to the Minister and the C&AG. It emerges that the designation of the CEO as Accounting Officer, a measure which was intended to strengthen the powers of the HSE, has burdened it with onerous double accounting responsibilities and has also had the effect of weakening the board's control of its CEO.

In recognition of this, the Minister was obliged to introduce an amendment to the Act, stating the Board 'shall inform the Minister of any matter that it considers requires the Minister's attention.' Minister for State at Health, Brian Lenihan, introduced this amendment, explaining:

Given the accounting officer's responsibilities, there is always the possibility of a conflict between the board and the chief executive officer. In such circumstances, the chief executive officer has the option of seeking written directions from the board and notifying the Comptroller and Auditor General. This is an important aspect of the checks and balances that will operate within the executive. I propose that if such circumstances arise, the board will be under an obligation to inform the Minister about the matter.[39]

Effect of Accounting Officer decision on the management of the health service

The decision to give the HSE a separate Vote has undesirable, practical consequences for the management of the health service. When the Dáil votes expenditure, this is almost set in stone. A Department or body like the HSE, which is in receipt of a Vote, must not exceed this spending. If it looks like doing so, the Dáil must vote a supplementary estimate. This places severe restrictions on how the HSE may manage its finances, which the Department of Finance has communicated to it in detail:

- The HSE has no power to borrow funds.
- Any unspent funds must be returned to the Exchequer at year-end.
- It must keep all its bank accounts in credit at all times.
- It must, however, minimise cash in hand at end-month and end-quarter because that is when Finance calculates Exchequer spending and borrowing.
- Institutions which are now wholly owned by the HSE, like the former health board hospitals, may also not exceed their allocated expenditure for the year.
- If public hospitals earn additional, unexpected revenues, e.g. from private or public patient charges, they must return these funds to the Exchequer. The Minister for Health even appeared to envisage that this requirement might extend to car park charges and canteen receipts.[40]
- If spending on any programme is specified in a sub-heading of the Vote, then it must not be exceeded. The HSE must receive

the permission of the Department of Finance to move spending from one heading to another.

- This means that the HSE is now obliged to track precisely and not exceed allocated spending on hospital and counselling services for people who contracted Hepatitis C from blood products, since this is covered by a separate sub-heading.

Formerly, the Department of Health received a Vote, from which it funded the health boards and voluntary hospitals. The Department could hold back funds which it would allocate to the health boards to fund new programmes or meet over-runs during the year. Health boards and hospitals could also raise and spend additional sources of income, like patient charges. Under this system, a hospital had an incentive to increase revenues since it would keep them. Now, former health board hospitals have lost that incentive, whereas voluntary hospitals, which are funded but not owned by the HSE, retain their incentive to increase revenues. It is quite clear from internal Department of Finance documents that these consequences of assigning a Vote to the HSE were unforeseen and unintended when the government took that decision. These strictures place an enormous administrative burden on the HSE, as well as considerable limitations on its ability to manage the health service.

Legislate in haste, repent at leisure

The passage of the Health Act 2004 would appear to be a case of 'legislate in haste, repent at leisure'. The authors consider it inevitable and desirable that the government should amend the Act. Given the clear Department of Finance view that the Department of Health should negotiate the estimates and intermediate between it and the HSE, and given the many unforeseen and undesirable consequences of assigning a separate Vote to the HSE and the Accounting Officer role to its CEO, the authors recommend that the government revisit this decision, restore the Vote to the Department of Health and the Accounting Officer role to its Secretary General. The CEO of the HSE should then be designated an 'Accountable Person' for its spending, as envisaged in the Composite and Brennan Reports.

Democratic accountability

The dissolution of the health boards and their replacement by the HSE has given rise to understandable concerns about the democratic accountability of this new structure. In health and social care, decisions by government or administrators and the behaviour of professionals can have intimate consequences for the lives of citizens. Democratic societies agree that it is important not only that justice should be done, but that it should be seen to be done, which is why the courts conduct their business in public. Similarly, the decisions which shape a health care system and which determine the allocation of resources between individuals or between locations should be taken transparently and subject to public scrutiny. Delay or denial of care, inadequate or negligent treatment can be a matter of life and death.

The Irish health services are largely Exchequer funded. Even nominally private care benefits substantially from Exchequer subsidy. Health is a central part of the business of government. No democrat should seek to remove politics from health, or health from politics.

The operation of the health service and its relationship to the political system should be transparent. Citizens should know how decisions about health care are taken and by whom. The community as a whole should have ownership and control of such decisions through their elected representatives. The decision-makers in health should ultimately be democratically accountable.

The discussion above about the establishment of the HSE has highlighted some of the grey areas which persist about responsibility and accountability in this new structure. The following discussion examines the operation of democratic accountability under a series of headings.

National democratic accountability: the role of the Oireachtas

The Minister determines health policy and is accountable to the Oireachtas. The CEO of the HSE as Accounting Officer is answerable to the PAC. The board of the HSE is accountable to the Minister. The annual report of the HSE, which includes a report on the implementation of its corporate, service and capital plans, must be submitted to the Minister, who must then lay it before the Houses of the Oireachtas. The HSE's service plan must be laid before the Oireachtas and must be published. An Oireachtas Committee may require the chief executive of the HSE to appear before it to give an account of 'the general administration' of the HSE.

The Minister for Health, Mary Harney, stated that the HSE would have a parliamentary division but told the Dáil 'it is not possible to write into legislation the detail of how the executive should deal with queries from Members of the Oireachtas.'[41] The Health Act 2004 provides for the Minister to make regulations governing the HSE's 'dealings' with members of the Oireachtas. These regulations were finally made in December 2005, 12 months after the passage of the Act.

Experience in the UK would suggest that it is not a clear-cut exercise to assign responsibility for answering parliamentary questions between the Minister and the HSE. After responsibility for answering parliamentary questions was passed to agency chief executives there, there was concern that the replies would not be published. Eventually, they were published in Hansard (in the same way that Minister's answers to Oireachtas members' written questions are published in Irish *Dáil Debates* volumes). But some viewed this as a dilution of ministerial responsibility.[42]

The authors consider the answering of Oireachtas members' questions about the HSE a crucial part of the apparatus to ensure the democratic accountability of the HSE and transparency in its operations. In the 2005 report, which was an earlier version of this book, the authors recommended that if the government decided that the CEO of the HSE should directly answer parliamentary questions, these answers should be published in the *Dáil Debates* volumes, and the Minister should be made aware of their contents prior to their being returned to the questioners. The Minister should be ultimately accountable for the contents of these answers, as for the operation of the health service as a whole. In the event, the December 2005 regulations were minimal. They did not assign responsibility to the CEO of the HSE to answer parliamentary questions. Instead they laid out a framework to ensure that the HSE would be expected to 'deal with any correspondence and requests for access for information from a member of either House of the Oireachtas as expeditiously as may be in accordance with a proper level of customer service.'

The regulations further stated that 'Nothing in these regulations shall be read as implying that a lesser level of customer service is to apply as regards the dealings with a member of either of the Houses of the Oireachtas or any other person.'[43]

This relegation of enquiries to the HSE from Oireachtas members to the status of enquiries from general members of the public offers no reassurance that the Oireachtas will achieve oversight over the operations of the HSE. The authors recommend that these regulations be revised to require that the HSE's parliamentary division answer enquiries from Oireachtas members with as much despatch as the Department formerly answered their parliamentary questions. If this would require that their questions should be parliamentary questions directed to the CEO of the HSE, then this should be the means employed. As an organisation responsible for nearly one-third of Exchequer current spending and for the delivery of health and social services, this would seem an appropriate level of democratic oversight.

A further important measure to ensure accountability and transparency in this new structure is the requirement that when the Minister issues written directions to the HSE, these must be laid before the Houses of the Oireachtas within 21 days. The authors recommend that this provision be further strengthened to require the Minister to publish directions when they are made.

While the HSE board is required to inform the Minister of any matter that it considers requires the Minister's attention, there is no requirement in the Act that this should be made public. The authors recommend that the Minister should be obliged to so inform the Dáil.

Given the important role assigned to Oireachtas committees in ensuring democratic oversight of the HSE, the authors recommend that committee debates and hearings should be available on the Oireachtas website as immediately as full Dáil debates. The role of the Oireachtas Committee on Health and Children should be strengthened. It should be resourced to analyse the activity of the HSE and should meet more often to review its operations.

Local democratic accountability: regional health forums

Representational health boards' public meetings were an opportunity for a regular, transparent calling to account of health administrators for the performance of the health care system. They also provided a public occasion at which the local implications of central decisions could be teased out.

With the dissolution of the boards, this transparency and accountability has been lost to the health care system. When the HSE took a family of children with autism from the care of their parents in March 2005, there was a sense that a faceless and unaccountable organisation had taken this intimate decision. The interim chief executive of the HSE, Kevin Kelly, later told the Oireachtas Committee on Health and Children that he had been 'personally involved in terms of being briefed in detail on the background of the case. I am extremely satisfied with the professionalism with which it was dealt.'

But as Liz McManus, Labour Party deputy leader and health spokesperson, has observed: 'The biggest change – it is an important one – that has occurred is that there is practically no accountability in the system. When children were taken from their parents in the former Northern Eastern Health Board area, there was no accountability system in place to which public representatives, community leaders or whoever could react.'[44]

Kevin Kelly responded, 'We are close to setting up the four regional offices. It is through those offices that there will be liaison and dialogue with public representatives. As to what form this will finally take, that is still being discussed.'

The regional forums, which are provided for in the Health Act 2004, with members appointed by local councils, could restore some transparency and accountability to regional decision making. It would have been preferable for the members of the forums to be directly elected rather than appointed by councils. If the current concerns about a democratic deficit in the operations of the HSE continue after the forums have been in operation for some time, there should be amending legislation to provide for direct elections.

The requirements governing their establishment, composition and operation depend on regulations made by the Minister for

Health in December 2005, 12 months after the passage of the Act. Once again, these were minimal regulations. The forums may not meet more than six times a year; their committees may not meet more than four times. They have no power to require officials of the HSE to attend their meetings to respond to their concerns.[45] The authors recommend that the forums should meet more regularly and publicly and that regional and national officials of the HSE should be required to attend them where necessary. These forums could and should ensure that the HSE, its officers and its decision-making processes become as familiar to local communities and local media as the former health boards.

While the Act provides for the HSE to consult local communities through advisory panels, this is very much a discretionary matter for the HSE, and unlike the forums, does not require the involvement of people with a democratic mandate to speak for local communities.

Organisational accountability: the appointment of the HSE board

The Health Act 2004 provides for the Minister to appoint to the HSE board people 'who, in the Minister's opinion, have sufficient experience and expertise relating to matters connected with the Executive's functions to enable them to make a substantial contribution to the performance of those functions.' In other words, the Minister has complete freedom in whom she chooses, except she may not appoint elected politicians. The Minister rejected an opposition proposal that some members of the board should be directly elected, saying: 'The board is not going to be representational in any sense...I do not think elections always produce the wrong people, but they do not always produce the right people...We cannot have some people elected and others appointed. That is not a good principle in this situation.'[46]

This was a curious position for the Minister to take, given the well-established practice of elected worker directors sitting on the boards of major semi-state companies such as the ESB, RTÉ, Bord na Móna, Bord Gais, Bus Éireann, Dublin Bus and An Post. Employee representatives sat on the health boards. Other semi-state companies like FÁS and the Irish Aviation Authority have directors nominated by unions. While the HSE board has responsibility for not just one but many institutions and services, this does not seem a valid reason to exclude some provision for representational directorships. Although the members of the first HSE board are people of considerable knowledge in a number of spheres, there has been concern among health service employees and others about the paucity of frontline clinical experience among their members. Some provision for elected directors could ensure that there would always be a spread of knowledge on the board of the very diverse areas within the HSE's remit.

It is not good practice for the Minister to have such unconstrained powers in the selection of board members. The Prospectus report observed that international best practice in health organisation governance was that 'there should be clear rules for the composition of the board, for criteria of eligibility, and for the selection and appointment of Board members.' Prospectus reported that the UK, New Zealand and a number of Canadian provinces had centralised, standardised appointment systems in order to promote transparency and accountability.

The HSE is the single most important semi-state organisation, with the highest turnover, largest number of employees and greatest impact on the welfare of the public. The authors recommend that the people who govern it – its directors – must reflect stakeholder interests, including those of employees. It is not adequate that the directors' appointment should be entirely in the hands of the Minister, without any obligation that their appointment should satisfy objective eligibility criteria or ensure a balanced board composition.

Stakeholder consultation: nationally and locally

The Health Act empowers the Minister to appoint a national consultative forum to advise her. Although the Minister told the Dáil that 'the idea is to have all the stakeholders involved' and 'we want this to be as broadly based and representative as possible', she has total discretion in deciding whether to appoint a forum, who should sit on it and how it should conduct its business. The forum is in no sense a mechanism which could hold the health care system or the political system to account.

However, the forum could be developed as a conduit for regular, formal consultation between the Department of Health and other stakeholders on national health policy. This was recommended by the National Primary Care Steering Group in 2004.[47] The Department of Health stated in September 2005 that a draft order providing for the convening of the forum was 'under preparation' in the Department. The authors recommend that the consultative forum should not be established until it can be assured that it will be representative of a comprehensive range of stakeholders in health. It should have the support of a secretariat and the capacity to commission policy studies. It should engage the expertise of effective existing advisory bodies, such as the National Council on Ageing, Women's Health Council, Crisis Pregnancy Agency and Office for Tobacco Control, which are being subsumed into the Department or HSE as part of the administrative reform.

The reader may be surprised to discover that there is no provision for Health interests to be represented on the National Economic and Social Council (NESC). The government has nominated the Secretaries General of five government departments to the NESC, but Health is unrepresented. The authors recommend that the Secretary General of Health and a senior official of the HSE should sit on the council and that the consultative forum should also appoint a representative to the council.

There has been growing awareness nationally and internationally of the value of involving local communities and voluntary groups in the planning and delivery of care. The Primary Care Strategy promised to develop such involvement.[48] The Minister should direct the HSE to deliver on this commitment by developing local advisory panels, which would directly engage citizens and their representatives in local needs identification, planning and decision making. The HSE should engage with local authorities, which have a statutory responsibility for many services that touch on health – physical planning, housing, environmental services, recreation, economic and social development and aspects of transport. The HSE delivers non-acute services through the former community care areas, now the Local Health Offices (LHOs), most of which coincide with local authority areas.

Whistleblowing

The Health Act 2004 has stringent provisions forbidding employees to disclose any information which the HSE defines as confidential. It has been pointed out in the Dáil that whistleblowers have played an important role in protecting the interests of patients.[49] It is the authors' view that this provision of the Act must be balanced by a Whistleblowers' Charter, which protects individuals who can make a defensible case that they have disclosed information in the interests of patient safety.

Role of HIQA

A Health Information and Quality Authority (HIQA) was a key component of the reform programme announced by the government in 2003. This had been proposed in the 2001 Health Strategy.[50] In 2004 the Department of Health published a National Health Information Strategy (NHIS), which described HIQA as 'the central driving force' behind its implementation. The NHIS recommended early establishment of HIQA and the publication of a Health Information Bill.[51]

The Composite Report had envisaged that HIQA would be an independent statutory agency, accountable to the Minister. It would provide independent review of quality and performance and inform policy development within the Department. It should publish a system-wide annual report, providing information on the performance of the system as a whole: 'Responsibility for delivery of health services will lie with the HSE; the DOHC will set the performance management framework. HIQA will assist in the development of the performance management framework and will provide the external review.'[52]

Although the Composite Report recommended that HIQA should be established early in 2004, legislation providing for its establishment had not been published at the time of writing. The Minister appointed an interim board for HIQA in January 2005, when the HSE was already established. The board did not meet until March 2005.

The authors understand that there has been some debate among health policy-makers about HIQA's remit. The

Composite Report advocated that it would extend to all health service providers in both the private and public sectors. It recommended that consideration should be given to the introduction of legislation to require all hospitals, both public and private, to be subject to registration/licensing and audit and quality control standards.[53] It is the authors' view that the absence of a national licensing system for hospitals is a glaring deficiency in Ireland's health care system that exposes citizens to unacceptable risk. We recommend that HIQA be statutorily empowered to require externally validated standards in Ireland's health care system. These standards should apply to hospitals – public, voluntary and private; primary care providers; long-stay care providers and all other health care facilities. HIQA should have statutory powers to inspect health care facilities and police these standards.

The Composite Report also recommended that HIQA should 'have a role in ensuring that health professionals and the public have access to information that enables them to make informed decisions.' While there are many areas in health care in which access to information is important, it has become especially apparent to the authors of this report that informed policy debate about health care in Ireland is hampered by the paucity of regularly published, transparently assembled, up-to-date data. Researchers should not be obliged to make FOI requests to access data which should be in the public domain. Health system data which should be regularly published include health accounts, the national bed count, discharge and treatment patterns of public and private hospitals and earnings of health care professionals (both public and private).

A national health accounting system

Debates concerning the proper level of health spending in Ireland have been confounded with debates concerning what the actual levels of health spending have been because Ireland has no national health accounting system. Figures commonly cited as representing Irish health care spending are widely known to include social spending. Reported current health expenditure is estimated to overstate actual health spending by more than 20 per cent. At the same time, there is no regular and comparable data on private health care spending. A further confusion concerns inconsistent treatment of medical education. The education of nurses appears as a health expenditure, while the education of doctors appears as an education expenditure.

There must be a new health accounting system, with the following properties:

- It must be consistent and comparable with those of leading countries and international organisations (OECD, WHO). This can be achieved by the adoption of the OECD method (see their manual, *System of Health Accounts*).
- It must distinguish clearly between health spending and social spending.
- It should include income as well as product or output accounts.
- It must include money spent from sources other than public sources.
- Expenditures on the education of all health professionals should be reported.

Conclusion: openness, integrity, accountability, clarity

We stated above that our assessment of the HSE would seek to judge it against the principles of openness, integrity and accountability, as well as clarity in roles and responsibilities. We believe there is insufficient clarity about the division of responsibilities between the Minister, her Department and the HSE. This is partly a consequence of deficiencies in the legislation, notably the appointment of the CEO of the HSE as Accounting Officer, but it also appears to reflect a governmental unwillingness to accept political responsibility for the health service, which it has taken unequivocally to itself with the abolition of the health boards. This needs to be understood. The Minister for Health is responsible for the health service, and not only the public health service which the HSE administers, but also the private health service. The standards of care pertaining in private health care, the relationship of private care to the public system, the financial climate in which the private system operates – all of these elements are within government, not HSE, control. The Minister's powers over the HSE – and therefore the public health system – are absolute within the new statutory framework. She appoints and can remove its board, which in turn appoints its CEO. She can direct and instruct it at every turn.

Such centralised power needs to be exercised within a framework of transparency, openness and accountability. That framework remains inadequate. New regulations governing Oireachtas members' questions and the establishment of regional forums offer too limited scope for oversight. HIQA has not been statutorily established. Improved provisions for transparency and accountability should be implemented without delay. The role of the Oireachtas Committee on Health and Children should be strengthened. It should be resourced to analyse the activity of the HSE and should meet more often to review its operations.

We have made a particular case for revisiting the HSE legislation because we believe that the assignment of a separate Vote to the HSE and of the role of Accounting Officer to its CEO has unfortunate consequences for the relationship between the CEO and his board, between the HSE and the Department of Health and for the day-to-day management of the health service. The Minister for Finance and his Department have made clear that, the separate Vote notwithstanding, they hold the Department of Health responsible for the overall financial management of the health service. The power which should accompany that responsibility should be restored to the Department and its Secretary General.

13

AN AGENDA FOR REFORM IN IRISH HEALTH CARE

A system in crisis

It is widely acknowledged that the Irish health care system is in crisis. It is under-resourced, inequitable and frequently chaotic. Changing it for the better will require advancing on a number of fronts together: improving resourcing of people and facilities, ensuring access according to need as a core value and reforming many aspects of how health and social services organise and deliver care.

The government's priority since 2003 has been to reorganise the administration of the health service. The establishment of the HSE in January 2005 was a major reform. Many aspects of this reform remain unclear and some critical elements appear ill considered. Even if it were running smoothly, transparently and with community buy-in, at the end of the day it is nothing more than the reform of an administrative structure. Reforming the Irish health care system is a much bigger enterprise – and it remains to be undertaken.

The 2001 Health Strategy, which purported to be the government's blueprint for reform, has been effectively abandoned. The government shows no signs of delivering on any significant element of it: acute bed capacity, the Primary Care Strategy or extended care and community care facilities for the elderly. The cap on public sector employment since 2002 has made a nonsense of the expansion promised in the strategy.

Yet every day there emerge more and more instances of under-resourcing. Because of a shortage of trained consultant specialists, most specialist care in acute hospital settings is provided by non-consultant hospital doctors (NCHDs) – physicians in training. Public patients and, increasingly, private patients must wait for appointments and care. There are indications of general practitioner (GP) shortages, both overall and in under-served rural and urban areas. Inadequate after-hours supply of GP services puts pressure on hospital accident and emergency (A&E) departments. Supply inadequacies in diverse professions and support services, such as social workers, speech and language therapists and home helps, exacerbate demands on hospitals. Inadequate provision for care of the elderly in the community and in long-stay institutions is a critical contributor to acute care crisis. The mentally ill are under-served whether they need acute or community care.

The public hospital sector has responded badly to the pressures on it. There are waiting lists for hospital services, including outpatient appointments, elective surgery or to see a doctor in an A&E department. Patients continue to be condemned to the purgatory of nights on trolleys in public spaces, finished with their A&E treatment but not yet admitted to hospital rooms and wards. Near-poor patients cannot always afford doctor visits or medicines, and many have lost Medical Card eligibility.

The government seems to be on an ideological crusade to chip away at public health and social services. Medical Card coverage has fallen to an historic low. The government has abandoned a promise of 850 beds in community nursing units but promotes private nursing homes with generous tax subsidies. It has delivered only a fraction of the acute beds promised in the 2001 Health Strategy, but proposes to keep its promise to add hospital beds for public patients, in part by providing tax incentives for the construction of private hospitals. A two-tier system of acute care in hospitals yields unacceptable waiting lists for public care. The government deals with the problem not by addressing the sources of inadequacy and inequity, but by making private patients of those on public waiting lists, in many cases enriching the consultants and rewarding the hospitals who failed the patients in the first place. Even though all are eligible for generous free or subsidised hospital care, half the population buy private health insurance to assure themselves of prompt, consultant-provided care.

Hospitals are not licensed and doctors do not face mandatory quality assurance, clinical audit or continuing medical education. Salaried public hospital consultants are not accountable, either clinically or administratively.

The system is replete with anomalous incentives which lead to inefficient behaviour. Methods of paying doctors and relative prices of aspects of medical care promote behaviours by doctors and patients which will not produce the best outcomes for health. Community-rated private health insurance expresses social solidarity, but delays and uncertainties regarding risk equalisation can yield fear of adverse selection by the VHI, providing it with an incentive to discriminate against aged customers. Hospital budgeting is arbitrary, fails to take account of demographic changes, is inconsistent with hospital autonomy, does not include incentives for efficient behaviour and yields inter-regional inequities.

These many problems take a toll on the health of the Irish people, who have shorter life expectancies and higher morbidities for many illnesses than is the average for Europe. The poor, who are much more likely to be sick, are much less likely to receive the care they need when they need it under the Irish system.

A moment of opportunity

In spite of this litany of problems and concerns, it can also be said that the present moment is one of enormous opportunity for Irish health care. There are three sources of notable strength upon which to build.

Firstly and centrally, Ireland is blessed with an endowment of well-trained and skilled health service staff: GPs, consultants, nurses and allied health personnel. Even though there is a cap on employment, training places have increased in a number of key health care professions. While the system they are located in is in important ways dysfunctional, the human component of the health care system is a strong base upon which to build.

Secondly, the Irish economy is strong. After more than a decade of rapid economic growth, Ireland can have a health care system which is appropriate to its wealth and which its people deserve. Not every required reform is costly, but some of them clearly are. Poverty is no longer a reason not to provide needed care on an efficient and equitable basis.

However, economic strength is, perhaps ironically, a double-edged sword. The Irish economy is currently operating at or near full capacity. There is a labour shortage, one met in part by returning Irish emigrants and by immigrants. In an economy operating at capacity, the health care system can grow rapidly only if other sectors are reduced in size. Adding doctors, other clinicians, primary care centres and hospital beds can be done with ease only if expansion occurs in a planned way over time. This limitation does not apply to changes in the way existing care is financed, e.g. to added Medical Cards, relief for low-income non-Medical Card holders or universal health insurance, unless those financing changes bring about changes in the real size of the health care system.

Thirdly, Ireland can benefit from four years of extraordinarily deep and insightful examinations of the health care system – among them the Brennan Report on financial management, the Deloitte & Touche report on value for money, the Hanly Report on hospital organisation, physician training and a consultant-provided specialist service, and not least of all, the Health Strategy and its spin-off, the Primary Care Strategy. Rarely, one suspects, has a country of any size seen such an extensive and intensive examination of its health care system. One need not agree with every point in every report to admire the scholarship, ingenuity and wisdom of this multi-volume work. It is a firm foundation for reform.

In this chapter we recapitulate the recommendations for change made by the authors throughout this report. The rationale for our proposals appears not so much here as in the appropriate chapters from which the recommendations are drawn. Some of the proposed changes are costly. We do not flinch from recommending costly changes, even in the short run.[1] The changes we propose are important in the lives of people. They affect standards of living, health, even life itself. We then conclude by looking at the big picture. We describe the kind of health care system we believe Ireland can and should move towards in the coming years.

Recommendations for change

Spending

- Debate on health spending should take place in a climate of honest appraisal, and a national system of health accounts should be developed as a matter of urgency to facilitate informed debate.
- Current and capital spending on health and social care needs to increase to fund the capacity deficits identified in the 2001 Health Strategy – in primary, continuing, community and acute care.
- This increase in spending should be implemented in a planned and paced manner, and within the framework of the 2003 Hanly Report, of reform in how hospital doctors work and are remunerated and in how patients access care.
- The costing of the 2001 Health Strategy by the Department of Health should be revisited. Its statement of capacity needs should be reassessed and revised if necessary in light of population growth and the more developed understanding which is emerging of the relationships between the acute care and other sectors.
- There should be a comprehensive and realistic analysis of the investment needs of health and social services over the next 10 years, followed by a planned, phased commitment of investment.

Privatisation

- The government should abandon its plan to permit and encourage private hospitals to be constructed on the grounds of public hospitals.
- The VHI should continue to be a state company so that it can continue to serve national rather than private or parochial interests. Whatever is the future of the VHI, it should not become a for-profit company.

Incentives

- The Irish health care system has within it many anomalies in economic incentives, leading to inefficient and inequitable results.
- Hospital consultants should treat all patients, public and private, in the same way. Hence, they should be paid in the same way for all patients. To avoid over- and under-provision of care, this should be a hybrid system, part salary and part fee per item of service. This change would be a major move in attacking the two-tier system of care.
- GPs should also treat all patients, public and private, in the same way. Hence, they should be paid in the same way for all patients. Ideally, this should be a hybrid system, part capitation and part fee per item of service.
- Hospitals should be paid in the same ways for public and private patients to remove any incentives for them to differentiate between them in ways that favour private patients.
- Hospital budgeting should be reformed. Hospital budgets should be set in large part on the basis of their case loads, but should also have a significant discretionary component set by the HSE.
- Economically non-neutral devices such as the doctor-only Medical Card should be avoided.
- GPs should receive capitation rates set according to risk. Rates favouring people living greater distances from GPs' offices and favouring 70-and-overs who do not receive Medical Cards on the basis of need should be re-examined and changed.

Financing

- Public hospitals should set charges for private patients at the level of true economic cost.
- GPs should receive the same capitation rate for all 70-year-olds and over. The present premium rate for 70-plus recipients creates inequity among GPs and discourages GPs from locating in low-income areas.
- The DPS programme caps drugs expenditures for households at €85 per month, or €1,020 per year, which is too high. The DPS system should be reformed to reimburse a percentage of

all prescription drug purchases by non-Medical Card holders at the point of sale, and that percentage should be higher for people on lower incomes.

- Risk equalisation should be effected between Bupa and VHI, and in any circumstance in which competing insurance companies have significantly different risk profiles.

Primary care

- Access to free primary care should be restored immediately to its 1997 level and extended soon to the entire population.
- Medical Card eligibility on the basis of need should be restored immediately to the traditional proportion of the population, which is in the range of 35 to 38 per cent. After that change, Medical Card guidelines should be indexed to the median income of production workers or the median earnings of Irish workers, so that they change continuously rather than intermittently and so that the level is set automatically rather than politically.
- A new form of eligibility should be created for those low-income people who are not eligible for Medical Cards but whose incomes place them in the bottom half of the Irish income distribution. The rise in medical costs associated with a rise in income that makes people or families ineligible for Medical Cards is enormous; a form of eligibility which buffers the shock of this difference, perhaps through a demi-Medical Card which provides half-benefits, is needed now.
- The organisation and infrastructure of Irish primary care needs modernisation. This may be the single most important change needed now in the Irish health care system. The needed changes are along the lines of the Primary Care Strategy and the ICGP/IMO *Vision*. Flaws in these and the widespread view that the Primary Care Strategy is dead require a new, credible plan. The plan must include commitment of adequate resources over a long period of time, beginning immediately. The plan should achieve multi-disciplinary, public-private primary care teams in technologically modern primary care centres, built with state support.

- There should be legislation requiring universal patient registration as an immediate step toward modern care and public-private integration.

Hospitals: capacity

- Acute hospital bed capacity is insufficient and should be expanded in a planned and honest manner. The HSE should produce a plan for expanded hospital capacity. This should begin with a transparent bed count validated by HIQA. It should also include an assessment of the actual ratio of beds to population in each region, and it should be reconciled with the regional reorganisation of acute hospital services.
- Investment in extra acute beds should take place against a backdrop of explicit identification of which hospitals should grow, which should change function and of changes in how hospitals are staffed, managed and financed.
- If the government, the HSE or official policy-makers are no longer convinced of the merit of the assessment of capacity needs in the Acute Hospital Bed Capacity Review, the government should initiate a further review as a matter of urgency. This review should take into account the considerable increase in population and population growth forecasts since the 2001 review.

Hospital-acquired infections

- The growing problem of hospital-acquired infections reinforces the case for greater investment in hospitals in order to increase capacity, increase the number of single rooms and the space around beds in wards and to modernise outdated facilities.
- The authors endorse the Infection Control Sub-Committee's strategy for the control and prevention of MRSA and point out that while improved hygiene has an important role to play, the sub-committee was clear that present staffing and hospital facilities are inadequate to control MRSA.

Hospitals: equity

- There should be a common waiting list for patients in public hospitals, but with care to be provided promptly so that few patients appear on waiting lists and none stays long.

- Public hospitals may offer patients who choose to pay for them enhanced, private rooms, but must provide them with the same care as all other patients. In other words, there should be no private and public patients in public hospitals.
- Public hospitals with unused capacity should be funded to treat more patients within the public system, not via the National Treatment Purchase Fund (NTPF).
- If public hospitals are not funded to operate at full capacity, they should be permitted to compete to supply NTPF-funded treatments on the same footing as private hospitals.
- The NTPF's annual report should contain precise details of how many procedures have taken place respectively in public and private hospitals, in Ireland and abroad and of the cost per procedure in each of these hospitals.

Hospitals: A&E, long-stay and community care

- Any existing public long-stay capacity which is not open should be reopened immediately.
- In the short term, public purchases of private nursing home care, flexibility in working practices and better hospital team-working can play a role in easing A&E pressures.
- The acute medical units (AMUs) for Tallaght, Beaumont and St Vincent's should be fast tracked by the government.
- AMUs should be developed in all acute hospitals with A&E departments.
- The government should invest in increasing capacity and services in public long-stay institutions, staffing and services in community care and in acute care bed capacity.
- The government should as a matter of urgency develop public community nursing units for older people, as envisaged in the Health Strategy. The units should offer services and facilities for assessment/rehabilitation, respite, extended care, care of the elderly, mentally infirm and convalescence. Day centres for the elderly should be combined with the community nursing units. The first of these units should be developed without

delay in Dublin, where inadequate extended care facilities place great pressure on acute hospitals.

- Community care supports for people at home should complement, but not substitute for, the expansion of extended care facilities planned in the Health Strategy.
- The state should take responsibility for providing a secure, well-funded and high-quality system of long-term care for frail elderly, severely disabled and others unable to care for themselves, to be provided by or funded by the state, either from taxation or social insurance, or with a co-payment element, which is proportionate to the income and assets of the beneficiary but is neither an unpredictable private charge nor an effective confiscation of the income of pensioners, as is currently the case.

Mental health services

- The Department of Health and the HSE must develop a modern mental health strategy with a national minimum standard of care.
- Mental health services should be planned, expanded and funded in response to analysis of unmet need.
- Additional psychiatric inpatient units should be developed.
- Community care and rehabilitative services should be expanded.
- The numbers of psychiatrists, psychotherapists, family therapists, clinical psychologists and occupational therapists should be increased.
- An outpatient team specialising in eating disorders should be established to provide a regional service with an inpatient facility.

Hospital specialist care

- Ireland needs mandatory physician quality assurance, clinical audit and continuing medical education. The Medical Practitioners Act should be revised without delay in order to give a statutory basis to these reforms.
- The consultants' contract must be reformed. It is central to inequity in access to hospital care and is an obstacle to rational

management in Irish hospitals. The authors appreciate that revising the contract will be a difficult and time-consuming process. A reformed contract should provide for clinical and administrative accountability; should require all consultants to treat patients according to need, drawn from a common waiting list; and should require all consultants to work as rostered members of teams, answerable to a head of department or clinical director, who is in turn answerable to the hospital/hospital group's CEO.

- The option of a public-only contract should be available to all consultants and should be mandatory for newly appointed consultants.
- The Category II contract permitting off-site private practice should no longer be offered.
- Hospital consultants should be paid in the same way for all patients, whether public or private. Ideally, it should be a hybrid method. There should be a salary component which reflects not only public care but also private care. That can be achieved by mandating monthly contributions from insurance companies in relation to patient numbers. There should be a fee component for both public and private patients. That can be achieved through state payment of fees.

Hospitals: organisation

- Hospital services should be reorganised to ensure a consultant-delivered service for all patients, to ensure supervised and genuine training for all NCHDs and, above all, to ensure that patients, wherever they live, receive high and consistent standards of treatment and care. To achieve these objectives will inevitably require some smaller hospitals to cease offering A&E and acute surgery services. They will have to become satellite hospitals to larger regional centres. Every region should develop a genuine centre of excellence.
- Reorganisation of hospital services should not be viewed in isolation from the many other factors which affect patients' access to and experience of care. These include primary care, community care, ambulance services, the capacity and quality

of existing regional hospitals, travel distances to hospitals and the quality of roads, the quality and availability of public transport, population projections, spatial planning and the commitment of investment.

- Smaller hospitals should not discontinue services until extra capacity and staffing have been provided in the regional centre to meet their needs.

Hospital management
- Major Hospitals and affiliated Local (and General) Hospitals in a region should constitute an organisational entity, with a governing board and significant local and regional representation for each hospital network.
- The governing board should act as an interface between the HSE and the hospital. It should represent a variety of interests – the state (the Department of Health, the HSE), local and regional economic interests, the trade union movement, non-governmental organisations (NGOs) and patients – and should eventually have the power and responsibility to appoint the CEO, approve budgets and capital plans, hear audit reports and otherwise function as a governing board functions.
- Hospitals/hospital groups should have a single budget, should be led by a single CEO and should share consultant staff, some of whom would rotate among the hospitals to provide care.
- Hospital doctors should be managed within a modified version of the clinical directorate in which budget and planning powers are retained by CEOs. Clinical directors should be chosen by hospital CEOs, or at the very least, with the concurrence of hospital CEOs.
- Hospitals should be paid in the same ways for public and private patients in order to remove any incentives for them to discriminate in favour of private patients.
- Hospital budgets should be set in large part on the basis of their case loads, but should also have a significant discretionary component set by the HSE. This component should permit budgets to reflect circumstances that vary from hospital to hospital and provide a continuing payment to hospitals to

reflect the service they provide to their communities through their mere existence and availability.

Health service staffing

- The cap on employment in the health services has been harmful and inefficient from the start and should be lifted so that health staffing can grow to meet unmet needs. The cap was created when the Department of Health still ran the health services, and would be inconsistent with the integrity of the HSE even if there were no unmet demand.
- Planning for future staffing needs should become an integral part of the operations of the Department of Health and the HSE.
- Planning should be based on assessments of need across care areas and disciplines and should be informed by regular monitoring.
- Decisions on the number of educational and training places for health and social service staff should be based on evidence of need, analysis of the inter-relationships of health care staff and population growth projections.
- Ireland needs increases in the numbers of both GPs and hospital consultants. It will take years to achieve the needed and desired numbers, especially if Irish nationals are to fill most of the needed posts. But the long process must begin now. The cap on Irish (and other EU) students in Irish medical schools must be drastically raised, as the Fottrell Report recommended. The authors also endorse adding a post-graduate stream in Irish medical education. The numbers of places in specialist training programmes in general practice in Ireland must be increased. Further, the authors urge implementation of the comprehensive recommendations of the Hanly Report on specialist training.
- The Department of Health should commission and publish a specialist study on the type of work typically undertaken by nurses in Ireland and in countries at a comparable level of development to Ireland in order to assess the feasibility, safety and efficiency of the government's policy of employing more

health care assistants as complements to and/or substitutes for nurses.

- Health care assistants should have mandatory training and nurse supervision.
- The Department of Health should undertake a survey which quantifies unmet need for the services of social workers in hospitals, primary and community care.

Administration of the health services

- The Minister for Health should be democratically and transparently accountable for the health service and its associated social services.
- The government should amend the Health Act 2004 to restore the full Health Vote to the Department of Health and the Accounting Officer role to its Secretary General. The CEO of the HSE should then be designated an 'Accountable Person' for the HSE's spending, as envisaged in the Composite and Brennan Reports.
- Regulations governing the answering of Oireachtas members' questions about the HSE are inadequate and should be strengthened. If the government decides that the CEO of the HSE should directly answer parliamentary questions, these answers should be published in the *Dáil Debates* volumes and the Minister should be made aware of their contents prior to their being returned to the questioners. The Minister should be ultimately accountable for the contents of these answers, as for the operation of the health service as a whole.
- When the Minister issues written directions to the HSE, the Minister should be required to publish these directions at the time they are made.
- While the HSE board is required to inform the Minister of any matter that it considers requires the Minister's attention, there is no requirement in the Act that this should be made public. The Minister should be obliged to so inform the Dáil.
- Given the important role assigned to Oireachtas committees in ensuring democratic oversight of the HSE, the authors recommend that committee debates and hearings should be available on the Oireachtas website as immediately as full Dáil debates.

The role of the Oireachtas Committee on Health and Children should be strengthened. It should be resourced to analyse the activity of the HSE and should meet more often to review its operations.

- The regional forums provided for in the Health Act 2004, with members appointed by local councils, could restore transparency and accountability to regional decision making. They should ensure that the HSE, its officers and its decision-making processes become as familiar to local communities and local media as the former health boards. However, the Minister's regulations governing their establishment are too restrictive. These regulations should be revised to provide for the forums to meet more regularly and to require regional and national officials of the HSE to attend them where necessary.
- If the current concerns about a democratic deficit in the operations of the HSE continue after the forums have been in operation for some time, there should be amending legislation to provide for direct elections.
- The national consultative forum should be established as a conduit for regular, formal consultation between the Department of Health and other stakeholders on national health policy once there is assurance that it will be representative of a comprehensive range of stakeholders.
- The consultative forum should have the support of a secretariat and the capacity to commission policy studies. It should engage the expertise of existing effective advisory bodies, such as the National Council on Ageing, Women's Health Council, Crisis Pregnancy Agency and Office for Tobacco Control, which are being subsumed into the Department of Health or HSE as part of the administrative reform.
- The Secretary General of Health and a senior official of the HSE should sit on the National Economic and Social Council (NESC), and the consultative forum should also appoint a representative(s) to the Council.
- The Primary Care Strategy promised to develop the involvement of local communities and voluntary groups in the planning and delivery of care. The Minister should direct the HSE to deliver on this commitment by developing local advi-

sory panels, as provided for under the Health Act 2004, which would directly engage citizens and their representatives in local needs identification, planning and decision making. The HSE should engage with local authorities.

- Appointment of directors to the HSE's board should not be entirely in the hands of the Minister. Their appointment should satisfy objective eligibility criteria and ensure a balanced board composition. The directors must reflect stakeholder interests, including those of employees.
- The confidentiality provisions of the Health Act 2004 should be balanced by a Whistleblowers' Charter that protects individuals who can make a defensible case that they have disclosed information in the interests of patient safety.
- The authors endorse the recommendations of the Brennan Commission for key positions in health administration to be filled by open competition and for further review of the common recruitment pool.
- We recommend that the government should offer early retirement and voluntary redundancy packages to former health board staff who do not wish to remain in the HSE.

Patients' rights

- There should be a statement of principles affirmatively expressing patients' rights, along the lines of the European Charter of Patients' Rights. It is not necessary, and given the litigious character of Irish society, not desirable, that the charter be enforceable in courts of law, unless there is specific legislation regarding any of its contents. The charter should guide the HSE, the government, lawmakers and others who write statutes and make policy. It should also guide clinicians, administrators and other personnel who make decisions affecting patients. No one should forget that the patient is the beginning and the end – the *raison d'être* for the health care system.

HIQA

- Legislation creating the Health Information and Quality Authority (HIQA) should be passed without further delay.

- HIQA should be statutorily empowered to require externally validated standards in Ireland's health care system. These standards should apply to all hospitals – public, voluntary and private, primary care providers, long-stay care providers and all other health care facilities. HIQA should have statutory power to inspect health care facilities and police these standards.
- HIQA should regularly publish health system data, including health accounts, the national bed count, discharge and treatment patterns of public and private hospitals and earnings of health care professionals (both public and private).
- HIQA should have responsibility for the collection, collation and timely publication of hospital bed data. HIQA should require the Department of Health and the NHO to report regularly on when and where actual new beds have been funded, commissioned and made available for the treatment of patients.
- HIQA should have responsibility for maintaining, verifying and publishing waiting list data. HIQA should examine the reasons why patients decline the NTPF's offer of treatment.

Irish health care: attainable objectives

The authors' vision of the future Irish health care system is not a utopia but rather an attainable system appropriate to this country, which can be reached in a decade or less if appropriate first steps are taken now. While we have listed many recommendations, here we emphasise the major objectives which any reform should aim to achieve.

Access

- Free primary care for all.
- A common waiting list for patients in public hospitals, but with care to be provided promptly so that few patients appear on waiting lists and none stays long.
- Public hospitals may offer hotel-like private rooms to patients who choose to pay for them, but should provide them with the same care as all other patients. In other words, there are no private and public patients in public hospitals.

- A state-provided or guaranteed long-term care system for frail elderly, severely disabled and others unable to care for themselves.

Resources

- More Irish medical students.
- More GPs.
- More hospital consultants.
- More allied professionals.
- More community care services.
- More modern long-stay and community care facilities.
- A planned expansion of acute hospitals.

Quality

- A modern primary care system, with GPs, practice nurses, public health nurses, physiotherapists, social workers and others working in teams from modern, well-equipped, computerised primary care centres in every community and large urban neighbourhood.
- A consultant-provided specialist service in acute hospitals.
- Reduced numbers of NCHDs, but sufficient in specialist training to provide an adequate continuing stream of new consultants.

Management

- Improved accountability and control, including clinical accountability, for all doctors and hospitals and other clinicians as well.
- Transparent and rational allocation of resources, including a reformed method of financing hospitals.
- Standardised health accounts comparable with those of other states, comprehending all care, public and private.

Priorities and timing

Investment priorities

There are many investment needs, all of which call out for immediate funding, but it is not possible to address them all at once. Even if unlimited funds were available, policy-makers would not be wise attempting major change simultaneously along manifold inter-related fronts. They would err or stumble because the limits on human ability to focus and to anticipate consequences are also finite.

Among the alternative investment priorities, the authors have chosen two to advance for immediate action.

One is the modernisation of primary care. This is a past-due reform and its full achievement will take a decade or more. It requires a new plan and immediate investment to begin the long but exciting task of building a patient-centred, technologically advanced inter-disciplinary primary care system.

The other is expansion of long-stay and community facilities for the ageing population, not only in Dublin, where it is desperately needed, but throughout the state.

The authors believe that expansion of acute hospital capacity is also urgently needed, but as we have described in this report, that investment should be developed with care and driven by planning. It should be paced and should take place first in hospitals which can show that they are using their existing capacity in the most effective manner possible, and which are well integrated with local community, primary and long-stay services. This planning and vetting process should take no more than a year. In the meantime, both primary care modernisation and expansion of long-stay and community facilities for the ageing will relieve pressure on the acute system. Private hospitals on public sites should not and cannot substitute for the expansion of public acute hospitals.

Access priorities

Particular populations in Ireland have urgent access needs which must be addressed immediately as the first priorities. First is the low-income population just above the current Medical Card eligibility threshold. Two steps need to be taken to relieve their burdens. Firstly, full Medical Card eligibility should be restored to the 35 to 38 per cent level which was traditionally followed until recently. Secondly, the remaining 12 to 15 per cent of the population in the bottom half of the income distribution should be given partial Medical Card benefits, with the 'demi-Medical Card' as an example.

In the acute system, there should immediately – tomorrow! – be a common waiting list for public and private patients.

Are there any measures that can be taken now to improve the situation in A&Es this winter?

Yes. Despite the government's emphasis on the A&E problem, it is surprising that some measures have not been taken more quickly. The HSE should take whatever steps are necessary to reopen immediately any available public long-stay facilities. The cap on health sector employment should be lifted, even though it does not apply to the Minister's 10-point plan, because it is still a constraint on fast and effective problem solving by health sector managers.

The government should make it a priority to publish proposals for the funding of a system of long-term care which guarantees care to all citizens in need and for which the cost is shared across the community. This measure will not immediately improve A&E, but it will provide reassurance to many older people and their families about their future care. If such a system were in place, with community support, in 12 months' time, discharge planning from public acute hospitals would be transformed.

A further measure, which will take time to bear fruit but which will also reassure older people and health sector and hospital managers, would be the immediate putting out to tender for the 17 community nursing units planned by Micheál Martin and vetoed by the Department of Finance.

How important are the consultants' contract negotiations?

All reform-minded people will be watching over the shoulders of the people's representatives in their negotiations on a new consultants' contract. We would wish them to enter into negotiations determined to deliver the reforms described in the section on hospital specialist care above.

These negotiations have the potential to deliver an historic reform. Their outcome could control our ability to reform the acute care system for years to come. The negotiations cannot be addressed in isolation. They must be seen in the context of a holistic need to reform the Irish health care system. Without contract reform, the system will remain inequitable, unsafe and unmanageable.

How threatening to the public hospital system is the private hospitals plan?

The plan to erect publicly subsidised private hospitals on public hospital grounds is a crossroads issue. If it goes forward, a changed Irish acute care system, one difficult to reverse or reform, may soon be in place. Along with the priorities for modernisation of primary care, for restoring Medical Cards, for nursing homes and community care, there is the priority to stop the private hospital plan. Indeed, the latter may be more crucial than the former in the coming days, because soon the private hospitals' scheme will be a *fait accompli* and we will be talking about undoing it rather than preventing it.

We have not stated that we are opposed to private hospitals per se. There are fine and equitable health care systems in which a private hospital sector plays a role. But what is peculiar to Ireland is the mix of the public and private – how private hospitals are largely staffed by public salaried consultants, how they operate without the overheads of pensions for their key staff and largely without junior doctors or multi-disciplinary care. Within the health care system at present, they draw resources from the public hospitals and perform only those procedures which are straightforward and predictable. The existing private hospitals linked to public hospitals do not, by and large, take acutely ill patients from their sister hospitals, not even patients with private insurance.

Ultimately, every resident of Ireland needs the security of a well-resourced, well-functioning public acute system. That is where patients go in acute emergencies. That is where older people receive care for the illnesses of later life. Private hospitals offer elective care, not crisis care. If they are further encouraged to proliferate, especially with the existing consultants' contract, and especially on the sites of public hospitals, they will undermine our public institutions. It is difficult enough for hospital chief executives to manage consultants who may conduct their own private business on site or off. How much more difficult will it be if those consultants are working for another employer on the very same campus, who can offer them the incentive of private fees? Or, worse still, if public consultants stand to gain as shareholders from the profits of the on-site private hospital? If much of elective care is drawn from the public to the private institution, how will medical students and junior doctors gain a rounded education? How will private patients recovering from elective care benefit from the multi-disciplinary after-care that public hospitals can offer?

Stand-alone private hospitals with their own staff, not public hospital staff, could have a role in selling their services to an equitable public system. It would be more reassuring for the patient if they were not-for-profit. Private companies could contract to build capacity for the public system. To say that the private sector designs and builds faster is no reason to hand the health care system over to the private sector.

It is in the interests of Irish society to develop an integrated, equitable, universal health care system. Private hospitals that compete on fair terms and may no longer employ public staff could be part of that.

Changing the system of funding

Health insurance for all?

Many observers have advocated a universal health insurance (UHI) system for Ireland, with everyone mandated to have cover, and with state subsidies towards the cost according to the incomes of individuals and households. We neither single it out as the sole pathway to reform nor do we oppose UHI. It has both advantages and disadvantages for Ireland.

The central attraction of UHI to its advocates is that it provides a clear path to enhanced equity. If consultants and public hospitals privilege private, fee-paying patients over non-fee-paying public patients, one way to provide seemingly instant equity is to pay fees for all patients, and a very straightforward way to achieve that is to provide health insurance for all. To achieve equity, it will be easier to provide health insurance to those who do not have it than to take it away from those who do. To achieve equity, it will be easier to pay fees for public patients than to switch to an all-salaried consultant system and pay salaries in respect of private care.

There are other advantages to UHI:

- By subsidising insurance instead of the costs of particular types of care, the state can use allocationally neutral subsidies.
- Health care resource allocation decisions can increasingly be put in the hands of doctors and patients instead of the Department of Health or the HSE.
- If care prices are proportional to economic costs, doctors and patients will automatically be able to compare benefits with social costs in deciding on care.
- Money will automatically follow patients.
- If primary care is included in the insurance system, as it should be, there would automatically be needed burden relief for low-income patients.
- If primary care is included, there would be an injection of resources into the primary care system, which could help in the primary care modernisation process. If drugs are included, there would automatically be burden relief for low-income patients.
- Insurance premiums will be higher than currently, covering the economic costs of care and the addition of primary care and drugs. Increased premiums for upper-income individuals can inject more money into the health care system without a tax increase.
- Private and public hospitals could supply care on an equitable basis to all patients.

UHI requires either a single insurance provider, ideally a state or semi-state body such as the VHI, covering all people or a system of risk equalisation to create equity amongst competing insurers and to avoid fear of adverse selection. If there is a single insurance provider, insurance could be funded by new pay-related social insurance (PRSI) contributions related to income rather than by premiums. An amount of income should be free from liability for such PRSI to exempt low-income people from contributing, and to inject progressivity into the structure. Funding through PRSI would also require employers to make contributions. Many employers already contribute to their employees' VHI schemes. This approach would have the attraction of being a social partnership approach, with individuals, businesses and the state having a shared interest in the health of the health care system.

Disadvantages of UHI

Universal health insurance typically makes the greatest use of fee-for-service medicine of any model of health care system. The authors have tried to mitigate these effects by suggesting hybrid payments systems for both GPs and consultants. But with UHI it would be difficult to avoid increased use of user charges, prices and fees. The reason is that, with insurance, the public will buy many kinds of care with insurance cover instead of seeing it provided directly by the state. There would be a fee component in public GP care and a fee component in public consultant care. It is known that the economic effect of such instruments is to increase utilisation throughout the system. Thus, a UHI system is predisposed to higher levels of utilisation and hence health care expenditure than other systems.

UHI systems generally look to a variety of other methods to control costs, e.g. spending caps, pre-utilisation review, supply-side care rationing, etc. to offset the expansionary effects of fees. Such devices are helpful, but not perfect.

The list of benefits of UHI is imposing. The disadvantages are real, but they may seem small in comparison to the benefits. What is needed is a public debate concerning the best way for Ireland to reach the objectives of neutrality, transparency, efficiency and equity.

Alternatives to UHI?

There are equitable and efficient alternatives to UHI, achieved through reforms of the existing tax-funded system. Without UHI there could be free primary care in which the state would pay GPs by salary, capitation, fees or a mixture of methods. Without UHI the state could ban private practice in public hospitals and invest in public care so that the majority would opt to be treated in one-tier public hospitals. Without UHI, consultants could be paid by a hybrid of salaries and fees. Such a system would move towards that in the UK or Denmark, which are much more mainstream internationally than the existing Irish system. The VHI would then revert to insuring a much smaller proportion of the population for elective care in the small number of private hospitals. Provided the state invested sufficiently in the public system, the nascent private hospital industry would probably lose its appeal. However, if the state did not invest sufficiently in the public system, there would be a risk that patients and doctors would take flight into the private system and the two-tier divide would not only fail to disappear, but actually widen and deepen.

Reform advocates have turned to UHI because it avoids some of these risks. It creates a system in which all must participate. The distinction between public and private patients ends. Private hospitals contract to treat patients within the state system. The VHI remains large and possibly grows further as part of the new system.

Payment of an insurance premium for each individual for a defined package of benefits provides an earmarked fund for health care. Consultants can be paid a combination of salary and fees, economically a better arrangement than all of one or the other, and politically possibly easier to achieve than an all-salary system. In states where doctors are paid by fees, there are alternative cost-control measures like capping their incomes or freezing their rates of pay. No system is perfect, and realistically, no system will end the struggle between states and doctors over who owns and controls health care.

Paying for an improved health care system

Improved health and social services cannot be achieved without sustained investment and increased current spending. Reform need not necessarily require additional resources for health care. Free primary care, for instance, obviates the need for much private spending on health and represents a rechanneling of payments by individuals (from private fees to tax or PRSI), not an additional cost to Irish society, except in so far as services grow and need to be funded in the sector. The benefit of such a universal, free at point of use system is that instead of flat fees which hit poorer families hard and hit people hardest when they are sickest, there is a predictable annual contribution, progressively levied and shared across the community. But achieving a health care system which meets the expectations of Ireland today will also require growth in services. That means that Irish society must fund additional spending, whether by means of extra taxation or social insurance or by reduced tax incentives or state spending elsewhere.

It has not been our brief to describe how the future financing of health care might be achieved – which sectors of society should contribute more or less, now or in the future. However, we would support its achievement by equitable and progressive means. The existing state subsidies and tax incentives and the existing organisation of the health care system frequently subsidise private care and discriminate against those who depend on the public system. We argue for an equitable, universal health care system, with care delivered according to need and funded according to ability to pay. In Appendix 5 we indicate the dimensions of the investment required to deliver a better-resourced system, and explain which reforms would represent a rechanneling of payment and which would require additional resources for health care.

Conclusion

The analysis contained in this report and the recommendations based on that analysis seek four objectives:
- To address as a matter of urgency the current crisis in the Irish health care system, which has too often failed to meet patients' needs and whose chaotic problems are constantly on the front pages in recent times.
- To advance the principle of social solidarity, which weaves together in a single, strong fabric the young and the old, the rich and the poor and the well and the sick with a single, central idea: that care goes to those who need it.
- Because resources are finite and medical need is not, to organise the Irish health care system according to principles of economic and administrative efficiency.

- To advance the principles of clarity, transparency, accuracy, thoroughness and timeliness of information concerning health and health care.

Though health and longevity reflect many factors, individual and social, other than medical care, they remain the final test of the health care system. The health care system, first of all, must do no harm. Among other things that means that hospital patients should not acquire infections in hospital. Further, a modern system of primary and community care must assure that, in so far as possible, Irish people remain free from preventable illnesses. When they become ill, the system should assure early detection and intervention. Admission to hospital should not be a first resort but rather a last line of defence, much like a goalkeeper in a football match. When patients come to the acute care system they should be treated impartially, according to best medical practice, not according to their incomes or public-private patient status. They should be free from lengthy waits for care. Whatever their health status and medical treatment, they should be treated with respect.

When the aged become frail and unable to care for themselves in every respect without aid, they should as a matter of right expect to be cared for in safe, comfortable, convenient and dignified accommodations, whether in their own homes with outside help, in nursing homes or in some other suitable arrangement.

The authors have not approached the problem of the Irish health care system as if they had a blank piece of paper on which to write. The analysis and recommendations presented here reflect the history and current structure of the system and build upon these.

Those of us – the authors and our readers – who try to influence policy must guard against dogmatism about the means towards the end. Other states have achieved greater equity and efficiency than Ireland in uniquely different ways. Ireland should have confidence in designing its own solution, while taking the best from other states. What is required is clarity about the destination: free and well-resourced multi-disciplinary primary care; equitable access to public hospitals; an end to the dishonest public-private mix within public hospitals, on public hospital campuses or between public and private hospitals; a well-resourced system, primary, acute, community and long-stay; and a democratically accountable and transparent health administration.

Appendix 1: Research Brief for the Authors from the Irish Congress of Trade Unions

Health service – scoping paper

The continuing failure of the health service to meet the needs of the public is of such importance that it needs a resolve on the part of government and social partners equal to that applied to public finances in 1987. Partnership means that the people working in the system have ownership of the problem as well as government and the objective of this review will be to give priority to finding solutions which transcend the representational interests of unions in the sector in favour of the common good. The review will take *Quality and Fairness* as the de facto blueprint for the health service and will inquire into the factors preventing its full implementation.

1. The immediate measures necessary to improve the functioning of accident & emergency departments with reference to the government's 10-point plan.
2. The impediments to implementing the Primary Care Strategy.
3. The extent to which increased investment has improved the health service, the amount taken by medical inflation and increase in population and service, the impact of lifestyle changes relating to alcohol and drugs, the effectiveness of the use of the balance of the investment and the amount still required to achieve the objectives outlined in *Quality and Fairness*.
4. The extent to which organisational structures and existing methods of working in hospitals and elsewhere are a barrier to efficiency and how they might be improved.
5. The increasing incidence of infections in hospitals and the extent to which this is related to standards of hygiene.
6. The appropriate standards necessary to ensure that chronically ill, recuperating or elderly patients are not discharged into care arrangements which are inadequate or unsuitable to their needs.
7. Any policy decisions relating to the mix of public and private care having regard to economic efficiency, standards of patient care and the desirability of building capacity into the public system in the interests of sustainability.

8. The implications for political accountability inherent in the new health structures in the context of one-third of all public expenditure now being controlled by the HSE.
9. The options for funding health care into the future, including the potential costs of an ageing population and the importance of insurance risk equalisation in that context.
10. The extent to which psychiatric health services have been impacted by reduced expenditure.

Appendix 2: The Cost to the Exchequer of Tax Incentives for Private Hospitals

An example of how this relief is given:

Assume €100 million of construction cost of a hospital qualifies for tax relief.

Assume the hospital's promoters attract an investor who pays tax at top 42 per cent rate plus 2 per cent levies and has substantial rental earnings which s/he wishes to shield from tax.

Percentage of cost allowable against tax:

| | Years 1 to 6 | 15% |
| | Year 7 | 10% |

	Year 1	Year 2	Year 3	Year 4	Year 5	Year 6	Year 7	Total
% of total cost	15%	15%	15%	15%	15%	15%	10%	100%
Tax rate	44%	44%	44%	44%	44%	44%	44%	
Value of tax relief to investor	€6.6m.	€6.6m.	€6.6m.	€6.6m.	€6.6m.	€6.6m.	€4.4m.	€44m.

How the deal might be constructed:

Hospital promoters and investor agree to split the value of the tax relief.

Assume they split 50/50 (close to the market norm).

How the tax relief gains are divided between hospital and investor:

The Exchequer gives the investor €44 million in tax relief on other earnings over a seven-year period.

The investor contributes €22 million (50 per cent of €44 million) up front to the hospital's construction.

The investor gains a net €22 million over seven years.

How much does the tax relief cost the government - and all of us?

The exchequer gives €44 million in tax relief over seven years. Of this 50 per cent has gone to the investor and 50 per cent to the hospital. The cost to the Exchequer in present value terms of this tax relief can be calculated based on alternative rates of return (in government gilts, for instance) at some €39.4 million.

Is this a good way of getting value for money for state investment in Irish health care?
Absolutely not. The government has paid the equivalent of €39.4 million of Exchequer funds for a €22 million investment in a private, for-profit institution, in which it has acquired no stake or control. This hospital will choose to perform the most profitable procedures for the patients who pay most. Meanwhile, a wealthy individual will receive €44 million over seven years or €39.4 million in present value, in return for providing €22 million now. It would have been much cheaper for the government to have grant-aided the private hospital the €22 million. It would have been a better use of state funds to invest in a public hospital, an institution which the state controls and to which the government could ensure all citizens gain equal access based on need. The only argument in favour of this arrangement is if the government cannot find the capital to invest in hospitals now. But that is not the case. The government could borrow this money more cheaply on the money markets than by this arrangement.

But won't the government gain a €100 million hospital for its €39.4 million investment?
No. The government does not gain the hospital, nor do public patients. This is a private, for-profit institution. It might decide to concentrate on treating rich people from overseas. In 10 years, it could be sold off as apartments or a hotel and the investor would still keep his or her tax relief. (At the time of writing, the Finance Bill 2006 proposed to require the extension of its use as a hospital from 10 to 15 years.)

Is this how the government plans to fund more beds for public patients?
Yes. The government is seeking private for-profit hospitals to set up on public hospital campuses.

And will this arrangement fund more beds for public patients?
Some private patients would move from public hospitals to care in private hospitals on the public campus and free up some public beds. But because private hospitals don't provide comprehensive care not all private patients would be able to move. And the presence of the private hospital will draw the most senior clinicians away from the public hospital and public patients' care, just as existing off-site private hospitals do. So the net effect will be to provide more private beds in private, for-profit institutions at the state's expense while public hospitals are starved of the investment and the senior staffing that they need.

Appendix 3: Restoring Medical Card Coverage to its 1996 Level			
Year and basis for coverage	Persons covered	Population	Percentage of population
1996 all persons covered on means-tested basis	1,252,384	3,626,100	34.5%
2005 persons covered on means tested and age basis	1,150,551	4,130,700	27.9%
Persons aged 70 and over covered on non-means-tested basis in 2005*	112,839	4,130,700	2.7%
Persons covered only on means-tested basis in 2005	1,037,712	4,130,700	25.1%
Coverage at 34.5% of population in 2005	1,425,092	4,130,700	34.5%
Additional persons to restore means-tested coverage to 34.5% of population in 2005	387,380	4,130,700	9.4%

*Sources: GMS Payments Board Reports to November 2005, Central Statistics Office Population Forecasts, as of April 2005. *Over-70s figure for November 2005 supplied by GMS Payments Board. Authors' calculations.*

		1997	2004	Increase
Appendix 4				
What have increases in health spending delivered in the years 1997 to 2004?				

Appendix 4

What have increases in health spending delivered in the years 1997 to 2004?

	1997	2004	Increase
THE POPULATION OF IRELAND:			
Population	3,664,300	4,043,800	10%
Births	52,775	61,684	17%
Deaths	31,581	28,151	-11%
PUBLIC ACUTE HOSPITALS:			
Spending on public and voluntary acute hospitals €m (in 1995 prices)*	1,503.92	2,582.01	72%
Patients treated in public hospitals	680,245	982,925	44%
Inpatient treatments	473,704	558,544	18%
Day case treatments	206,541	424,381	105%
Numbers of public hospital consultants	1,327	1,947	47%
Numbers of non-consultant hospital doctors	2,827	4,170	48%
Number of public acute hospital inpatient beds	11,861	12,375	4%
MEDICAL CARD SCHEME:			
Spending on GMS €m (in 1995 prices)	338.47	738.07	118%
Numbers covered by Medical Cards	1,219,852	1,148,914	-6%
Number of items prescribed	19,944,000	35,030,000	76%
Cost per item (unadjusted for any inflation measure)	€11.20	€21.35	91%
Numbers of GPs in GMS	1,641	2,210	35%
Spending on other drug subsidy schemes €m (in 1995 prices)	113.48	256.66	126%
OTHER PROFESSIONS AND CARE:			
Number of consultant psychiatrists	200	295	48%
Number of NCHDs in psychiatry	310	485	56%
Number of social workers	1,164	1,975	70%
Physiotherapists	593	1,133	91%
Nurses (working in all sectors, WTE)	25,611	34,313	34%

continued overleaf

CHILD PROTECTION**:	1996	2001	Increase
Spending on child protection €m (in 1995 prices)	72.26	169.03	134%
Children in care	3,668	5,517	50%
CARE OF THE ELDERLY:	**1997**	**2004**	**Increase**
Spending on public extended care in district hospitals, long-stay hospitals and welfare homes. €m (in 1995 prices)	190.77	314.18	65%
Subventions to patients in private nursing homes €m (in 1995 prices)	46.04	90.29	96%
CARE OF THE DISABLED:**	**1996**	**2004**	**Increase**
Spending on disability programme	332.99	773.98	132%
Staff working in intellectual disability services (WTE)	6,024	10,610	76%
Facilities for intellectually disabled (National Disability Database):			
Nos availing of centre-based respite services	891	4,004	349%
Nos receiving regular part-time care	94	175	86%
Nos being supported to live semi-independently	105	264	151%
Supported employment placements	329	1,580	380%
High-support day places	400	556	39%
Intensive day places	116	273	135%
Day programmes for the elderly	277	629	127%
Nos attending activation centres	4,326	5,067	17%

Note: Department of Health System Achievements Report published October 2005 reports that 1,700 additional residential places, 2,950 new day places and 465 dedicated respite places were provided for the intellectually disabled between 1997 and 2002.

*Sources: Department of Health HIPE data, Department of Health Health Statistics, Department of Health Health System Achievements Report October 2005, Consultant Staffing Reports including Consultant Staffing in the Mental Health Services, Comhairle na nOspidéal, GMS Payments Boards Reports, 2005 Annual Report of the National Disability Database Committee. *All spending figures have been adjusted by an index of prices for purchases of goods and services by public authorities to calculate the real or volume increase in health care. **In these categories limited availability of data requires change in the years compared.*

Appendix 5

Appendix 5.1

How much would it cost to solve the Irish health care crisis?

1. What did the Department of Health estimate as the cost of the 2001 Health Strategy? In 2001 the Department of Health estimated that implementing the Strategy over 10 years would cost (in 2001 prices) €7.7 billion in capital investment and would have increased current spending from €7 billion by €5 billion annually with full implementation at the end of 10 years. Following a Freedom of Information request, the Department later released the detailed estimates which underlay these global figures. The full €7.7 billion in capital spending is detailed here and €4.3 billion of the envisaged additional current spending. A further €450 million current spending on strategy programmes was already provided for in the 2002 estimates, the Department calculated. These were the Department's detailed estimates in October 2001.

Conversion rate from Irish pounds: 1.2697

Strategy	Capital cost (€million)					Current cost				
	Total	2002	2003 to 2005	2006 to 2008	2009 to 2011	Total	2002	2003 to 2005	2006 to 2008	2009 to 2011
Acute Care:										
2,800 additional inpatient beds, 200 day beds	1,269.7	50.8	266.6	476.1	476.1	482.5	50.8	215.8	215.8	284.4
Cancer services: BreastCheck centres, clinical radiotherapy	190.5	25.4	83.8	60.9	20.3	289.5	25.4	111.7	114.3	
Cardiovascular rehab	63.5	6.3	57.1			194.3	15.2	137.1	41.9	
Primary Care:										
Primary Care Model: 550 units to support teams	1,466.5	12.7	127.0	507.9	819.0	614.5	2.5	127.0	200.6	284.4
Primary Care 24 Hour GP Co-ops	31.7	12.7	19.0			31.7	12.7	19.0		
Primary Care Diagnostics and ICT to support teams	44.4	6.3	19.0	19.0		31.7	3.8	27.9		
Upgrade existing community health infrastructure	444.4	12.7	203.2	228.5						
Dental services	127.0	6.3	60.3	60.3		70.7	6.3	32.2	32.2	
Women's health screening; laboratories and colposcopy clinics	12.7	1.3	11.4			20.3		20.3		
Expansion of Medical Card eligibility						76.2	76.2			
Mental Health Services:										
Child/adolescent inpatient/outpatient units, 20 consultant-led teams	88.9	12.7	38.1	38.1		39.4	5.1	20.3	14.0	
10 psycho-geriatric units, psychiatrics ICUs for disturbed patients	69.8	6.3	25.4	38.1						
Community residences with 3,000 new places	292.0	25.4	152.4	76.2	38.1	82.5	7.6	47.0	27.9	
Day hospitals, day centres, mental health centres	25.4	6.3	6.3	12.7						

Disability Services:										
Intellectual disability services and facilities	253.9	38.1	139.7	76.2		127.0	31.7	69.8	25.4	
Physical disability services and facilities	190.5	25.4	88.9	76.2		253.9	25.4	121.9	106.7	
Training and sheltered work	57.1	2.5	22.9	31.7		63.5	12.7	38.1	12.7	
Autism	31.7	6.3	12.7	12.7						
Care of the Elderly:										
Assessment and rehab units, extended care and community nursing units, day hospitals and specialist services	1,476.7	19.0	253.9	660.2	543.4	677.7	38.1	380.9	258.7	
Palliative Care:										
1,250 additional staff, specialist centres, 350 beds	158.7	6.3	101.6	50.8		56.2	5.1	25.5	25.5	
Children's Services:										
High support, crisis intervention, accommodation services for homeless and at risk children	146.0	25.4	76.2	44.4		164.4	38.1	78.1	48.2	
Asylum Seekers:										
Seven new centres to support asylum seeker and refugee health needs	3.8	0.4	1.5	1.9		11.4	1.3	4.4	5.7	
Health Research:										
Centres, equipment, IT	114.3	9.6	79.2	25.4		246.6	2.5	159.9	84.2	
Equipment Maintenance and Replacement:										
Range of needs in acute and non-acute sectors, urgent refurbishment	952.3	190.5	380.9	380.9						
Information Technology:										
ICT to support change management, value for money, health information, primary care initiative, health agency IT systems	257.7	38.1	139.7	80.0		39.1	3.8	20.9	14.4	
Other additional staffing and training:										
Bacon Report						102.8	19.0	42.0	42.0	
Nurse training						63.5	6.3	19.0	19.0	19.0
103 A&E advanced nurse practitioners						5.0	2.0	1.5	1.5	1.6
Human Resources						173.3	31.7	141.6	141.6	
Recruitment and retention (medical and dental)						73.0	15.2	28.9	28.9	
Training and education (medical and dental)						298.4	38.1	130.1	130.1	
TOTAL	7,769.3	547.1	2,366.8	2,958.4	1,896.9	4,289.2	474.9	2,021.7	1,449.8	305.1

Appendix 5.2
The Cost of Implementing the 2001 Health Strategy

The 2001 Health Strategy was envisaged as an investment plan in facilities and staffing, which would be spread over 10 years. It was intended to meet the growing health and social care needs of an increasing and ageing population. Since it was to be funded over 10 years, the investment cost would be spread over that time. The gradually increasing current costs would be funded from a growing economy and the increased tax revenues generated by a growing employed labour force. An assessment of the cost of the Health Strategy must therefore be set within a framework of medium-term growth forecasts.

Table A.5.2 below shows how health spending would have grown as a proportion of national income had the 2001 Health Strategy been implemented within the growth and inflation forecasts of the ESRI's 2003 *Medium-Term Review*.[1]

Operating on the assumption that the strategy had been implemented from 2001 and that the costs had been as then forecast by the Department of Health, by 2011 total health spending would have stabilised at approximately 9.9 per cent of GNP, below the current level in France or Germany and below the level contemplated as necessary to fund the NHS. Total health spending peaks at 10.6 per cent of GNP six years into the 10-year investment programme and subsequently falls. Private spending is assumed to fall as a proportion of total spending as the quality of the public health care system improves.

Of course, the Health Strategy proposed investment in social services, explicitly excluded here but nonetheless likely to continue to be funded from the Health Vote. Its exclusion here is by no means an argument that it is any less necessary than investment in health care. What this analysis suggests is that if this society chooses to fund the health care capacity needs identified in the 2001 Strategy, in the long run Irish health care spending need not be out of line with that of neighbouring states.

As we have seen throughout this study, the strategy has not been implemented. The investments targeted for the acute, primary and extended care sectors have not taken place to any significant degree. The latest available Department of Health estimate at the time of writing was that in 2004, public health spending was 8.3 per cent of GNP and total health spending (public and private) was 10.4 per cent of GNP. However, if the Department's calculations are adjusted to take into account the 20 per cent of health spending allocated to social programmes, then public health spending in 2004 was 6.6 per cent of GNP and total health spending 8.7 per cent. (See Table A.5.3.) This compares with the forecasts, had the Health Strategy been implemented and funded, of public health spending (less social spending) at 8.1 per cent of GNP and total health spending at 10.1 per cent in 2004. (See Table A.5.2.)

Table A.5.2: Growth of health spending as a proportion of national income with implementation of 2001 Health Strategy					
	Public health spending (current & capital) as % GNP	Less 20% of health budget allocated to social services	Public health spending (excluding social spending) as % GNP	Private health spending as % of GNP	Adjusted total health spending as % GNP
2002	8.0	-1.6	6.4	2.0	8.4
2003	9.2	-1.8	7.4	2.0	9.4
2004	10.1	-2.0	8.1	2.0	10.1
2005	10.5	-2.1	8.4	2.0	10.4
2006	10.7	-2.1	8.5	2.0	10.5
2007	10.7	-2.1	8.6	2.0	10.6
2008	10.7	-2.1	8.5	2.0	10.5
2009	10.1	-2.0	8.1	2.0	10.1
2010	10.0	-2.0	8.0	2.0	10.0
2011	9.9	-2.0	7.9	2.0	9.9

Source: Derived by assuming growth in health spending as provided for in the Department of Health's underlying estimates of the cost of the 2001 Health Strategy, phased as the Department envisaged (see Appendix 5.1) and by applying the GNP and price growth forecasts of the ESRI's Medium-Term Review *(2003).*

Table A.5.3: Growth of health spending as a proportion of national income 1990–2004

As % of GNP	1990	1991	1992	1993	1994	1995	1996	1997	1998	1999	2000	2001	2002	2003	2004
-Total Public Health Spending	6.1	6.5	6.9	7.0	6.9	6.9	6.6	6.4	6.1	6.5	6.9	7.4	8.2	8.4	8.3
-Total Private Health Spending	2.0	2.1	2.4	2.2	2.3	2.2	2.3	2.2	2	2.1	2.4	2.2	2.1	2.1	2.1
Total Health Spending	8.1	8.5	9.2	9.2	9.2	9.2	8.9	8.5	8.1	8.5	9.2	9.6	10.3	10.5	10.4

Source: Department of Health calculations, 2004, an estimate.

As % of GNP	1990	1991	1992	1993	1994	1995	1996	1997	1998	1999	2000	2001	2002	2003	2004
Public Social Spending	1.2	1.3	1.4	1.4	1.4	1.4	1.3	1.3	1.2	1.3	1.4	1.5	1.6	1.7	1.7
Public Health Spending excluding Social Spending	4.9	5.2	5.5	5.6	5.5	5.5	5.3	5.1	4.9	5.2	5.5	5.9	6.6	6.7	6.6
Total Health Spending excluding Social Spending	6.9	7.2	7.8	7.8	7.8	7.8	7.6	7.2	6.9	7.2	7.8	8.1	8.7	8.8	8.7

Source: Authors' calculations, assuming that the share of the public health budget allocated to social programmes remains constant at 20 per cent.

Appendix 5

What would the Strategy cost to implement today?

In effect, the calculations above answer that question. Implementing the health strategy at the pace envisaged by its planners would have brought total health spending to some 10 per cent of GNP in 2004. Public health spending combined with social spending, funded by the health budget, would also have been 10.1 per cent of GNP. What actually happened in 2004 was that public health and social spending totalled €10.1 billion, or 8.3 per cent of GNP. Had spending increased as the Department planned in 2001, then the public health and social care budget in 2004 would have been close to €12.3 billion, nearly €2.2 billion, or over 21 per cent above its actual level in the year.

A further way to look at the cost today of implementing the Health Strategy is to calculate how price changes would have affected the aggregate costs calculated by the Department of Health in 2001 prices. (See Table A.5.4.) This table takes the aggregate 2001 costs and applies to them the increases in prices in construction and equipping, recorded by the Department's Hospital Planning Office. Construction prices have risen by surprisingly little, 6.8 per cent, in the four years since 2001, whereas in the four preceding years, they rose by nearly 60 per cent, a significant contributory factor to the poor value for money for the increases in health investment in the years 1997 to 2001. In sum, this highly aggregated exercise suggests that were the Health Strategy to be implemented from 2005, its capital investment costs would come to some €8.4 billion over 10 years and on completion it would have increased current spending by €6.2 billion over its current level. Capital investment in health care in 2005 was budgeted at €584 million.[2] The 2001 Health Strategy's planned investment for 2005 was €852 million in 2005 prices. It can be seen from this exercise that the capital costs associated with implementing the Health Strategy would not be prohibitive. At €852 million, this would have increased health investment by €268 million, which would represent a 46 per cent increase in the health capital budget but only a 4 per cent increase in the overall public capital budget for the year. Health's share would have increased from 9.6 to 13.4

per cent but would still be dwarfed by the massive transport budget, at 27 per cent of this expanded total. (See pie charts in Chapter 2.)

Table A.5.4: Effect of price changes on Health Strategy costing			
	Aggregate cost in 2001 prices €m	Rate of price Increases* %	Aggregate cost in 2005 prices €m
Capital costs: Construction	6,559	6.8%	7,005
Equipping**	1,210	12%	1,355
Total capital	7,769		8,360
Current costs	5,000	23.3%	6,165

*Note: This table calculates the effect of price changes on the costings of the 2001 Health Strategy as in Table A.5.1. *The rate of price increase used for construction is percentage increases in the Department of Health's Hospital Planning Office tender index between the last quarter of 2001 and the third quarter of 2005. For equipping, the percentage increase in the HPO's equipping tender index is used. For current spending, the rate of increase in the index of prices of goods and services purchased by public authorities is used as the best available measure of price increase in the absence of an index of Irish health care prices. **The authors have separated spending on the more obvious equipping areas (IT, equipment maintenance and research) but information available to the authors under most investment headings did not distinguish between construction and equipping.*

What are current costs for health care facilities?

The calculations above are all based on aggregations. It is also possible to look at the individual costs for some of the specific facilities, which have been discussed in this study.

Acute care

When the Department of Health forecast in 2001 that the cost of 3,000 additional beds (2,800 inpatient, 200 day) would come to €1,269.7 million over 10 years, an internal document (released under FOI) noted that 'it is difficult to be more precise'. The Department official observed that the Acute Bed Capacity Review had not gone into detail on where additional beds should be located nor how they should be split by specialty. The Department envisaged that its 2001 acute hospital investment forecasts would need to be revised 'in light of decisions to be taken on locations and specialties'. The Department planned to conduct that assessment over the following year in discussion with the health boards. In the absence of government commitment to fund these beds, it would appear that this work still remains to be done by the HSE.

These same caveats must still apply to any exercise in costing additional acute beds. The costs would vary greatly depending on whether the beds were to be delivered in a new greenfield hospital, required in a region like the North-East, where Our Lady of Lourdes Hospital in Drogheda is too old, too small and on too constrained a site to serve as a Regional Hospital, as envisaged by Hanly; or whether the beds could be provided simply by adding wards to an existing hospital like Tallaght, constructed with scope for expansion.

The Department of Health's Hospital Planning Office (HPO) maintains a computerised estimating system of the costs of health care facilities, which is supported by expert analysis of actual health care facilities costs, market factors and historical cost movement and inflation projections. Prices are also adjusted for policy and statutory changes. In November 2005, the HPO estimated that the total project cost per bed (excluding site purchase) in a major teaching hospital ranged from €550,000 to €600,000 and in a major acute regional hospital ranged from €500,000 to €550,000.[3]

The HPO points out that costs per bed, particularly in acute hospitals, has limited usefulness as a unit of measurement. 'With ever increasing reliance on day procedures the ratio of capital to bed numbers is increasing and is likely to continue to do so, given the rapid advances in ICT in delivery of healthcare. Acute hospitals also vary significantly in cost per bed depending on the mix of specialties and teaching requirements.

Inner city locations can also add dramatically to the construction costs.'

In calculating the cost of adding acute beds, it is necessary not only to bear in mind these caveats, but to recall that rising population and the redefinition of some beds as non-acute may have added to the need for additional beds since 2001. Based on the HPO's range of project costs, it can be stated that, in 2005 prices, the cost of adding 3,000 acute beds, divided evenly between major teaching hospitals and major regional hospitals, would range from €1,575 million to €1,725 million, excluding site purchase costs. Over 10 years, the annual cost would range from €157.5 to €172.5 million, that is, 2.6 to 2.8 per cent of gross voted capital in 2005.

It has been evident from delays in authorisation of capital spending in health in 2005 that the government and the Minister for Health are more concerned about the current costs associated with running and staffing hospitals than the investment costs, described above. The Department of Health calculates running costs based on its casemix system for costs of procedures. The average cost per bed day was €589, or €4,123 per week in 2003, according to the Department of Health. This figure is based on audited costs and activity for 2003, the latest year for which data were available at the time of writing, and excludes day cases, outpatient services, A&E cost and activity, and capital depreciation. Adjusted for price increases in purchases by public authorities (our conservative index of health care prices), this would translate into an average cost per bed day of some €658 in 2005 and a weekly cost of €4,606.

This average cost per bed day figure provides a measure of the average operating cost that would apply to additional beds in an existing hospital but does not give a measure of the operating costs associated with providing beds in a new hospital, which must also fund an A&E department, outpatients clinics, etc. Given that caveat, it can be calculated that adding an additional 3,000 beds to the existing NHO hospital stock would cost a minimum of €720 million per annum in 2005 prices, the equivalent of increasing the NHO budget by 16 per cent. This is self-evidently an understatement of the increased operating costs associated with such an expansion in bed capacity, since this would require the development of new hospitals, with outpatient and A&E departments. On the other hand, this expansion would take place over a period of years, in which the capacity of the economy to fund it could grow.

Existing bed-day costs are based on the existing skills mix and patterns of hospital working and levels of staff remuneration. We have argued in this study for the implementation of the Hanly Report recommendations for consultant-provided care and team-working by consultants and we have pointed out that the rate of remuneration of hospital doctors in Ireland is high by European standards. Were this expansion in acute bed capacity to be accompanied by reform in medical staffing and hospital networks, it might be achieved at a reduced cost per bed day.

Primary care

The Department of Health's estimate in 2005 prices of the total project cost of a primary care centre of average size is €3 million. This represents construction and equipping costs and excludes site purchase costs. It is the cost of a centre of some 800 square metres in size. Primary care centres can range in size from a small rural centre, of 200 square metres in area, housing two GPs and ancillary staff, to a large, well-equipped urban centre of 2,000 square metres in size, accommodating some 12 GPs and diverse other primary care professionals. Instances of both already exist. A significant number of GPs work from dedicated primary care centres, albeit not all in the model of team-working provided for in the Primary Care Strategy. Already up to half of all GPs in the North-West (Counties Donegal, Sligo and Leitrim) work from purpose-built accommodation, mostly provided by the health board in the last 10 years.[4]

Based on the Department's 2005 costing, providing 550 average primary care centres would cost €1,650 million. In 2001 the Department estimated that providing 550 centres would cost €1,466.5 million. The Primary Care Strategy's target was to provide 400 to 600 such centres within 10 years. Site costs could vary greatly but many primary care centres could be built on existing HSE land. In a booming county town, the site might cost some €1 million. Inner-city Dublin costs would probably be higher than elsewhere.

These are capital costs only, not current costs. Employing additional health care professionals would increase current spending, but what this exercise reveals is that accommodating them in well-equipped, purpose-built centres, which facilitate team-working, greater intensity of diagnosis and treatment, and ease of public access, should not be a daunting exercise for the state/HSE to undertake. Had this 10-year investment commenced in 2005, at €165 million annually, it would have constituted 2.7 per cent of voted capital for the year.[5]

Extended care facilities

The Department of Health HPO estimated in November 2005 that the total project cost (excluding site purchase) of providing extended care facilities could be expressed as a cost per bed ranging from €200,000 to €225,000 for a facility with minimum rehabilitation/day care provision, and ranging from €225,000 to €250,000 for facilities with enhanced rehabilitation/day care provision. This costing could be applied to the 800 additional extended care places for the elderly, which the Health Strategy proposed to provide annually over a seven-year period to reach a total of 5,600 beds. If these were facilities with minimum rehabilitation provision, the cost of providing 800 beds would range from €160 to €180 million in 2005 prices. The cumulative cost over seven years of providing the Strategy's 5,600 beds would range from €1,120 million to €1,260 million. For facilities with enhanced provision of rehabilitation and day care, the cost of 800 beds would range from €180 million to €200 million and the cost of 5,600 beds over seven years would range from €1,260 million to €1,400 million.

The Department estimates the 2005 running cost of a bed in a public long-stay facility at €1,270 a week for core service provision. This translates into an annual cost per bed of €66,000. An additional 800 beds would cost €52.8 million to run annually in 2005 prices. An additional 5,600 beds would cost €370 million.

2005 prices	Capital cost				Weekly cost per bed	Annual operating cost
	Total cost		Annual cost			
	Low	High	Low	High		
	€m	€m	€m	€m	euro	€m
Table A.5.5: Summary cost of major Health Strategy targets						
To be provided over 10 years:						
3,000 acute beds	1,575	1,725	157.5	172.5	4,606	720
550 primary care centres	1,650	1,650	165	165		
To be provided over 7 years:						
5,600 public long-stay beds	1,120	1,400	160	200	1,270	370
Total	4,345	4,775	483	538		1,090

Source: Department of Health, including Hospital Planning Office and Casemix Unit. Calculations the authors'. Note: Capital costs do not include site purchase. See text for caveats about limitations of costing, in particular in relation to acute operating costs.

Funding major Health Strategy targets

Table A.5.5 summarises the above discussion. It emerges that implementing these three major Health Strategy targets in acute, primary and continuing care could require in the region of €500 million in additional capital investment annually over the next seven to 10 years. This would represent close to a doubling of the 2005 capital budget for health care, bringing it to over €1,100 million. Had this increase taken place in 2005, health would have accounted for 16.9 per cent of the gross voted capital budget, as compared to 9.6 per cent.

Subject to the caveats above about the limitations of the casemix data as a means of calculating running costs for acute hospitals, and about the varied manner in which beds might be added to the system, this exercise suggests that current spending at the end of the 10 years could have risen by €1,090 million in 2005 prices, or by 9.6 per cent on the 2005 outturn.

Just as the Department of Health experienced in 2001 when it set out to cost the Health Strategy, we have been limited in our attempts at costing by the absence of any published government plan for how acute capacity should expand, in which locations and in which specialties. The purpose of this costing appendix is, however, to make clear that it is possible to cost for expanding Irish health care provision, that tools are available to the Department of Health to do so, and that costing – whether in aggregate, or by sector – reveals that the magnitude of investment and increased current spending required are well within the resources of Irish society. The most realistic costing exercises are those which, as in Table A.5.2, place the costs of meeting future health care needs within the framework of the national income that a growing population and labour force will generate.

How much would it cost to change the health care system?

We have argued in this study that the Irish health care system needs both investment and reform. We have discussed above how investment needs might be costed. But how does one cost reform? The following sections analyse the costs of the major reforms we have advocated: increased access to and eventually universal free access to primary care; a common waiting list in public hospitals; the Hanly agenda for medical staffing reform; and finally, Universal Health Insurance. It should be noted that we do not attempt to estimate changes in utilisation and hence spending which might result from behaviour change arising from the changed incentive structure associated with our proposed reforms. These supply and demand changes are quite complex and are as likely to bring negative as positive spending changes. For example, one might perhaps expect a change to free primary care to result in greater demand for that care. However, at present everyone resident in Ireland has access to free or nearly free care in acute hospitals, but the large majority must pay, and pay dearly, for GP care. A shift to free primary care could result in a shift in demand from costly hospital care to less costly primary care. Many of our reform proposals are specifically intended to bring about more efficient behaviour.

Expanded or free primary care

We explained in Chapter 13 that reform need not necessarily require additional resources for health care. Free primary care would obviate the need for much private spending on health, and represents a rechanneling of payments by individuals (from private fees to tax or PRSI), not an additional cost to Irish society, except in so far as services grow and need to be funded in the sector. Table A.5.6 uses as a measure for costing free primary care the costs per patient to the Exchequer under the Medical Card scheme. It applies the latest available published per capita doctor and prescription drug costs, which relate to 2004, to progressive expansion of the scheme, first to 40 per cent of the population, then to the entire population.

In calculating the cost to the Exchequer of paying for all drug purchases for the entire population, this table subtracts the other state payment or subsidy schemes for drugs, which would then have been superceded. The total of €1.5 billion in additional drug costs is almost certainly an overstatement, however. Existing Medical Card holders are the poorest and oldest members of the population, who are also those with greatest health care and medication needs. Assuming that their average drug costs per capita would be applicable to the entire population in a universal scheme is implausible. Equally, the sum allocated to additional doctor payments probably represents more than the state would or should wish to pay for a universal scheme, because the patients added to the scheme would be less likely to avail of it than those already covered.

This table costs entirely free access at the point of use to doctors and prescription drugs. Clearly, it would have to be funded from general taxation or PRSI. The benefit of such a universal, free at point of use system is that instead of flat fees which hit poorer families hard and hit people hardest when they are sickest, there is a predictable annual contribution (tax or PRSI), progressively levied and shared across the community. An alternative would be to give universal free access to medical care and introduce a reformed Drug Payments Scheme that subsidises the cost of drug purchases for all at a rate related to ability to pay.

This analysis does not assume universal health insurance, but UHI could fund access to free primary care.

Table A.5.6: A method of calculating the cost of expanding access to free primary care (2004 prices)						
	Numbers covered	Percentage of population	Per capita doctor cost 2004 euro	Total doctor cost €m	Per capita drug cost 2004 euro	Total drug cost €m
Medical Card holders in November 2005	1,150,551	27.9%	261.53	301	664.4	764.4
Extra Medical Card holders for 40% cover*	499,815	12.1%	261.53	131	664.4	332.1
Extra Medical Card holders for universal cover	2,480,334	60%	261.53	649	664.4	1,211.2
Universal coverage	4,130,700	100%		1,080		2,308
Added cost of universal coverage				779		1,543

*This table applies the 2004 GMS Payments Board per capita cost data to expansion of coverage from November 2005 levels. This method overstates added cost because the members of the population who are most likely to suffer ill-health are those already covered. (See text.) *This study has argued that Medical Card coverage should initially be expanded on a means-tested basis to 35 to 38 per cent of the population. In November 2005, 2.7 per cent of the population held medical cards on an age basis. Increasing coverage to 40 per cent achieves a means-tested coverage of 37.3 per cent of the population. Source: 2004 GMS Payments Board Report for costs and GMS monthly coverage figures.*

Common waiting list

We include a common waiting list here merely in order to make the point that this is a reform with no cost to the state.

Hanly agenda

The Hanly Report costed its own proposals. It estimated that by 2013, when it envisaged full implementation of a consultant-provided service, the additional cost would be €111 million in 2003 prices. The Report did not cost the 3,000 additional beds announced in the 2001 Health Strategy, although it considered them necessary to accommodate its proposals. Nor did it cost medical education and training requirements, effects on primary care, capital costs or IT costs. The taskforce took the view that these costs did not arise solely from its recommendations.[6]

Universal health insurance

We discussed in Chapter 13 how UHI could lead to higher levels of health care utilisation and therefore require a variety of methods to control costs. Assuming the same level of utilisation, however, how might UHI change the manner in which Irish health care is funded? We observed in Chapter 5 that in 2003 tax-payers paid 78 per cent of the costs of the health care system, private insurance contributed less than 7 per cent and individuals paid more than 13 per cent in out-of-pocket fees and purchases. The remaining few percentage points of total health spending were made up of private capital investment.

A UHI system with universal cover and no co-payments might combine today's private insurance payments, out-of-pocket payments and taxpayers' contributions to Exchequer-funded health care into one health insurance fund. It would be preferable for contributions to such a fund to be levied in proportion to ability to pay. If the contributions were to come through Pay Related Social Insurance, there could also be an employer contribution to the fund, as there is in social insurance-funded European systems.

For Irish society as a whole, this change of system would not mean an added burden of cost. It would mean a change in how individuals contribute to health care costs and it could also mean a change in the balance between who contributes more or less. If, for instance, the system were PRSI-funded, individuals' tax payments would fall but their PRSI payments would rise. In combination, individuals' tax and PRSI would probably rise, unless employers' contributions obviated the need for greater employee payments, or unless other sources of Exchequer revenue were to subsidise this PRSI funding. Individuals would, however, gain in many ways: they would no longer have to pay private health insurance premiums (the VHI might be the vehicle for this state scheme); they would no longer have to pay fees to GPs or consultants' outpatient fees; they would no longer have to pay fees to other health care professionals like physiotherapists; and their drug costs might be covered in whole or part. UHI might also fund most or all of long-term or community care for the elderly. In return for higher annual contributions to health care over their lifetime, individuals would have cover for their times of need. UHI is simply the application of the insurance principle across an entire society in an equitable manner.

NOTES

Preface

[1] The scoping document is reproduced in Appendix 1.

Executive Summary

[1] *OECD Health Data 2005, A Comparative Analysis of 30 Countries* (CD), Paris: OECD.

1. The Health of the Irish People

[1] 'EU15' is used throughout the text to denote the 15 member states of the European Union prior to enlargement (Austria, Belgium, Denmark, Finland, France, Germany, Greece, Ireland, Italy, Luxembourg, the Netherlands, Portugal, Spain, Sweden, the United Kingdom).

[2] Source: *OECD Health Data 2005*. The OECD extracts the number of deaths according to sex and selected causes from the World Health Organization Mortality Database. Age-standardised death rates per 100,000 population for selected causes are calculated by the OECD Secretariat using the total OECD population for 1980 as the reference population. The age-standardised death rates are necessary for comparing the level of mortality across countries and over time since they take into account the differences in age structure of the populations.

[3] *Cancer in Ireland 1994–2001 – Incidence, Mortality and Treatment*, National Cancer Registry, June 2005.

[4] *National Service Plan 2005*, Health Service Executive, 2005.

[5] *Reach Out: National Strategy for Action on Suicide Prevention 2005–2014*, Health Service Executive, 2005.

[6] *Homeless in Cork*, Cork Simon, 1998.

[7] *Inequalities in Health in Ireland – Hard Facts*, The Department of Community Health and General Practice, Trinity College, Dublin, 2001; *Better Health for Everyone, A Population Health Approach for Ireland*, Annual Report of Chief Medical Officer, Department of Health, 2001; *Inequalities in Mortality 1989–1998*, Institute of Public Health in Ireland, 2001; *Health in Ireland – An Unequal State*, Public Health Alliance, 2004.

[8] R. Wilkinson, *Unhealthy Societies: The Affliction of Inequality*, London: Routledge, 1996.

[9] T. Callan, M. Keeney, B. Nolan and B. Maître, *Why is Relative Income Poverty So High in Ireland?*, Dublin: Economic and Social Research Institute, Policy Research Series No. 53, September 2004.

[10] *People Living in Tallaght and their Health – A Community Based Cross-Sectional Survey*, report prepared for the Adelaide Hospital Society by the Department of Community Health and General Practice, Trinity College, Dublin, 2002.

[11] *Just Caring – Equity and Access in Healthcare, A Prescription for Change*, an Adelaide Hospital Society Policy Paper, May 2005.

[12] *Obesity: The Policy Challenges – Report of the National Taskforce on Obesity 2005*, Department of Health and Children, 2005.

[13] S. Friel, O. Walsh and D. McCarthy, *Cost of Healthy Eating in the Republic of Ireland*, Centre for Health Promotion Studies, NUI, Galway, 2004.

[14] *OECD Health Data 2005*.

[15] *Reach Out: National Strategy for Action on Suicide Prevention, 2005–2014*, Health Service Executive, 2005.

[16] *Suicide in Ireland: A National Study*, published by the Departments of Public Health on behalf of the Chief Executive Officers of the Health Boards, 2001.

[17] *Reach Out: National Strategy for Action on Suicide Prevention, 2005–2014*, Foreword, Health Service Executive, 2005.

[18] *The Stark Facts – The Need for a National Mental Health Strategy, as well as Resources*, Irish Psychiatric Association, 2003.

[19] *The Black Hole – The Funding Allocated to Adult Mental Health Services: Where is it Actually Going?*, Irish Psychiatric Association, 2005.

[20] *Irish Journal of Psychological Medicine*, March 2005 (Editorial).

[21] *A Better Future Now – Position Statement on Psychiatric Services in Ireland*, Occasional Paper OP 60, Irish College of Psychiatrists, 2005.

[22] Ibid.

2. Spending on Health

[1] J. FitzGerald, C. McCarthy, E. Morgenroth and P.J. O'Connell (eds.), *The Mid-Term Evaluation of the National Development Plan and Community Support Framework for Ireland, 2000 to 2006* (ESRI 2003) recommended that expansion of physical capacity should only take place once funding to utilise existing infrastructure was assured, pointing out that large numbers of beds had been closed due to staff shortages and funding deficits. It did not express a view on the Health Strategy's assessment of capacity needs. The chief executive of the HSE, Professor Brendan Drumm, has expressed scepticism about the need for additional acute beds, but this so far appears to be a personal view unsupported by any published analysis. (We assess his reported position in Chapter 7.)

² *OECD Health Data 2005*, updated 14 October 2005.

³ *OECD Health Data 2004* had assessed Ireland's per capita current health spending as 98.4 per cent of the EU average in 2002. The change in Ireland's position in that year to 94.5 per cent of the average primarily reflects revisions upwards in other states' spending.

⁴ *Report of the National Task Force on Medical Staffing*, chaired by David Hanly, Department of Health, 2003.

⁵ The social programmes excluded from the health budget would still have to be funded. However, their inclusion under the health heading reinforces the impression that health spending takes up a greater share of national output than its typical performance indicators would warrant.

⁶ The OECD has observed that the main growth of long-term care spending takes place during the initial phase of setting up new social programmes in relation to Germany, Japan and Luxembourg. Where a system is in place for a longer period of time, no cost explosion relative to acute care spending has occurred. (See *Long-term Care for Older People*, OECD, 2005.)

⁷ Pie charts are from Revised Estimates for Public Services 2005, Department of Finance. The current spending chart is based on gross current spending.

⁸ The 2004 outturn for health spending was supplied by the Department of Health on the traditional pre-HSE programme basis.

⁹ The rate of increase in prices of Irish public authorities' spending on goods and services averaged 5.4 per cent in the five years 1998 to 2002, compared to a 3.8 per cent annual average rise in consumer prices, a difference of 1.6 percentage points. In 1999 the Department of Health identified that average prices for medical goods and services had increased annually since 1988 by 2.9 per cent above the CPI. (Source: *Health Inflation: Cost Pressures Within the Health Services*, paper prepared for the Public Accounts Committee, Dublin, Department of Health, 1999.)

¹⁰ The OECD reported in 2004 that spending on health and health care in most OECD countries had risen dramatically over the previous five years. Combined with lower economic growth, the increase in health spending had driven the share of health expenditure as a percentage of GDP up from an average 7.8 per cent in 1997 to 8.5 per cent in 2002. 'This is in sharp contrast to the period 1992–1997, when the share of GDP spent on health remained almost unchanged.' In a report on *OECD Health Data 2004*, the OECD stated that this database update 'shows that U.S. health expenditure grew 2.3 times faster than GDP, rising from 13 per cent in 1997 to 14.6 per cent in 2002. Across other OECD countries, health expenditure outpaced economic growth by 1.7 times. In the United States, health spending reached $5267 per capita in 2002, almost 140 per

cent above the OECD average of $2144 and around 10 times more than Mexico and Turkey, which spent $553 and $446 respectively. This growth in health expenditure was, in part, a deliberate policy in some countries, such as the United Kingdom and Canada, which realised that cost containment during the mid-1990s had strained their healthcare systems…Rapid advances in medical technologies, population ageing and rising public expectations were largely responsible for the health spending growth, which was particularly notable in the area of pharmaceuticals. Between 1992 and 2002, spending on pharmaceuticals grew, on average, 1.3 times faster per year than total health expenditure, rising to account for between 9 and 37 percent of total health spending in OECD countries in 2002.' (Source: www.oecd.org/health.)

[11] *The State of Implementation of the OECD Manual: A System of Health Accounts*, Paris: OECD, 2002.

[12] M.A. Wren, *Unhealthy State*, Dublin: New Island, 2003.

[13] See discussion in M.A. Wren, 'Health Spending and the Black Hole', Economic and Social Research Institute, *Quarterly Economic Commentary*, September 2004.

[14] Assumptions underlying Table 3, p. 43, *Quality and Fairness*, Department of Health (2001), supplied by Department of Health in 2002.

[15] In contrast to Table 1 of M.A. Wren, 'Health Spending and the Black Hole', Economic and Social Research Institute, *Quarterly Economic Commentary*, September 2004.

[16] *OECD Health Data 2005.*

[17] Ibid.

[18] *Commission on Financial Management and Control Systems in the Health Service*, Dublin: Stationery Office, 2003.

[19] *International Classification for Health Accounts*, Paris: OECD, 2000.

[20] V. Timonen, *Health and Social Services – Integration vs. Division of Management, Delivery and Funding*, Department of Social Studies, Trinity College, Dublin, unpublished manuscript, 2003.

[21] Financial Statement of the Minister for Finance, Brian Cowen, TD, 1 December 2004 (www.finance.irlgov.ie).

[22] 'While spending has increased by 125 per cent between 1997 and 2002, inpatient discharges have gone up by only 4 per cent.' This comparison juxtaposed the increase in unadjusted spending for the entire health and social services budget with the increase in hospital inpatients. S. Barrett, 'The Task of Irish Health Service Reform', *Irish Banking Review* (Winter 2003).

[23] Public Health Expenditure Figure for *OECD Health Data 2005*, released by Department of Health under Freedom of Information (FOI).

[24] Statement from the Department of Health in response to a query from

the authors about the basis on which non-health programmes are excluded from Irish health spending returns for the OECD, October 2005.

[25] J. FitzGerald, C. McCarthy, E. Morgenroth and P.J. O'Connell (eds.), *The Mid-Term Evaluation of the National Development Plan and Community Support Framework for Ireland, 2000 to 2006*, Dublin: Economic and Social Research Institute, 2003; J. Lawlor and C. McCarthy, 'Browsing Onwards: Irish Public Spending in Perspective', *Irish Banking Review* (Autumn 2003). Discussed in M.A. Wren, 'Health Spending and the Black Hole', Economic and Social Research Institute, *Quarterly Economic Commentary*, September 2004. 'On a per capita basis Irish health spending, at €2,304 per person, is the third-highest in the EU, with only Luxembourg and Denmark ahead of us. To put things in context, our public expenditure per person on health is 8 per cent higher than France, 9 per cent higher than Germany, 37 per cent higher than the Netherlands and 70 per cent higher than Italy…Every single statistic used in this article I have drawn from a single short paper published recently by John Lawlor and Colm McCarthy…' The Tánaiste, Mary Harney, *The Irish Times*, 15 October 2003.

[26] *The Developmental Welfare State*, NESC Report No. 113, National Economic and Social Council, 2005.

[27] Bennett *et al.*, *Population Ageing in Ireland and its Impact on Pensions and Healthcare Costs*, Report of Society of Actuaries Working Party on Population Studies, Society of Actuaries in Ireland, 2003, cited in NESC (2005) above.

[28] *Long-Term Care for Older People*, OECD, 2005.

[29] Ibid.

[30] C. Normand and B. Graham, *Proximity to Death and Acute Health Care Utilisation in Scotland, Final Report to the Chief Scientist's Office of the Scottish Executive Department of Health*, 2001.

[31] K. McGrail *et al.*, 'Age, Costs of Acute and Long Term Care and Proximity to Death: Evidence for 1987/88 and 1994/95 in British Columbia', *Age and Ageing*, 29 (2000), 249–53.

[32] *Long-term Care for Older People*, OECD, 2005.

[33] Ibid. This study also compares countries' percentages of older people receiving long-stay care in an institution, but notes that comparisons should be made with great caution because of differing definitions of institutions.

[34] *Population and Migration Estimates April 2005*, CSO, 14 September 2005.

[35] Hospital activity data from Department of Health Hospital Inpatient Enquiry (HIPE).

[36] These arguments were developed at greater length in Wren (2004).

37 C. O'Reardon, 'Improving Irish Public Services', *Irish Banking Review* (July 2004), also discussed in Wren (2004).

38 'Surgeon resigns over restricted access to theatres', *The Irish Times*, 20 July 2004.

39 *Health Inflation: Cost Pressures within the Health Services*, paper prepared for the Public Accounts Committee, Dublin: Department of Health, 1999.

40 *Report of the National Task Force on Medical Staffing* (2003).

41 M.A. Wren, *Unhealthy State*, Dublin: New Island, 2003.

42 Discussed further in Chapters 9 and 10.

43 Calculations in detail in Wren (2004).

44 This exercise calculated Irish spending as a proportion of GNP and compares with other states' as a proportion of GDP, for the reasons stated in the note to Table 2.2.

45 The social programmes excluded from the health budget would still have to be funded. However, their inclusion under the health heading reinforces the impression that health spending takes up a greater share of national output than its typical performance indicators would warrant.

46 The OECD has observed in relation to Germany, Japan and Luxembourg that the main growth of long-term care spending takes place during the initial phase of setting new social programmes up. Where a system is in place for a longer period of time, no cost explosion relative to acute care spending has occurred. (See *Long-term Care for Older People*, OECD 2005.)

3. Solidarity, Decentralisation and Privatisation

1 *Equity of Access to Hospital Care*, Forum Report No. 25, Dublin: National Economic and Social Forum, 2002.

2 A reference to a 1999 strategic plan to reform the social insurance system in Y. Imai, S. Jacobzone and P. Lenain, *The Changing Health System in France*, OECD Economics Department Working Papers No. 269, Paris: OECD, 2000.

3 At the same time, however, GP care is supplied to non-Medical Card holders by self-employed GPs working in a free market, with a number of the negative consequences attributed above to free markets.

4 J. Figueras, R. Robinson and E. Jakubowski (eds.), *Purchasing to Improve Health Systems Performance*, European Observatory on Health Systems and Policies Series, Open University Press, 2005.

5 It might be argued that the Eastern Regional Health Authority (ERHA) was an experiment in this direction. It commissioned but did not deliver care. Since most of the acute hospitals in the east are voluntary or not-for-profit hospitals, the ERHA spent a lot of time negotiating service agreements with them. See M.A. Wren, *An Unhealthy State*, p. 101.

⁶ The European Charter of Patients' Rights (ECPR), developed by the Active Citizen Network at a conference in Brussels on 1 March 2005 (www.activecitizenship.net/projects/project_europe_chart.htm), has no special standing in Ireland and is referred to here as an example. The 14 points of the ECPR are: (1) *Right to preventive measures*: Every individual has the right to a proper service in order to prevent illness. (2) *Right of access*: Every individual has the right of access to the health services that his or her health needs require. The health services must guarantee equal access to everyone, without discriminating on the basis of financial resources, place of residence, kind of illness or time of access to services. (3) *Right to information*: Every individual has the right of access to all kinds of information regarding their state of health, the health services and how to use them and all that scientific research and technological innovation makes available. (4) *Right to consent*: Every individual has the right of access to all information that might enable him or her to actively participate in the decisions regarding his or her health; this information is a prerequisite for any procedure and treatment, including the participation in scientific research. (5) *Right to free choice*: Each individual has the right to freely choose from among different treatment procedures and providers on the basis of adequate information. (6) *Right to privacy and confidentiality*: Every individual has the right to the confidentiality of personal information, including information regarding his or her state of health and potential diagnostic or therapeutic procedures, as well as the protection of his or her privacy during the performance of diagnostic exams, specialist visits and medical/surgical treatments in general. (7) *Right to respect of patients' time*: Each individual has the right to receive necessary treatment within a swift and predetermined period of time. This right applies at each phase of the treatment. (8) *Right to the observance of quality standards*: Each individual has the right of access to high-quality health services on the basis of the specification and observance of precise standards. (9) *Right to safety*: Each individual has the right to be free from harm caused by the poor functioning of health services, medical malpractice and errors, and the right of access to health services and treatments that meet high safety standards. (10) *Right to innovation*: Each individual has the right of access to innovative procedures, including diagnostic procedures, according to international standards and independently of economic or financial considerations. (11) *Right to avoid unnecessary suffering and pain*: Each individual has the right to avoid as much suffering and pain as possible in each phase of his or her illness. (12) *Right to personalised treatment*: Each individual has the right to diagnostic or therapeutic programmes tailored as much as possible to his or her personal needs. (13) *Right to complain*: Each individual has the right to complain whenever he or she has suffered a harm and the right to receive a response or other feedback. (14) *Right to compensation*: Each individual has the right to receive sufficient compensation within a reason-

literature, see H. Luras (ed.), *Four Empirical Essays on GP Behaviour and Individual Preferences for GPs*, Health Economics Research Programme, University of Oslo, 2004, especially Chapter 2, 'A brief review of the literature', pp. 4–6. See also A. Dale Tussing, *Irish Medical Care Resources: An Economic Analysis*, Paper 126, Dublin: Economic and Social Research Institute, November 1985, pp. 43–4.

[2] T. Iverson and H. Luras, 'The Effect of Capitation on GPs' Referral Decisions', *Health Economics*, 9 (April 2000), 199–210.

[3] Phelps, *op. cit.*, pp. 189–90.

[4] Consultants' Contract (1997 version) para 5.1; also para 5.1 in 1991 version. This description, which was explicitly not then intended as 'an attempt at a legal definition', was recommended by the Working Party on a Common Contract, established in 1977 in its interim report, which the Irish Medical Association printed as an appendix to the first 1981 version of the common contract.

[5] Of course, this supposes that there are other doctors in the vicinity, and that they would take on a patient dissatisfied with a peer doctor.

[6] C.A. Ma and T.G. McGuire, 'Optimal Health Insurance and Provider Payment', *American Economic Review*, 87 (1997), 685–704.

[7] A.D. Tussing, 'Pay method key to health reform', *The Irish Times*, 1 February 2001.

[8] This point was called to our attention by Professor Miriam Wiley of the ESRI.

[9] *Composite Report* (*Health Service Reform Programme*), Department of Health and Children website (www.dohc.ie/publications/comprep.html), June 2004, p. 74. This document summarises the views of several departmental action committees on reforms proposed by external working groups. For our discussion of the report, see Chapter 12.

[10] Comptroller and Auditor General, *Annual Report, 2004*, Dublin, 2005, p. 136.

[11] As another example of the same principle, Minister for Health and Children, Mary Harney, has stated that if and as public hospitals lose private revenues when private beds are closed and private care is shifted to private hospitals on public hospital campuses, the budget allocation to those public hospitals would simply be increased to compensate them for their losses. (Source: Mary Harney, op-ed, *The Irish Times*, 24 August 2005.) The clear implication is that in the budget process, private revenues do not really matter. Budget totals are decided upon, then expected private revenues are subtracted and the allocation is simply a residual.

[12] M. FitzGerald, 'The Lack of Competition and its Impact on the Supply of Acute Healthcare' in R. Kinsella (ed.), *Acute Healthcare in Transition in Ireland: Change, Cutbacks, and Challenges*, Cork: Oak Tree Press, 2003.

5. Financing of Health Care

[1] HIPE Discharges 2004, supplied by the Department of Health.

[2] Total health expenditures by source of funds, 2003, supplied by the Department of Health. This analysis is based on OECD methodology.

[3] M.A. Wren, *Unhealthy State*, Dublin: New Island, 2003, p. 207.

[4] *The Irish Times*, 29 October 2004.

[5] This charge was set to increase to €60 in 2006.

[6] *The Private Health Insurance Market in Ireland*, Insight Statistical Consulting for the Health Insurance Authority, 2005. This survey, conducted in 2005, found that 52 per cent of those surveyed had private health insurance, 26 per cent had Medical Cards and 3 per cent had both, leaving 25 per cent with neither.

[7] Figure for November 2005 supplied by the GMS Payments Board.

[8] Median income is mid-range, not average, income.

[9] A doctor-only Medical Card might in fact help solve the problems of this group, but the result would be an anomalous incentives system, as discussed in Chapter 4, so partial aid toward the entire range of primary care costs is preferable.

[10] General Medical Services (Payments) Board, 2004 annual report.

[11] *The Irish Times*, 16 August 2005.

[12] However, it has been shown that GP utilisation by Medical Card patients did not change significantly after 1989, when remuneration changed from FFS to capitation, even though a priori one would expect a difference. D. Madden, A. Nolan and B. Nolan, 'GP Reimbursement and Visiting Behaviour in Ireland', Working Paper, Dublin: Economic and Social Research Institute, November 2004.

[13] An exception occurs where fees for a public patient in a private hospital are paid by the National Treatment Purchase Fund, as discussed elsewhere in this report.

[14] To be increased to €60 in 2006.

[15] 'Credit unions lent €30m in 2004 for medical expenses', *The Irish Times*, 30 May 2005.

[16] B. Nolan and M. Wiley, *Private Practice in Irish Public Hospitals*, Dublin: Oak Tree Press and the ESRI, 2000.

[17] Commission on Financial Management and Control Systems in the Health System, *Report*, Dublin: Stationery Office, 31 January 2003.

[18] D. Watson and J. Williams, *Perceptions of the Quality of Care in the Public and Private Sectors in Ireland*, Report to the Centre for Insurance Studies, Graduate School of Business, University College, Dublin, 2001.

[19] Nolan and Wiley, *op. cit.*

[20] *A Report on the Experiences and Expectations of People of the Health Services*, Eastern Regional Health Authority, 2002.

21 *Equity of Access to Hospital Care*, Report No. 25, Dublin: National Economic and Social Forum, July 2002.

22 Comptroller and Auditor General, *Annual Report, 2004*, Dublin, 2004, p. 136.

23 Letter to the Editor, *The Irish Times*, 30 August 2005.

24 Comptroller and Auditor General, *op. cit.*

25 In 2003, NCHDs averaged 75 hours of work per week. Under the European Working Time Directive, this was required to fall in phased reductions to 58 hours per week until August 2007, at which time the maximum falls to 56 hours. In August 2009, the maximum weekly working time for NCHDs will be 48 hours.

26 *Report of the National Task Force on Medical Staffing*, 2003.

27 Wren, *op. cit.*, pp. 167f.

28 *Consultant Staffing 2005*, National Hospitals Office/Comhairle, HSE, 2005.

29 A.D. Tussing, 'Pay method key to health reform', *The Irish Times*, 1 February 2001.

30 A.D. Tussing, *Irish Medical Care Resources: An Economic Analysis*, Paper 126, Dublin: Economic and Social Research Institute, November 1985.

31 The Health Insurance Act 1994 and the Health Insurance Regulations 1996.

32 F. Colombo and N. Tapay, *Private Health Insurance in Ireland: A Case Study*, Health Working Papers 10, Paris: OECD, 2004.

33 Ibid., p. 28.

34 A.D. Tussing and M.A. Wren, *The Health Report: An Agenda for Reform in Irish Health Care*, Irish Congress of Trade Unions, November 2005.

35 Sometimes given as CPT, for the Irish, *cuideachta phoiblí theoranta*.

36 Companies (Amendment) Act 1983.

37 *Report of the National Task Force on Medical Staffing*, 2003.

6. Primary Care

1 Professor Ivan Perry, address to Bupa Health Summit, Dublin, 24 May 2005. Professor Perry argues that private GP patients actually do not pay enough for primary care because they do not pay for the infrastructure 'which is available to us twenty-four seven'.

2 A small number of people get partial primary care cover through private insurance, thus constituting a third group. (See Chapter 5.)

3 Many countries with essentially public primary care systems nonetheless charge patients a nominal co-pay at the point of use. For example, France has introduced a €1 charge per visit, while Norway charges most patients €10. The present report is not the place to recount the positions of those who favour and those who oppose nominal co-pays for primary care. We favour a GP service free at the point of use, but would regard a system with

nominal co-pays for non-Medical Card patients as far preferable to the existing system.

[4] A doctor-only Medical Card might in fact help solve the problems of this group, but the result would create anomalous incentives, with some types of care free at the point of use and other types priced at full cost. For efficiency reasons, it is better to have prices at the point of use proportional to costs.

[5] For example, see B. Starfield, 'Is primary care essential?', *Lancet*, 344 (1994), 1129–33; and N. Starey, 'Primary Care Health Policy' in M. Lakhani and R. Charlton (eds.), *Recent Advances in Primary Care*, London: Royal College of General Practitioners, 2005.

[6] The Primary Care Strategy proposes a 'framework for quality assurance' (*PCS*, p. 39) to be achieved by the end of 2004 (p. 43). The discussion of peer review and quality assurance in *PCS* never becomes more specific than that. Little if any progress appears to have been made in this area.

[7] *OECD Health Data 2005, A Comparative Analysis of 30 Countries* (CD), Paris: OECD. For Irish GP data, the OECD uses membership in the Irish College of General Practitioners (ICGP). The ICGP in turn estimates that 95 per cent of Irish GPs are members. Adjusting the Irish total upward by 5 per cent would not change the ratio for Ireland in Table 6.1.

[8] Ratio calculated by totalling 1,824 approved consultant posts, 197 private specialists, 4,000 NCHDs, 2,560 GPs and 650 others.

[9] *Healthcare Skills Monitoring Report*, Dublin: FÁS, 2005.

[10] *Medical Education in Ireland: A New Direction*, Report of the Working Group on Undergraduate Medical Education and Training, Department of Health and Children, 2006 (Fottrell Report).

[11] *Report of the National Task Force on Medical Staffing*, Dublin: Department of Health, June 2003.

[12] Professor Perry (*op. cit.*) argues that to solve the shortage of GPs, it will be necessary to 'provide a range of flexible contracts, including salaried posts with terms and conditions comparable to those available in the hospital sector.'

[13] A.D. Tussing, *Irish Medical Care Resources: An Economic Analysis*, Paper 126, Dublin: Economic and Social Research Institute, November 1985, pp. 92–8.

[14] Disclosure: The Irish Medical Organisation is a sponsor of the present report (see preface).

[15] Irish Medical Organisation/Irish College of General Practitioners, *A Vision of General Practice – Priorities 2001–2006*, Dublin, 2001. Hereafter called *Vision*.

[16] *Primary Care – A New Direction*, Dublin: Department of Health, 2001. Hereafter called *PCS* (Primary Care Strategy).

[17] *Quality and Fairness: A Health System for You – Health Strategy*, Dublin: Department of Health, 2001.

18 *PCS*, pp.16–17.
19 Ibid., p. 56.
20 Ibid., p. 16.
21 Ibid., p. 56.
22 Ibid., p. 17.
23 *Vision.*
24 Ibid., pp. 1, 5, 6, 7.
25 Ibid.
26 *PCS*, p. 25.
27 *Vision*, p. 4.
28 Ibid., p. 1.
29 *PCS*, p. 28
30 Ibid., p. 8.
31 *Vision*, pp. 5–6.
32 *The Irish Times*, 19 July 2005. Houston writes of 'seven of the 10 pilot schemes pretty much dead in the water and a clear failure to fund even these to a level outlined in the strategy document, never mind expand the strategy nationally.'
33 Letter from Fergal Goodman, Principal, Primary Care, Department of Health, 6 October 2005.
34 The Department (ibid.) states that the Primary Care Strategy 'remains Government policy. However, it has always been the view of the Minister and Department that its successful implementation is about much more than the provision of additional funding. It is first and foremost about developing new ways of working and of reorganizing the resources already in the system (both those in the employment of the statutory sector and those contracted to provide services) in line with the service model described in the strategy. It is in that context that additional resources can be deployed to best effect.'
35 *PCS*, pp. 32–3.
36 *Quality and Fairness, A Health System for You: Action Plan Progress Report 2004*, Dublin: Department of Health and Children, May 2005.
37 *The Irish Times*, 18 November 2005; Health Service Executive, *National Service Plan 2006*, 2005.
38 *Op. cit.*
39 E. Edwards, 'Will patients lose out to profit?', *The Irish Times*, 11 October 2005.

7. Hospitals: Capacity and Access

1 Announced in July 2005 by the Minister for Health, Mary Harney.
2 In the three hospital networks of the National Hospitals Office (NHO) in the Greater Dublin Area, there are 18 acute hospitals, of which 15 are voluntary.

[3] Average number of beds available for use in publicly funded acute hospitals, August 2005. (Source: Integrated Management Returns (IMR), Department of Health.) This official Department bed count excludes beds closed for any reason, e.g. cutbacks, refurbishment, etc.

[4] The hospitals which the Department has included in its count of acute beds but which are not included in the NHO list are NRH Dún Laoghaire (119 inpatient beds in August 2005), Peamount (60 beds), St Mary's Baldoyle (50 beds), Orthopaedic Clontarf (96 beds) and Manorhamilton, County Leitrim (56 beds). The NHO does, however, include 21 acute rheumatology beds in Manorhamilton in its count. The NHO list also counts hospitals as one: Cashel and Clonmel are the South Tipperary General Hospital, and St Finbarr's in Cork is counted as part of Cork University Hospital (CUH).

[5] *The Irish Examiner*, 3 March 2005.

[6] *Consultant Staffing January 2005*, National Hospitals Office/Comhairle.

[7] *Cheering up the Patient: Opportunities for Private Sector Investment in the Irish Healthcare Sector*, Ian Hunter, Goodbody Stockbrokers, April 2005, p. 54.

[8] Source: *OECD Health Data 2005*. EU average for 2001 and 2002, incomplete data for 2003. When the Department of Health returns acute bed numbers to the OECD for the purpose of international comparison, it excludes extended care beds. The latest OECD data for Ireland shows 11,789 acute beds in 2003, 96 per cent of the official IMR inpatient bed count. The OECD counts hospital beds available for acute care, defined as 'curative care' as per the OECD Manual *A System of Health Accounts* (2000). Acute care beds are 'beds accommodating patients where the principal clinical intent is to do one or more of the following: manage labour (obstetric), cure illness or provide definitive treatment of injury, perform surgery, relieve symptoms of illness or injury (excluding palliative care), reduce severity of illness or injury, protect against exacerbation and/or complication of an illness and/or injury which could threaten life or normal functions, perform diagnostic or therapeutic procedures.'

[9] *The Irish Times*, 8 October 2005.

[10] *The Irish Times*, 10 October 2005.

[11] *Delivering the NHS Plan*, UK Department of Health, 2002.

[12] *NHS Improvement Plan*, UK Department of Health, NHS, 2004.

[13] Eastern Regional Health Authority *Bed Capacity Review*, 25 January 2001. This review calculated that when referrals from outside the Eastern region were taken into account, the East had 2.45 beds available per 1,000 population compared to a national ratio of 3.11 for people residing outside the East.

[14] Department of Health and Children, *Quality and Fairness*, Dublin: Stationery Office, 2001, pp. 102, 108.

[15] *Acute Hospital Bed Capacity – A National Review*, Department of Health and Children, Dublin: Stationery Office, 2002, p. 10.

[16] *Quality and Fairness*, p. 151.

[17] *Population and Labour Force Projections, 2001–2031*, Central Statistics Office 1999, cited in Government of Ireland, *Acute Hospital Bed Capacity Technical Report*, Dublin: Stationery Office, 2002.

[18] Department of Health and Children, *Quality and Fairness*, Dublin: Stationery Office, 2001, p. 102.

[19] This summary of the Codd Report was based on an IMR count of beds of 11,862 for 2000, which was subsequently revised upwards to 11,891. (The IMR is the Department of Health's integrated management returns.) The official department bed count excluding beds closed for any reason, e.g. cutbacks, refurbishment, etc. From these returns the Department derives a series for the average number of beds available for use in publicly funded acute hospitals.

[20] Hospital Inpatient Enquiry (HIPE) provisional data for 2004, returns to end-August 2005, supplied by the Department of Health.

[21] Review of Acute Hospital Bed Designation, Acute Hospitals Division, Department of Health, 18 September 2003. Released under FOI.

[22] An Agreed Programme for Government between Fianna Fáil and the Progressive Democrats, June 2002, pp. 21–2.

[23] Critics have suggested use of multivariate instead of bivariate analysis.

[24] Dr Robert Cunney, consultant microbiologist with the Health Protection Surveillance Centre, *The Irish Times*, 24 August 2005.

[25] Beaumont Hospital has declined to publish MRSA rates at the hospital until there is a standardised national framework on the collection of data, and has said that the EARSS data are not standardised, have not been validated and do not allow for differences between hospitals' casemix. Letter to *The Irish Times*, Liam Duffy, chief executive, Beaumont, 30 August 2005. The Health Protection Surveillance Centre has stated that care should be taken when interpreting international data, as it would be possible to under- or over-estimate the problem in some countries if the population covered by testing were not considered.

[26] Trends in antimicrobial resistance in Europe: report from EARSS, Nienke Bruinsma, Institute for Public Health and the Environment (RIVM), Bilthoven, the Netherlands, on behalf of all EARSS participants, *Eurosurveillance Weekly*, 8/51 (16 December 2004); and *A crude comparison of MRSA bacteraemia data from countries reporting to European Antimicrobial Resistance Surveillance System (EARSS) in 2003*, Health Protection Surveillance Centre website, www.ndsc.ie.

[27] Bruinsma, *op. cit.*

[28] Trends in MRSA in Ireland reported to the EARSS, Health Protection Surveillance Centre website, www.ndsc.ie.

[29] *Control and Prevention of MRSA in Hospitals and in the Community*, A Strategy for the Control of Antimicrobial Resistance in Ireland, Health Protection Surveillance Centre/HSE, 2005.

[30] S. Creedon, 'Healthcare workers' hand decontamination practices: compliance with recommended guidelines', *Journal of Advanced Nursing*, 51/3 (August 2005).

[31] Established as part of the Strategy for the Control of Antimicrobial Resistance in Ireland (SARI).

[32] *Control and Prevention of MRSA in Hospitals and in the Community*, op. cit.

[33] *The Irish Times*, 16 September 2005.

[34] Letter to *The Irish Times*, 2 February 2005.

[35] Hospital Inpatient Enquiry (HIPE) data for 2004, as received to end-August 2005, not yet complete, supplied by Department of Health. In 2003 private patients were 32.4 per cent of elective inpatients, 23 per cent of emergency inpatients, 23.7 per cent of day cases and 24.9 per cent of all cases (HIPE 2003). HIPE includes some data for the Mater and St Vincent's Private Hospitals which have been excluded in these percentages.

[36] R. Breen, *Review of Acute Hospital Bed Designation*, Acute Hospitals Division, Department of Health, 18 September 2003 (released by the Department of Health under FOI).

[37] J. Cregan, Report on Public/Private Activity in Acute Public Hospitals, Acute Hospitals Division, Department of Health, 13 August 2003 (released by the Department of Health under FOI).

[38] Letter to Department of Health from Sean Hurley, CEO, Southern Health Board, 27 June 2003 (released by the Department of Health under FOI).

[39] Letter to Department of Health from Tim Kennelly, chief executive, St John's Hospital, Limerick, 24 April 2003 (released by the Department of Health under FOI).

[40] According to a survey conducted for the Health Insurance Authority by Insight Statistical Consulting between March and April 2005, available as *The Private Health Insurance Market in Ireland – A Market Review* at www.hia.ie.

[41] B. Nolan and M. Wiley, *Private Practice in Irish Public Hospitals*, Oak Tree Press and the ESRI, 2000, p. 105.

[42] Watson and Williams, p. 33.

[43] *A Report on the Experiences and Expectations of People of the Health Services*, ERHA 2002, p. 21.

[44] Announcement by the Tánaiste and Minister for Health at the launch of the NTPF annual report, 25 May 2005.

[45] *The Private Health Insurance Market in Ireland*, Insight Statistical Consulting for the Health Insurance Authority, 2005.

[46] Van Doorslaer, X. Koolman and F. Puffer, *Equity in the use of physician visits in OECD countries: has equal treatment for equal need been achieved?*, OECD conference proceedings 'Measuring Up: Improving Health Systems Performance in OECD Countries', OECD Health Conference on Performance Measurement and Reporting, 2001.

[47] R. Layte and B. Nolan, 'Equity in the Utilisation of Hospital Care in Ireland', *The Economic and Social Review*, 35/2 (Summer/Autumn 2004). The authors are currently refining this analysis using complementary data sources.

[48] P.A. McCormick, M. O'Rourke, D. Carey and M. Laffoy, 'Ability to Pay and Geographical Proximity Influence Access to Liver Transplantation Even in a System With Universal Access', *Liver Transplantation*, 10/11 (November 2004).

[49] Study by John McManus in his Bray GP practice, reported at *The Irish Times*/Royal Academy of Medicine lecture, 23 October 2001.

[50] *National Patient Perception of the Quality of Healthcare 2002*, Irish Society for Quality and Safety in Healthcare, 2003.

[51] Nolan and Wiley, *op. cit.*

[52] Released under FOI.

[53] Fall in waiting times, statement released by the Department of Health, 4 May 2004.

[54] *A Report on the Patient Treatment Register*, National Treatment Purchase Fund, 2005.

[55] Government of Ireland, *Annual Report of the Comptroller and Auditor General 2004*, Dublin: Stationery Office, 2005, Chapter 14.

8. The Accident and Emergency Crisis: Solutions Within and Outside Hospitals

[1] In 2001, the Medical Manpower Forum reported that 'frontline services are mainly provided by non-consultant hospital doctors, many of whom are in the early stages of their training or not in formal training posts.' *Report of the Forum on Medical Manpower,* Department of Health, 2001.

[2] *Acute Medical Units*, Comhairle na nOspidéal, 2004.

[3] Trolley counts available on the INO and HSE websites: www.ino.ie and www.hse.ie.

[4] Cited in V.M. Bradley, 'Placing Emergency Department Crowding on the Decision Agenda', *Nursing Economics*, 23/1 (2005).

[5] *Acute Medical Units*, Comhairle na nOspidéal, 2004.

[6] Ibid., p. 3.

[7] By August 2005 there were 196 additional beds available compared to the 2004 average. Over the year to August there were on average 150 additional beds available compared to 2004 (see Table 7.6 in Chapter 7).

[8] *Summary of immediate initiatives required to address overcrowding in accident and emergency departments*, Irish Nurses Organisation, Submission to Minister for Health, October 2004.

[9] *Acute Medical Units*, Comhairle na nOspidéal, 2004.

[10] Ibid., p. 7.

[11] The chief executive of the National Hospitals Office (NHO), Pat McLoughlin, told the Joint Oireachtas Committee on Health in April 2005, 'At any one time, up to 400 beds are blocked, particularly in the Eastern region, with patients who could be cared for elsewhere.' This can represent as many as 10 per cent of beds in one hospital but only represents 3 per cent of the national acute inpatient bed stock, showing the degree to which this is a Dublin problem.

[12] Deloitte & Touche, *Value for Money Audit of the Irish Health System*, 2001.

[13] Department of Health, *Quality and Fairness*, Dublin: Stationery Office, 2001, p. 151.

[14] Announcement by the Minister for Health, 29 July 2002.

[15] Referred to as DBOF – Design, Build, Operate, Finance.

[16] *Acute Medical Units*, Comhairle na nOspidéal, 2004.

[17] *Dáil Debates*, 14 April 2005.

[18] *Baseline Study of the Provision of Hospice and Specialist Palliative Care Services in Ireland*, Irish Hospice Foundation, 2005.

[19] Speaking at a plenary session of the National Economic and Social Forum (NESF), *The Irish Times*, 29 September 2005.

[20] *Long-term Care for Older People*, OECD, 2005, p. 41. The OECD also compares the percentage of 65-and-overs receiving long-term care in an institution, but advocates great caution in comparing this measure across countries because of differences in the definition of care institutions.

[21] *One Island – Two Systems. A comparison of health status and health and social service use by community-dwelling older people in the Republic of Ireland and Northern Ireland*, prepared by the Healthy Ageing Research Programme (HARP) Steering Group, Dublin: The Institute of Public Health in Ireland, 2005.

[22] V. Timonen, *Evaluation of Homecare Grant Schemes in the NAHB and ECAHB*, ERHA, 2004.

[23] Ibid.

[24] Home help numbers returned by Health Service Executive area, Department of Health.

[25] Timonen (2004), *op. cit.*

[26] OECD, *op. cit.*

[27] OECD, *op. cit.*

[28] *Study to Examine the Future Financing of Long-Term Care in Ireland*, Mercer Ltd, for the Department of Social and Family Affairs, 2003.

[29] In the *Annual Report of the Ombudsman 2004* (Office of the Ombudsman 2005), the Ombudsman wrote: 'The current controversy has focused solely on the question of patients in public institutions. It does not deal with the issue of those patients, both medical card holders and non medical card holders, who had been directed by the health boards towards private care, without in any way acknowledging their own responsibilities in the area. I remain of a similar view to my predecessors in relation to the legal situation in this regard, viz. everybody resident in the State is eligible to be provided with in-patient services, where necessary, by the HSE. The services can be provided directly by the HSE in one of its own hospitals, in another publicly funded hospital, or by way of a contracting out arrangement between the HSE and a private institution.'

[30] *Commission of Enquiry on Mental Illness*, Department of Health, 1966.

[31] F. Keogh, A. Roche, and D. Walsh, *'We Have No Beds...'*, Health Research Board, 1999. While there has been no subsequent study, so few of the recommendations in this report have been implemented that psychiatrists believe this picture to be largely unchanged.

[32] M.A. Wren, *Unhealthy State*, Dublin: New Island, 2003, p. 234.

[33] A Study of the Number, Profile and Progression Routes of Homeless Persons before the Court and in Custody (2005), pre-publication account of its findings in *The Irish Times*, 29 August 2005.

[34] *World Health Report – Mental Health: New Understanding, New Hope*, Geneva: WHO, 2001.

[35] *Mental Health Commission Annual Report 2004*, p. 121.

[36] *A Vision for Change*, Report of the Expert Group on Mental Health Policy, Dublin: Stationery Office, 2006; Minister's remarks at launch, 24 January 2006, www.dohc.ie.

9. Specialist Care in the Acute Hospital Setting

[1] *Healthcare Skills Monitoring Report*, Dublin: FÁS, 2005.

[2] In 2003, NCHDs averaged 75 hours of work per week. No record is kept of consultant hours (see Chapter 5).

[3] *Report of the National Task Force on Medical Staffing*, 2003.

[4] Ibid.

[5] *Preparing Ireland's Doctors to meet the Health Needs of the 21st Century*, Report of the Postgraduate Medical Education and Training Group, Department of Health and Children, 2006 (Buttimer Report).

[6] Irish data are authors' own calculations. *OECD Health Data 2005* for EU15 average.

[7] *Medical Education in Ireland: A New Direction*, Report of the Working Group on Undergraduate Medical Education and Training, Department of Health and Children, 2006 (Fottrell Report).

[8] *Value for Money Audit of the Irish Health System, Main Report,* June 2001.

[9] Ibid., p. 169.

[10] *Op. cit.*

[11] E. Donnellan, 'A clash of cultures', *The Irish Times,* 8 October 2005.

[12] *The Irish Times,* 19 October 2005.

[13] *The Irish Times,* 4 October 2005.

[14] F. Lennon, 'Medical profession failed patients', *The Irish Times,* 29 September 2003.

[15] See their website at www.medicalcouncil.ie/.

[16] There are exceptions to this rule. An unregistered doctor may practise unless he or she claims to be 'a registered medical practitioner' or offers certain certificates, or dispenses or prescribes controlled drugs. Plastic medicine and alternative medicine are areas where unregulated doctors are said to practise, and possibly do harm.

[17] *Healthcare Skills Monitoring Report,* Dublin: FÁS, 2005.

[18] Under Part V of the Medical Practitioners Act 1978.

[19] Medical Council, www.medicalcouncil.ie.

[20] Ibid.

[21] The transition from the previous system resulted in controversy. Irish doctors had traditionally bought cover by becoming members of one or the other of two UK-based medical defence unions, organised as mutual societies. These are not really insurance companies. They are not obliged to indemnify members in case of a court loss; rather, they offer indemnification at the discretion of their governing boards. One of these companies, the Medical Defence Union (MDU), has declined to indemnify Irish physicians against claims arising from the period before the creation of the Clinical Indemnity Scheme. The Irish government has been in talks with the MDU endeavouring to ensure it covers some proportion of these historic liabilities. The government has offered verbal assurance of protection to physicians, but physicians want a legally binding contract. The authors do not take a position on this issue, which is still under discussion as the time of writing, and may well be settled in the courts.

[22] D.H. Mills, J.S. Boyden, D.S. Rubsamen and H.L. Engle, *Report on Medical Insurance Feasibility Study,* San Francisco: California Medical Association, 1977; Harvard Medical Practice Study, *Patient, Doctors, Lawyers: Medical Injury, Malpractice Litigation, and Patient Compensation in New York,* Cambridge, MA: Harvard University, 1990; E.C. Brennan *et al.,* 'Incidence of adverse events and negligence in hospitalized patients', *New England Journal of Medicine,* 325/6 (1991), 370–76; David M. Studdert *et al.,* 'Negligent care and malpractice claiming behaviour in Utah and Colorado', *Medical Care,* 38/3 (2000).

10. The Organisation of Acute Hospital Care

[1] *Report of the National Task Force on Medical Staffing*, Department of Health and Children, 2003.
[2] Ibid., p. 13.
[3] *Medical Manpower in Acute Hospitals – A Discussion Document*, Department of Health, Comhairle na nOspidéal and Postgraduate Medical and Dental Board, June 1993 (Tierney Report); and *Report of the Forum on Medical Manpower*, Department of Health and Children, January 2001.
[4] Hanly Report, p. 62.
[5] E. Donnellan, 'HSE to have four hospital networks', *The Irish Times*, 5 October 2005.
[6] *Report of the National Task Force on Medical Staffing*, pp. 102–104.
[7] Ibid., p. 103.
[8] Ibid., p. 103.

11. Health Service Staffing

[1] *Quarterly Economic Commentary*, Economic and Social Research Institute, December 2002.
[2] *Report of the Independent Estimates Review Committee to the Minister for Finance*, Department of Finance, 2002.
[3] *Sunday Tribune*, 18 May 2003.
[4] Department of Health Home Help Returns by Health Board Executive Area.
[5] 'Restrictions on staff numbers cost health board 1 million', *The Irish Times*, 31 August 2004.
[6] *Sunday Tribune*, 4 May 2004 and *The Irish Times*, 15 September 2004.
[7] Increase in nurse employment was effectively only 16 per cent between 1997 and 2001 if account is taken of the effect of student nurses' move into full-time education.
[8] *Commission on Financial Management and Control Systems in the Health Service*, Dublin: Stationery Office, 2003, p. 89.
[9] *Primary Care – A New Direction*, Department of Health, 2001, p. 33.
[10] Department of Health and Children, *Quality and Fairness*, Dublin: Stationery Office, 2001, p. 117.
[11] The Irish data returned to the OECD is the Department of Health public health employment census. It is overstated in so far as it includes employees in social programmes and understated because it excludes private sector employees. Sources: *OECD Health Data 2005*; *Definitions, Sources and Methods* (*OECD Health Data 2005*).
[12] The CSO's Quarterly National Household Survey count of numbers employed in health includes both public and private employees and does

not distinguish between full- and part-time employment. Source: CSO Employment and Unemployment Series.

[13] 'Martin says higher taxes needed for better healthcare', *The Irish Times*, 24 May 2003; 'Finance officials propose hike in income tax', *Sunday Tribune*, 15 June 2003.

[14] *Healthcare Skills Monitoring Report*, FÁS, 2005.

[15] Approximately 5 per cent below those in Table 7.5.

[16] Statement from John McGrath, Research Manager, Skills and Labour Research Unit, FÁS.

[17] Department of Health personnel census, which counts both absolute numbers (head counts) and wholetime equivalents.

[18] J. Buchan and L. Calman, *Skill-Mix And Policy Change In The Health Workforce: Nurses In Advanced Roles*, OECD Health Working Paper No. 17, February 2005.

[19] The ratio for 2003 would be 190 doctors to every 1,000 nurses. This does not alter Ireland's position in the ranking in Table 11.4.

[20] Table 11.3 overstates Irish doctor numbers. The actual Irish ratio in 2003 should be 2.3 doctors per 1,000 population.

[21] Derived from Department of Health personnel census.

[22] J. Needleman *et al.*, 'Nurse-Staffing Levels and the Quality of Care in Hospitals', *The New England Journal of Medicine*, 346/22 (30 May 2002).

[23] *Social work posts in Ireland*, NSWQB Report No. 2, National Social Work Qualifications Board, 2002. The figures here derive from a table in the report, with an adjustment for Irish population in 2001, when social work posts were surveyed.

[24] P. Bacon *et al.*, *Current and Future Supply and Demand Conditions in the Labour Market for Certain Health Professional Therapists*, Peter Bacon and Associates, Economic Consultants, Killinick, 2001.

[25] Data from the European Region of the World Confederation for Physical Therapy.

[26] *Submission to the Department of Health and Children on the Strategic Review of Disability Services*, Irish Association of Speech and Language Therapists, September 2005.

12. Accountability and Administration in Health

[1] These were the North-Western Health Board (NWHB), Western Health Board (WHB), Mid-Western Health Board (MWHB), Southern Health Board (SHB), South-Eastern Health Board (SEHB), Midland Health Board (MHB), North-Eastern Health Board (NEHB) and Eastern Regional Health Authority (ERHA), with three subsidiary boards – the Northern Area Health Board, South-Western Area Health Board and the East Coast Area Health Board.

[2] R. Barrington, *Health, Medicine and Politics in Ireland 1900–1970*, Dublin: IPA, 1987, *passim.*

[3] Department of Health and Children, *Quality and Fairness*, Dublin: Stationery Office, 2001, p. 125.

[4] Government announcement of reform programme, 18 June 2003.

[5] *Commission on Financial Management and Control Systems in the Health Service,* Dublin: Stationery Office, 2003, *passim.*

[6] Prospectus and Watson Wyatt, *Audit of Structures and Functions in the Health System*, Dublin: Stationery Office, 2003, p. 61.

[7] *Composite Report (Health Service Reform Programme)*, Department of Health and Children, June 2004.

[8] Two sections of the Health Act 2004 give effect to this. Section 20 states: 'The chief executive officer is the accounting officer in relation to the appropriation accounts of the Executive for the purposes of the Comptroller and Auditor General Acts 1866 to 1998.' Schedule 5, Section 7 (1) states: 'On the establishment day, there shall be established a Vote for the Executive, to be known as the Health Service Executive Vote, which shall be Vote 40.'

[9] *Dáil Debates*, Volume 10 Committee Satge (2 December 2004).

[10] *Dáil Debates*, Volume 9 Committee Stage (1 December 2004).

[11] Prospectus *op. cit.*, p. 147.

[12] Prospectus and Watson Wyatt, *Audit of Structures and Functions in the Health System*, Appendices Volume, Appendix E, p. 229.

[13] Statement from the Tánaiste, 19 November 2004.

[14] *Report of the Commission on Health Funding* (1989), p. 156.

[15] *Dáil Debates*, Joint Oireachtas Committee on Health and Children, Volume 39 (3 February 2005).

[16] *Dáil Debates*, Joint Oireachtas Committee on Health and Children, Volume 45 (14 April 2005).

[17] Ministerial announcement of 14 July 2005; letter to chairman of the board of the HSE, Liam Downey, from Michael Scanlan, secretary general of the Department of Health, with accompanying assessment framework.

[18] Ministerial announcement of 21 June 2005.

[19] *Financial Times*, 28 August 1996.

[20] Quoted in C. Polidano, 'The Bureaucrat Who Fell Under a Bus: Ministerial Responsibility, Executive Agencies and the Derek Lewis Affair in Britain', *Governance*, 12/2 (April 1999).

[21] *Ministerial Accountability and Responsibility*, Second Report, Public Service Committee, House of Commons, 1996.

[22] *Commission on Financial Management and Control Systems in the Health Service,* Dublin: Stationery Office, 2003 (Brennan Commission) p. 49.

[23] Graham Wilson, quoted in Polidano, *op. cit.*

[24] Polidano, p. 208.

[25] *Dáil Debates*, Volume 595 (9 December 2004).

[26] *Dáil Debates*, Volume 593 (23 November 2004).

[27] Internal Department of Finance e-mail, 10 January 2005.

[28] *Composite Report*, p. 20.

[29] Internal Department of Finance briefing note, 24 November 2004, released under Freedom of Information (FOI).

[30] Letter from the Minister for Finance, Brian Cowen, to Tánaiste and Minister for Health, Mary Harney, 29 November 2004. (FOI)

[31] Letter from the Minister for Finance, Brian Cowen, to Tánaiste and Minister for Health, Mary Harney, 17 December 2004. (FOI)

[32] Letter from Second Secretary General, Department of Finance, David Doyle, to Secretary General, Department of Health, Michael Kelly, but marked for the attention of Assistant Secretary, Dermot Smyth, 17 December 2004. (FOI)

[33] Draft internal memorandum from Michael Scanlan, then assistant secretary, Department of Finance, 10 December 2004. (FOI)

[34] *Report of the Working Group on the Accountability of Secretaries General and Accounting Officers*, Department of Finance, July 2002, para. 3.29. The high-level Working Group on the Accountability of Secretaries General and Accounting Officers was established by the Minister for Finance following a government decision of 30 May 2000. It was chaired by a former Secretary General of the Department of Finance, Paddy Mullarkey, and is sometimes referred to here as the Mullarkey Report, or 'Mullarkey'.

[35] Ibid., paras. 3.55–3.61.

[36] Ibid., para. 4.6.

[37] Ibid., para. 4.5.

[38] *Composite Report*, p. 69; *Commission on Financial Management and Control Systems in the Health Service*, p. 50.

[39] *Dáil Debates*, Volume 593 (23 November 2004).

[40] *Dáil Debates*, Committee Stages, Volume 10 (2 December 2004).

[41] *Dáil Debates* on Health Act 2004, Committee Stage (1 December 2004) and Report and Final Stages, (9 December 2004), Volumes 9 and 595.

[42] *Ministerial Accountability and Responsibility*, Second Report, Public Service Committee, House of Commons, 1996.

[43] Statutory Instrument, S.I. No. 798 of 2005, Health Act 2004 (Dealings with members of either House of the Oireachtas) Regulations 2005, Dublin: Stationery Office.

[44] *Dáil Debates*, HSE presentation to Joint Oireachtas Committee, Volume 45 (14 April 2005).

[45] Statutory Instrument, S.I. No. 797 of 2005, Health Act 2004 (Regional Health Forums) Regulations 2005, Dublin: Stationery Office.

[46] *Dáil Debates*, Committee Stage, Volume 9 (1 December 2004).

[47] *Guidelines for Community Involvement in Health*, Position Paper of the National Primary Care Steering Group, Department of Health, December 2004.

[48] Ibid. See also *Primary Care – A New Direction*, Department of Health, 2001; *Better Health for Everyone: A Population Health Approach for Ireland*, Annual Report of the Chief Medical Officer, Department of Health, 2001; *Just Caring – Equity and Access in Healthcare*, Adelaide Hospital Society, 2005.

[49] See discussion of Neary case, *Dáil Debates*, Volume 10, Committee Stage (2 December 2004).

[50] *Quality and Fairness*, Action 111, p. 172.

[51] *National Health Information Strategy*, Department of Health, 2004, pp. 11–12.

[52] *Composite Report*, p. 16.

[53] Ibid., p. 119.

13. An Agenda for Reform in Irish Health Care

[1] We estimate the cost of some proposals in Appendix 5.

Appendix 5: How Much Would it Cost to Solve the Crisis?

[1] J. Fitzgerald *et al., Medium-Term Review 2003-2010*, ESRI, 2003. The figures in this table were generated in 2004 and are discussed in M. Wren, 'Health Spending and the Black Hole', *Quarterly Economic Commentary*, ESRI, September 2004.

[2] Gross voted capital spending for Department of Health and HSE.

[3] According to the HPO, project costs include all outsourced capital costs to the contracting authority in the procurement of facilities excluding the cost of site purchase. The costs above are based on '"greenfield" sites with normal ground conditions, ample space for normal development and surface level car parking, reasonable access to nearby services and unhindered site access.'

[4] *Reflecting on the North Western Health Board 1970–2004*, North-Western Health Board, June 2004.

[5] 2006 Summary Public Capital Programme, Department of Finance, 2005.

[6] *Report of the National Task Force on Medical Staffing*, pp. 118-119, Department of Health, 2003.

SELECT BIBLIOGRAPHY

Books and monographs

Bacon, P. *et al.*, *Current and Future Supply and Demand Conditions in the Labour Market for Certain Health Professional Therapists*, Killinick: Peter Bacon and Associates, Economic Consultants, 2001.

Barrington, R., *Health, Medicine and Politics in Ireland 1900–1970*, Dublin: Institute of Public Administration, 1987.

Callan, T., Keeney, M., Nolan, B. and Maître, B., *Why is Relative Income Poverty So High in Ireland?*, Dublin: Economic and Social Research Institute, Policy Research Series No. 53, September 2004.

Feldstein, P.J., *Health Care Economics*, 5th ed., New York: Delmar Press, 1999.

Figueras, J., Robinson, R. and Jakubowski, E. (eds.), *Purchasing to Improve Health Systems Performance*, European Observatory on Health Systems and Policies Series, Open University Press, 2005.

Friel, S., Walsh, O. and McCarthy, D., *Cost of Healthy Eating in the Republic of Ireland*, Galway: Centre for Health Promotion Studies, National University of Ireland, 2004.

Johnson-Lans, S., *A Health Economics Primer*, Boston: Pearson Addison-Wesley, 2005.

Luras, H. (ed.), *Four Empirical Essays on GP Behaviour and Individual Preferences for GPs*, Oslo: Health Economics Research Programme, University of Oslo, 2004.

Nolan, B. and Wiley, M., *Private Practice in Irish Public Hospitals*, Dublin: Oak Tree Press and the Economic and Social Research Institute, 2000.

Phelps, C.E., *Health Economics*, 3rd ed., Boston: Addison-Wesley Press, 2003.

Tussing, A.D., *Irish Medical Care Resources: An Economic Analysis*, Paper 126, Dublin: Economic and Social Research Institute, November 1985.

Wilkinson, R., *Unhealthy Societies: The Affliction of Inequality*, London: Routledge, 1996.

Wren, M.A., *Unhealthy State*, Dublin: New Island, 2003.

Articles in periodicals and chapters in collections

Barrett, S., 'The Task of Irish Health Service Reform', *Irish Banking Review*, Winter 2003.

Bradley, V.M., 'Placing Emergency Department Crowding on the Decision Agenda', *Nursing Economics*, 23/1 2005.

Bibliography

Brennan, T.A., Leape, L.L. and Laird, N.M., *et al.*, 'Incidence of adverse events and negligence in hospitalized patients', *New England Journal of Medicine*, 325/6, 1991, 370–76.

Creedon, S., 'Healthcare workers' hand decontamination practices: compliance with recommended guidelines', *Journal of Advanced Nursing*, 51/3, August 2005.

Devereaux, P.J. and Schünemann, H.J., *et al.*, 'Comparison of mortality between private for-profit and private not-for-profit hemodialysis centers: a systematic review and meta-analysis', *Journal of the American Medical Association*, 288/19, 20 November 2002, 2449–57.

Devereaux, P.J. *et al.*, 'Payments for care at private for-profit and private not-for-profit hospitals: a systematic review and meta-analysis', *Canadian Medical Association Journal*, 170/12, 8 June 2004, 1817–24.

FitzGerald, M., 'The Lack of Competition and its Impact on the Supply of Acute Healthcare' in Kinsella, R. (ed.), *Acute Healthcare in Transition in Ireland: Change, Cutbacks, and Challenges,* Cork: Oak Tree Press, 2003.

Iverson, T. and Luras, H., 'The Effect of Capitation on GPs' Referral Decisions', *Health Economics*, 9, April 2000, 199–210.

Lawlor, J. and McCarthy, C., 'Browsing Onwards: Irish Public Spending in Perspective', *Irish Banking Review*, Autumn 2003.

Layte, R. and Nolan, B., 'Equity in the Utilisation of Hospital Care in Ireland', *The Economic and Social Review*, 35/2, Summer/Autumn 2004.

Lennon, F., 'Medical profession failed patients,' *The Irish Times*, 29 September 2003.

Ma, C.A. and McGuire, T.G., 'Optimal Health Insurance and Provider Payment', *American Economic Review*, 87, 1997, 685–704.

Madden, D., Nolan, A. and Nolan, B., 'GP Reimbursement and Visiting Behaviour in Ireland', *Health Economics*, 14, 2005, 1047–60.

McCormick, P.A., O'Rourke, M., Carey, D. and Laffoy, M., 'Ability to Pay and Geographical Proximity Influence Access to Liver Transplantation Even in a System with Universal Access', *Liver Transplantation*, 10/11, November 2004.

McGrail, K., Green, B., Barer, M., Evans, R., Hertzman, C. and Normand, C., 'Age, Costs of Acute and Long Term Care and Proximity to Death: Evidence for 1987/88 and 1994/95 in British Columbia', *Age and Ageing*, 29, 2000, 249–53.

Monsma, G., 'Marginal Revenue and Demand for Physicians' Services' in Klarman, H. (ed.), *Empirical Studies in Health Economics*, Baltimore: Johns Hopkins University Press, 1970.

Needleman, J., Buerhaus, P., Mattke, S., Stewart, M. and Zelevinsky, K., 'Nurse-Staffing Levels and the Quality of Care in Hospitals', *The New England Journal of Medicine*, 346/22, 30 May 2002.

Bibliography

O'Reardon, C., 'Improving Irish Public Services', *Irish Banking Review*, July 2004.

Polidano, C., 'The Bureaucrat Who Fell Under a Bus: Ministerial Responsibility, Executive Agencies and the Derek Lewis Affair in Britain', *Governance*, 12/2, April 1999.

Silverman, E.M., Skinner, J.S. and Fisher, E.S. 'The Association Between For-Profit Hospital Ownership and Increased Spending', *New England Journal of Medicine*, 341/6, 5 August 1999, 420–26.

Starey, N., 'Primary Care Health Policy' in Lakhani, M. and Charlton, R. (eds.), *Recent Advances in Primary Care*, London: Royal College of General Practitioners, 2005.

Starfield, B., 'Is primary care essential?', *Lancet*, 344, 1994, 1129–33.

Studdert, D.M., Thomas, E.J., Burstin, H.R., Zbar, B.I.W., Orav, E.J. and Brennan, T., 'Negligent care and malpractice claiming behavior in Utah and Colorado', *Medical Care*, 38/3, 2000.

Tussing, A.D., 'Pay method key to health reform', *The Irish Times*, 1 February 2001.

Woolhandler, S. and Himmelstein, D.U., 'When money is the mission – the high costs of investor-owned care', *New England Journal of Medicine*, 341/6, 5 August 1999, 444–6.

Wren, M.A., 'Health Spending and the Black Hole', Economic and Social Research Institute, *Quarterly Economic Commentary*, September 2004.

Conference papers and working papers

Bickerdyke, I., Dolamore, R., Monday, I. and Preston, R., *Supplier-Induced Demand for Medical Services,* Productivity Commission Staff Working Paper, Canberra, Australia, 2002.

Bruinsma, N., Institute for Public Health and the Environment (RIVM), Bilthoven, the Netherlands, Report on behalf of all EARSS (European Antimicrobial Resistance Surveillance System) participants, *Eurosurveillance Weekly*, 8/51 (16 December 2004).

Colombo, F. and Tapay N., *Private Health Insurance in Ireland: A Case Study*, Paris: Organisation for Economic Cooperation and Development Health Working Papers 10, 2004.

Timonen, V., *Health and Social Services – Integration vs. Division of Management, Delivery and Funding*, Department of Social Studies, Trinity College Dublin, unpublished manuscript, 2003.

Van Doorslaer, E., Koolman, X. and Puffer, F., *Equity in the use of physician visit in OECD countries: has equal treatment for equal need been achieved?*, OECD conference proceedings 'Measuring Up: Improving Health Systems Performance in OECD Countries', Organisation for Economic Co-operation and Development Health Conference on Performance Measurement and Reporting, 2001.

Bibliography

Irish official reports

A Report on the Experiences and Expectations of People of the Health Services, Eastern Regional Health Authority, 2002.

A Vision for Change, Report of the Expert Group on Mental Health Policy, Dublin: Stationery Office, 2006.

Acute Hospital Bed Capacity – A National Review, Department of Health and Children, Dublin: Stationery Office, 2002.

Acute Medical Units, Comhairle na nOspidéal, 2004.

Annual Report of the Comptroller and Auditor General 2004, Dublin: Stationery Office, 2005.

Annual Report of the Ombudsman 2004, Office of the Ombudsman, 2005.

Audit of Structures and Functions in the Health System, Prospectus and Watson Wyatt, Dublin: Stationery Office, 2003.

Audit of Structures and Functions in the Health System, Prospectus and Watson Wyatt, Appendices Volume, Dublin: Stationery Office, 2003.

Bed Capacity Review, Eastern Regional Health Authority, 25 January 2001.

Better Health for Everyone, A Population Health Approach for Ireland, Annual Report of Chief Medical Officer, Department of Health and Children, 2001.

Casemix Measurement in Irish Hospitals, A Brief Guide, Casemix Unit, Department of Health and Children, January 2005.

Commission on Financial Management and Control Systems in the Health Service, Dublin: Stationery Office, 2003 (Brennan Commission).

Composite Report (Health Service Reform Programme), Department of Health and Children, June 2004.

Control and Prevention of MRSA in Hospitals and in the Community, A Strategy for the Control of Antimicrobial Resistance in Ireland, Health Protection Surveillance Centre/Health Services Executive, 2005.

General Medical Services (Payments) Board Report for the year ended 31 December 2004, Health Service Executive/GMS(P)B, 2005.

Guidelines for Community Involvement in Health, Position Paper of the National Primary Care Steering Group, Department of Health, December 2004.

Healthcare Skills Monitoring Report, Foras Áiseanna Saothair (FÁS), 2005.

Medical Education in Ireland: A New Direction, Report of the Working Group on Undergraduate Medical Education and Training, Department of Health and Children, 2006 (Fottrell Report).

Medical Manpower in Acute Hospitals – A Discussion Document, Department of Health, Comhairle na nOspidéal and Postgraduate Medical and Dental Board, June 1993.

National Health Information Strategy, Department of Health, 2004.

National Service Plan 2005, Health Service Executive, 2005.

411

Bibliography

National Service Plan 2006, Health Service Executive, 2005.

Obesity: The Policy Challenges – Report of the National Taskforce on Obesity 2005, Department of Health and Children, 2005.

Population and Labour Force Projections, 2001–2031, Central Statistics Office 1999, cited in Government of Ireland, *Acute Hospital Bed Capacity Technical Report*, Dublin: Stationery Office, 2002.

Population and Migration Estimates April 2005, Central Statistics Office, 14 September 2005.

Preparing Ireland's Doctors to Meet the Health Needs of the 21st Century, Report of the Postgraduate Medical Education and Training Group, Department of Health and Children, 2006 (Buttimer Report).

Primary Care – A New Direction, Department of Health and Children, 2001.

Quality and Fairness: A Health System for You – Health Strategy, Dublin: Department of Health and Children, 2001.

Quality and Fairness, A Health System for You: Action Plan Progress Report 2004, Dublin: Department of Health and Children, May 2005.

Reach Out: National Strategy for Action on Suicide Prevention, 2005–2014, Health Service Executive, 2005.

Reflecting on the North Western Health Board 1970–2004, North-Western Health Board, June 2004.

Report of the Commission on Health Funding, Dublin: Stationery Office, 1989.

Report of the Forum on Medical Manpower, Department of Health and Children, January 2001.

Report of the Independent Estimates Review Committee to the Minister for Finance, Department of Finance, 2002.

Report of the National Task Force on Medical Staffing, Dublin: Department of Health and Children, June 2003 (Hanly Report).

Report of the Working Group on the Accountability of Secretaries General and Accounting Officers, Department of Finance, July 2002 (Mullarkey Report).

Study to Examine the Future Financing of Long-Term Care in Ireland, Mercer Ltd, for the Department of Social and Family Affairs, 2003.

Suicide in Ireland: A National Study, published by the Departments of Public Health on behalf of the Chief Executive Officers of the Health Boards, 2001.

Value for Money Audit of the Irish Health System, Deloitte & Touche and York Health Economics Consortium on behalf of the Department of Health, Dublin, 2001.

Other reports

Adelaide Hospital Society, *Just Caring – Equity and Access in Healthcare, A Prescription for Change*, an Adelaide Hospital Society Policy Paper, May 2005.

Bibliography

Bennett, *et al.*, *Population Ageing in Ireland and its Impact on Pensions and Healthcare Costs*, Report of Society of Actuaries Working Party on Population Studies, Society of Actuaries in Ireland, 2003.

Buchan, J. and Calman, L., *Skill-Mix and Policy Change in the Health Workforce: Nurses In Advanced Roles*, Organisation for Economic Cooperation and Development Health Working Papers 17, 2005.

Cork Simon Community, *Homeless in Cork*, 1998.

FitzGerald, J., McCarthy, C., Morgenroth, E. and O'Connell, P.J. (eds.), *The Mid-Term Evaluation of the National Development Plan and Community Support Framework for Ireland, 2000 to 2006*, Dublin: Economic and Social Research Institute, 2003.

Harvard Medical Practice Study Investigators. *Patients, Doctors, and Lawyers: Medical Injury, Malpractice Litigation, and Patient Compensation in New York*. The Report of the Harvard Medical Practice Study to the State of New York. Boston: Harvard University 1990.

Hunter, I., *Cheering up the Patient: Opportunities for Private Sector Investment in the Irish Healthcare Sector*, Goodbody Stockbrokers, April 2005.

Imai, Y., Jacobzone, S. and Lenain, P., *The Changing Health System in France*, OECD Economics Department Working Papers No. 269, Paris: Organisation for Economic Cooperation and Development, 2000.

Insight Statistical Consulting for the Health Insurance Authority, *The Private Health Insurance Market in Ireland*, HIA, 2005.

Institute of Public Health in Ireland, *Inequalities in Mortality 1989–1998*, 2001.

Irish Association of Speech and Language Therapists, *Submission to the Department of Health and Children on the Strategic Review of Disability Services*, September 2005.

Irish College of Psychiatrists, *A Better Future Now – Position Statement on Psychiatric Services in Ireland*, Occasional Paper OP 60, 2005.

Irish Hospice Foundation, *Baseline Study of the Provision of Hospice and Specialist Palliative Care Services in Ireland*, 2005.

Irish Medical Organisation/Irish College of General Practitioners, *A Vision of General Practice – Priorities 2001–2006*, Dublin, 2001.

Irish Nurses Organisation, *Summary of immediate initiatives required to address overcrowding in accident and emergency departments*, Submission to Minister for Health, INO, October 2004.

Irish Psychiatric Association, *The Black Hole – The Funding Allocated to Adult Mental Health Services: Where is it Actually Going?*, 2005.

Irish Psychiatric Association, *The Stark Facts – The Need for a National Mental Health Strategy, as well as Resources*, 2003.

Irish Society for Quality and Safety in Healthcare, *National Patient Perception of the Quality of Healthcare 2002*, 2003.

Keogh, F., Roche, A. and Walsh, D. *'We Have No Beds ...' An enquiry into the availability and use of Acute Psychiatric Beds in the Eastern Health Board region*, Dublin: Health Research Board, 1999.

Mental Health Commission, *Annual Report, 2004*.

Mills, D.H., Boyden, J.S., Rubsamen, D.S. and Engle, H.L., *Report on Medical Insurance Feasibility Study*, San Francisco: California Medical Association, 1977.

National Cancer Registry, *Cancer in Ireland 1994–2001 – Incidence, mortality and treatment*, June 2005.

National Economic and Social Council, *The Developmental Welfare State*, NESC Report No. 113, NESC, 2005.

National Economic and Social Forum, *Equity of Access to Hospital Care*, Report No. 25, Dublin: NESF, July 2002.

National Social Work Qualifications Board, *Social work posts in Ireland*, NSWQB Report No. 2, 2002.

National Treatment Purchase Fund, *A Report on the Patient Treatment Register*, 2005.

Normand, C. and Graham, B., *Proximity to death and acute health care utilisation in Scotland*, Final Report to the Chief Scientist's Office of the Scottish Executive Department of Health, 2001.

OECD, *International Classification for Health Accounts*, Paris: OECD, 2000.

OECD, *Long-Term Care for Older People*, OECD, 2005.

OECD, *OECD Health Data, 2004, 2005, Statistics and Indicators for 30 Countries*, CD-ROM, Paris: OECD and Irdes. With *Definitions, Sources and Methods* (OECD Health Data 2005).

OECD, *The State of Implementation of the OECD Manual: A System of Health Accounts*, Paris: OECD, 2002.

Public Health Alliance, *Health in Ireland – An Unequal State*, 2004.

Public Service Committee, House of Commons, *Ministerial Accountability and Responsibility*, Second Report, 1996.

The Healthy Ageing Research Programme (HARP) Steering Group, *One Island – Two Systems. A comparison of health status and health and by community-dwelling older people in the Republic of Ireland and Northern Ireland*, Dublin: The Institute of Public Health in Ireland, 2005.

Timonen, V., *Evaluation of Homecare Grant Schemes in the NAHB and ECAHB*, Eastern Regional Health Authority, 2004.

Trinity College Dublin, Department of Community Health and General Practice, *Inequalities in Health in Ireland – Hard Facts*, TCD, Dublin, 2001.

Trinity College, Dublin, Department of Community Health and General Practice, *People Living in Tallaght and their Health – A Community Based Cross-Sectional Survey*, Adelaide Hospital Society, 2002.

Bibliography

UK Department of Health, *Delivering the NHS Plan*, 2002.

UK Department of Health, *NHS Improvement Plan*, National Health Service 2004.

Watson, D. and Williams, J., *Perceptions of the Quality of Care in the Public and Private Sectors in Ireland*, Report to the Centre for Insurance Studies, Graduate School of Business, University College, Dublin, 2001.

World Health Organization, *Highlight on Health, France*, 2004.

World Health Organization, *World Health Report – Mental Health: New Understanding, New Hope*, Geneva: WHO, 2001.

Released under Freedom of Information and other unpublished documents

Breen, R., *Review of Acute Hospital Bed Designation*, Acute Hospitals Division, Department of Health, 18 September 2003 (FOI).

Draft internal memorandum from Michael Scanlan, assistant secretary, Department of Finance, 10 December 2004 (FOI).

Letter (e-mail) to authors from Fergal Goodman, Principal, Primary Care, Department of Health and Children, 6 October 2005.

Letter to Department of Health from Sean Hurley, CEO, Southern Health Board, 27 June 2003 (FOI).

Letter to Department of Health from Tim Kennelly, chief executive, St John's Hospital, Limerick, 24 April 2003 (FOI).

Letter from Second Secretary General, Department of Finance, David Doyle, to Secretary General, Department of Health, Michael Kelly, but marked for the attention of Assistant Secretary, Dermot Smyth, 17 December 2004 (FOI).

Letter from the Minister for Finance, Brian Cowen, to Tánaiste and Minister for Health, Mary Harney, 29 November 2004 (FOI).

Letter from the Minister for Finance, Brian Cowen, to Tánaiste and Minister for Health, Mary Harney, 17 December 2004 (FOI).

Report on Public/Private Activity in Acute Public Hospitals, Acute Hospitals Division, J. Cregan, Department of Health, 13 August 2003 (FOI).

Selected websites cited

Active Citizen Network
www.activecitizenship.net/projects/project_europe_chart.htm

Department of Finance
www.finance.irlgov.ie

Department of Health and Children
www.dohc.ie

Bibliography

Health Protection Surveillance Centre
www.ndsc.ie

Health Services Executive
www.hse.ie

Irish Nurses Organisation
www.ino.ie

Medical Council
www.medicalcouncil.ie

Organisation for Economic Co-operation and Development
www.oecd.org/health

INDEX

Index

Index

Index

Index

self-care 156
sexual abuse 51
SIPTU (Services, Industrial, Professional and Technical Union) 3
Sligo 375
Slovak Republic 289
social care 9, 26, 27, 54, 55, 65, 66, 70, 73, 74–5, 76, 82, 176, 215, 249, 273, 274, 275, 278, 279, 280, 290, 296, 320, 335, 368, 371
Social Partnership 1–2
social
  programmes 9, 53, 57, 65, 67, 73–4, 75, 82
  services 20, 53, 55, 58, 59, 65–71, 82, 83, 217, 263, 266, 273, 276, 280, 368
Social Services Inspectorate 235–6
social solidarity 10, 41, 85, 86–7, 91, 94–6, 106–107, 109, 146, 333, 356
social workers 28, 29, 30, 50, 154, 157, 164, 168, 169, 177, 217, 223, 234, 273, 281, 290, 291–2, 332, 344, 348, 364
South Tipperary General Hospital 396
South, the 48, 229, 230
South-East, the 48, 229, 230, 233
Southern Health Board 203
South-West, the 229
Spain 41, 61, 62, 63, 64, 158, 194, 199, 287, 289
specialist
  care 141–2, 151–2, 156, 206, 244, 226, 267
    in acute hospitals 243–58, 332
  services 23–5, 50, 80, 101
  shortage of 245, 246
  training 253, 255
Specialist Training Programmes 160
specialists 181, 332, 394
speech and language therapists 29, 164, 281, 293, 332
spending see health spending
St Finbarr's 396
St James's Hospital 180, 212, 226, 227, 268
St John's Hospital, Limerick 203, 204
St Luke's Hospital, Kilkenny 226
St Mary's Baldoyle 180, 396
St Vincent's Hospital 22, 51, 212, 219, 224, 227, 233, 242, 248, 339

staffing 26–30, 343–4
  cap on 274–7
  cutbacks 78
  doctors 282–3
  health skill needs 280–82
  Health Strategy deficits 53
  hospitals 78, 79, 176, 208, 217, 225–6, 227, 259, 261, 264, 272, 276
  increases 80, 82, 236, 283–94
  private 277–80
substance abuse 49, 66, 238, 359
suicide 7, 43, 45, 49–50, 51
surgical care 179
Sustaining Progress 302
Sweden 41, 61, 62, 63, 64, 158, 234, 286, 287, 289, 292
Switzerland 289

T

Tallaght hospital 22, 45, 180, 212, 218, 220, 224, 227, 242, 339, 373
tax incentives 2, 3, 38, 102, 106, 130, 169, 171, 230, 332, 356, 361
tax relief on medical expenses 150
team-based care 15, 51, 103, 163, 164–5, 173, 177, 217, 223, 224, 262, 264, 268, 271, 337, 339, 341, 348, 357, 375, 376; see also primary care teams
Timonen, Dr Virpi 66, 234, 235
Touchstone centre 171–2
trade unions 2, 3, 271, 302, 342
training places 26–7, 28, 29, 281, 282, 283, 292, 293, 294, 333, 343; see also medical school enrolment
Travelling community 44
treatment
  day 18, 179, 188, 202, 204, 206, 211, 364, 373
  elective 18, 98, 130, 176, 202, 222, 262, 332
  emergency 18, 202
  inpatient 204, 204, 205, 211, 364
  medical 211, 217, 222, 262
  outpatient 206
  surgical 211, 217, 222
trolleys, patients on 20, 23, 182, 188, 192, 195, 196, 203, 216, 218, 220, 221, 226, 241, 265, 332

Index